ALLERGY *in*
Primary Care

ALLERGY *in*
Primary Care

Leonard C. Altman, M.D.

Clinical Professor of Medicine,
Environmental Health and Oral Biology
Division of Allergy and Infectious Diseases
University of Washington School of Medicine,
Seattle, Washington
Chief, Allergy Division,
Harborview Medical Center
Seattle, Washington
Northwest Asthma and Allergy Center,
Seattle, Washington

Jonathan W. Becker, M.D.

Clinical Assistant Professor of Pediatrics
University of Washington School of Medicine,
Seattle, Washington
Northwest Asthma and Allergy Center,
Seattle, Washington

Paul V. Williams, M.D.

Clinical Professor of Pediatrics
University of Washington School of Medicine,
Seattle, Washington
Northwest Asthma and Allergy Center,
Seattle, Washington

W.B. SAUNDERS COMPANY

A Harcourt Health Sciences Company
Philadelphia   London   New York   St. Louis   Sydney   Toronto

W.B. SAUNDERS COMPANY
A Harcourt Health Sciences Company

The Curtis Center
Independence Square West
Philadelphia, Pennsylvania 19106

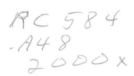

Library of Congress Cataloging-in-Publication Data

Allergy in primary care /edited by Leonard C. Altman, Jonathan W. Becker,
Paul V. Williams.—1st ed.

p.   cm.

ISBN 0–7216–8166–2

1. Asthma.   2. Allergy.   3. Primary care (Medicine).   I. Altman, Leonard C.
  II. Becker, Jonathan W.   III. Williams, Paul V. [DNLM: 1. Hypersensitivity.
  2. Primary Health Care. WD 300 A43422 2000]

RC591 .A48 2000   616.97–dc21

DNLM/DLC   99–048217

Editor: Ray Kersey
Developmental Editor: Dave Kilmer
Designer: Marie Gardocky-Clifton
Production Manager: Natalie Ware
Manuscript Editor: Tom Stringer
Illustrations Specialist: Bob Quinn

ALLERGY IN PRIMARY CARE   ISBN 0–7216–8166–2

Printed in the United States of America.

Last digit is the print number: 9   8   7   6   5   4   3   2   1

Contributors

Rafeul Alam, M.D., Ph.D.
Professor of Medicine, School of Medicine;
Director, Allergy and Immunology, University of
Texas Medical Branch, Galveston, Texas
   Basic Science (Eosinophils)

Leonard C. Altman, M.D.
Clinical Professor of Medicine, Environmental
Health and Oral Biology, Division of Allergy and
Infectious Diseases, University of Washington
School of Medicine; Chief, Allergy Division,
Harborview Medical Center, Northwest Asthma
and Allergy Center, Seattle, Washington
   Urticaria and Angioedema

Sandra D. Anderson, Ph.D., DSc.
Honorary Associate, Department of Pharmacology,
University of Sydney; Visiting Fellow, School of
Physiology and Pharmacology, University of New
South Wales; Principal Hospital Scientist,
Department of Respiratory Medicine, Royal Prince
Alfred Hospital, Camperdown, New South Wales,
Australia
   *Pulmonary Function Testing and Bronchial
   Provocation*

Gary A. Bannon, Ph.D.
Professor, Biochemistry and Molecular Biology,
University of Arkansas for Medical Sciences, Little
Rock, Arkansas
   Food Allergens

Vincent S. Beltrani, M.D.
Associate Clinical Professor, Department of
Dermatology, College of Physicians and Surgeons,
Columbia University, New York, New York;
Associate Clinical Professor, Department of
Medicine, Division of Allergy and Rheumatology,
UMDNJ, New Jersey Medical School, Newark, New
Jersey
   Atopic Dermatitis

Jonathan A. Bernstein, M.D.
Associate Professor of Medicine, Department of
Internal Medicine, Allergy Section/Immunology

Division, University of Cincinnati College of
Medicine, Cincinnati, Ohio
   Occupational Asthma

Wesley Burks, M.D.
Professor of Pediatrics, University of Arkansas for
Medical Sciences; Arkansas Children's Hospital,
Little Rock, Arkansas
   Food Allergens

Maité de la Morena, M.D.
Assistant Professor of Pediatrics, Division of Allergy
and Pulmonary Medicine, Immunology and
Rheumatology, Washington University School of
Medicine, St. Louis, Missouri
   Insect Allergy

Jordan N. Fink, M.D.
Professor of Medicine, Medical College of
Wisconsin, Milwaukee, Wisconsin
   Hypersensitivity Pneumonitis

Mitchell H. Friedlaender, M.D.
Head, Division of Ophthalmology, Scripps Clinic;
Adjunct Professor, The Scripps Research Institute,
La Jolla, California
   Conjunctivitis

Clifton T. Furukawa, M.D.
Clinical Professor of Pediatrics, University of
Washington School of Medicine, Seattle,
Washington
   Adverse Reactions to Food

Bruce C. Gilliland, M.D.
Professor of Medicine and Laboratory Medicine,
Divisions of Rheumatology and Immunology,
University of Washington School of Medicine,
Seattle, Washington
   *Basic Science (Introduction; Complement and Kinin
   Systems)*

David L. Gossage, M.D.
The Allergy, Asthma & Sinus Center, Knoxville,
Tennessee
   Airborne Allergens

v

Ricki Helm, Ph.D.

Associate Professor, University of Arkansas for Medical Sciences, Little Rock, Arkansas

Food Allergens

Golda Hudes, M.D., Ph.D.

Assistant Professor, Albert Einstein College of Medicine; Attending Staff, Montefiore Medical Center, Bronx, New York

Asthma: Diagnosis and Management

Michael S. Kennedy, M.D.

Clinical Associate Professor of Medicine, University of Washington School of Medicine; Northwest Asthma and Allergy Center, Seattle, Washington

Urticaria and Angioedema

Esther L. Langmack, M.D.

Assistant Professor, Department of Medicine, National Jewish Medical and Research Center, University of Colorado Health Sciences Center, Denver, Colorado

Basic Science (Lipid Mediators: Prostaglandins and Leukotrienes)

Mary V. Lasley, M.D.

Clinical Assistant Professor of Pediatrics, University of Washington School of Medicine; Northwest Asthma and Allergy Center, Seattle, Washington

Allergic and Nonallergic Rhinitides; Urticaria and Angioedema

Richard F. Lockey, M.D.

Professor of Medicine, Pediatrics and Public Health, Joy McCann Culverhouse Endowed Professor in Allergy and Immunology, University of South Florida, College of Medicine, Tampa, Florida

Insect Allergy

Mark M. Millar, M.D.

Division of Allergy-Immunology, Department of Medicine, Northwestern University Medical School, Chicago, Illinois

Anaphylaxis

Anthony Montanaro, M.D.

Professor of Medicine, Department of Internal Medicine, Oregon Health Science University, Portland, Oregon

Occupational Asthma

Laurie A. Myers, M.D.

Associate in Pediatrics, Division of Allergy and Immunology, Duke University, Durham, North Carolina

Skin Tests, In Vitro Tests

Hitoshi Okazaki, M.D.

Assistant Professor, University of Tokyo, Tokyo, Japan; National Institutes of Health, Bethesda, Maryland

Basic Science (Basophils and Mast Cells)

Nicholas Orfan, M.D.

Professor of Medicine, Washington County Hospital, Hagerstown, Maryland

Occupational Asthma

Dennis R. Ownby, M.D.

Professor of Pediatrics and Medicine, Allergy-Immunology Section, Medical College of Georgia Hospital and Clinics, Augusta, Georgia

Latex Allergy

Roy Patterson, M.D.

Chief, Division of Allergy-Immunology; Professor of Medicine, Department of Medicine, Northwestern University Medical School, Chicago, Illinois

Anaphylaxis

David L. Rosenstreich, M.D.

Professor, Albert Einstein College of Medicine, Montefiore Medical Center, Bronx, New York

Asthma: Diagnosis and Management

Lanny Rosenwasser, M.D.

NJCIKM, Head of Allergy, Denver, Colorado

Basic Science (Cytokines)

Gail G. Shapiro, M.D.

Professor, Clinical Pediatrics, University of Washington; Northwest Asthma and Allergy Center, Seattle, Washington

Asthma: Special Considerations

Reuben P. Siraganian, M.D.

Professor of Medicine, National Institutes of Health, Bethesda, Maryland

Basic Science (Basophils and Mast Cells)

Wayne A. Sladek, M.D.

Staff Allergist, Group Health Cooperative of Puget Sound; and Member, College of Allergy, Asthma, Immunology, Tacoma, Washington

Asthma: Pathophysiology and Epidemiology

Brian Alan Smart, M.D.

Clinical Assistant Professor of Pediatrics, University of Washington School of Medicine, Seattle, Washington

Basic Science (Antibodies; Lymphocytes)

Steve Stanley, Ph.D.

Assistant Professor, University of Arkansas for Medical Sciences, Little Rock, Arkansas

Food Allergens

Abba I. Terr, A.B., M.D., M.Sc.

Clinical Professor, Stanford University; Director, Allergy Clinic, Stanford University Medical Center, Stanford, California

Controversial Techniques in Allergy

Stephen A. Tilles, M.D.

Assistant Professor, Department of Internal Medicine, Oregon Health Sciences University, Portland, Oregon

Occupational Asthma

Ashok Vaghjimal, M.D.

Medical Associates of West Alabama, Tuscaloosa, Alabama

Asthma: Diagnosis and Management

Frank S. Virant, M.D.

Clinical Professor of Pediatrics, University of Washington School of Medicine; Attending Physician, Division of Allergy, Children's Hospital and Medical Center; Northwest Asthma and Allergy Center, Seattle, Washington

Sinusitis, Otitis Media, and Nasal Polyps

Ann M. Wanner, B.S.E., M.D.

Clinical Assistant Professor of Medicine, Department of Allergy and Immunology, University of Washington School of Medicine, Seattle, Washington; Staff Physician, Providence General Medical Center, Everett, Washington

Immunotherapy

Michael E. Weiss, M.D.

Clinical Associate Professor of Medicine, University of Washington School of Medicine; Northwest Asthma and Allergy Center, Seattle, Washington

Adverse Reactions to Drugs

Marshall P. Welch, M.D.

Clinical Assistant Professor, Department of Medicine, Division of Dermatology, University of Washington School of Medicine; Attending Physician, Medicine (Dermatology), Director, Contact Dermatitis Clinic, Harborview Medical Center, Seattle, Washington

Contact Dermatitis

Sally E. Wenzel, M.D.

Associate Professor, Department of Medicine, National Jewish Medical and Research Center, University of Colorado Health Sciences Center, Denver, Colorado

Basic Science (Lipid Mediators: Prostaglandins and Leukotrienes)

Michael C. Zacharisen, M.D.

Assistant Professor of Pediatrics and Medicine (Allergy), Medical College of Wisconsin, Milwaukee, Wisconsin

Hypersensitivity Pneumonitis

Preface

Allergy, asthma, and other immunologic diseases are very common health disorders, and recent evidence suggests that their incidence is increasing. Because these diseases affect all ages and nearly 20% of individuals, they comprise a large part of the patient population under the care of primary care physicians. Unfortunately, traditional medical education is often focused on hospital-based training, which provides inadequate exposure to allergic and immunologic diseases. For this reason, many physicians are uncomfortable with diagnosing and treating these patients. This is regrettable, especially because the treatment available for asthma, allergic, and immunologic conditions has improved dramatically in recent years and usually provides excellent treatment outcomes and very satisfied patients.

This book was written by basic immunologists and practicing allergy specialists in an effort to produce a practical, up-to-date reference text for all health professionals involved in the evaluation and treatment of patients with allergic, asthmatic, and immunologic diseases.

In the first chapter, many authors have combined their talents to give a succinct overview of the basic immunology needed to understand the pathogenesis of the diseases discussed in the remainder of the text. Chapters 2 through 5 discuss methods and materials used in the diagnosis of asthma and allergic disease. Chapter 6 cautions readers that a number of invalid or unproven diagnostic techniques and treatment methods exist in this field and must be rejected or be viewed with skepticism until proven. Chapters 7 through 9 concentrate on upper airway allergic diseases and their complications while Chapters 10 through 14 focus on asthma and hypersensitivity pneumonitis. Because of its complexity, potential morbidity, and increasing frequency of occurrence, asthma is discussed in four chapters each with a different focus. Chapters 15 through 17 give detailed and practical attention to the most common allergic skin disorders. Chapter 18 reviews adverse food reactions, making important distinctions between immunologic reactions and those caused by intolerance or other mechanisms. Chapter 19 is a discussion of anaphylaxis, and Chapters 20 to 22 discuss disorders that can cause anaphylaxis or less severe yet serious events. These are reactions to medications, insect stings, and latex products. Finally, Chapter 23 discusses immunotherapy, which is unique to the specialty of allergy as a form of therapy. This modality of treatment, which was developed empirically nearly 100 years ago with no knowledge of current immunologic mechanisms, is a very effective form of therapy for many patients with allergic diseases.

The editors are grateful to the individual authors of the chapters and to Holly Nigrelle for her continuous efforts in keeping the development and completion of this book on course.

LEONARD C. ALTMAN
JONATHAN W. BECKER
PAUL V. WILLIAMS

Contents

Chapter 1

Basic Science

Introduction

Bruce C. Gilliland

Allergic diseases are frequently encountered in primary care practice. A basic understanding of the causes and pathophysiology of allergic diseases is important in their recognition and treatment. Allergic diseases are characterized by an immune response to environmental antigens that lead to tissue inflammation and abnormal organ function. Allergic symptoms occur only when the previously sensitized individual is re-exposed to the antigen or allergen. The target of the allergic response may be a single organ or site, as occurs in allergic rhinitis, or several organ systems, as is observed in serum sickness or anaphylaxis. Not all individuals are allergic. Susceptibility to allergy is strongly determined by genetic factors, but these factors are not well understood.

Immunologically mediated inflammation in allergic diseases occurs by three different mechanisms; at times, more than one mechanism may be operative. In atopic diseases, the immune response to inhaled or ingested allergens results in the production of immunoglobulin isotype E (IgE) antibodies, which attach to specific receptors on mast cells and basophils. On re-exposure the allergen reacts with cell-bound IgE, resulting in the release of histamine and other mediators of inflammation. In other allergic diseases, the allergen stimulates the production of IgG or IgM antibodies, leading to the formation of immune complexes and their deposition in small blood vessels at various organ sites. Immune complexes activate complement-releasing chemotactic factors and anaphylatoxins that attract neutrophils and produce vascular permeability, respectively. Serum sickness and acute hypersensitivity pneumonitis are examples of allergic immune complex disorders. The third type of immune response is mediated by T lymphocytes. CD4 T lymphocytes that are previously sensitized to an allergen respond to re-exposure by secreting cytokines that attract and activate monocytes to the site of contact, for example, to the skin in poison oak exposure.

In this chapter, the basic immunology underlying allergic diseases is described to show its relevance to common clinical allergic disorders. B lymphocytes and their products, antibodies, are the main elements of humoral immunity. B lymphocytes go through several steps of differentiation, including gene rearrangement and somatic mutations, on their way to producing highly specific antibodies. These cells have the potential to make antibodies with an enormous variety of specificities. T lymphocytes stimulate and control production of antibodies by B lymphocytes and also function as cytotoxic cells. T lymphocytes differentiate into two major populations called CD4 and CD8 cells. CD8 cells are cytotoxic lymphocytes that kill cells such as tumor cells that express antigens they recognize. CD4 cells are further divided into two main subsets, T helper 1 (Th1) and T helper 2 (Th2). Th1

1

cells stimulate the cell-mediated cytotoxic function of CD8 cells, whereas Th2 cells stimulate production of antibodies and are important in the allergic response. Th1 and Th2 cells secrete different cytokines that are important in executing these immune responses.

Cytokines are low-molecular weight secreted proteins that affect growth, differentiation, and activation of many different types of cells. They may stimulate the cells from which they are secreted (autocrine function) or may affect adjacent cells of another type (paracrine function). Some cytokines, such as interleukin 1 (IL1) and tumor necrosis factor alpha (TNF$_\alpha$), produce generalized systemic symptoms of myalgias, arthralgias, fatigue, and fever. Cytokines also play a key role in allergic diseases by regulation of the IgE response and the activation and accumulation of eosinophils at sites of inflammation. In addition, they are involved in the development and activation of mast cells.

Eosinophils are key cells in many allergic reactions and are thought to play a critical role in host defense against parasitic infections. When eosinophils are activated, they secrete several products that produce inflammation and tissue damage. Among them is major basic protein, which causes bronchial epithelial desquamation and destruction of the basement membrane. These cells are implicated in the bronchial hyperreactivity of asthma. In addition, eosinophils also are the major source of leukotrienes, some of which cause bronchoconstriction and mucus secretion. These cells can induce mast cell degranulation, producing the release of histamine and other mediators.

When activated, basophils and mast cells release histamine, which causes vasodilatation and smooth muscle contraction at sites of involvement such as the lung, skin, and gastrointestinal tract. Arachidonic acid is released from cell membrane phospholipids and metabolized by cyclooxygenase to generate prostaglandins or by lipooxygenase to form leukotrienes, both of which have potent inflammatory properties. Cytokines are released from many cell types during allergic and other immunologic reactions and enhance inflammation and modulate the function of other cells. For example, interleukins 4 and 5 produced by Th2 cells regulate B lymphocyte synthesis of IgE and the recruitment of eosinophils. Activation of basophils and mast cells occurs in several ways. As mentioned previously, these cells have antigen-specific IgE on their surfaces, which reacts with a specific multivalent antigen, releasing histamine and other mediators. Eosinophils also induce mast cell degranulation. In addition biologically active cleavage products of complement activation, C3a and C5a referred to as anaphylatoxins, react with receptors on mast cells and basophils causing the release of histamine and other vasoactive mediators.

Prostaglandins and leukotrienes are lipid mediators that are synthesized from membrane phospholipids in response to cell stimulation by an allergen, infectious agent, or other initiator of inflammation. Certain prostaglandins cause pathologic bronchoconstriction and vasospasm whereas others are protective. Prostacyclin produces pulmonary vasodilation and protects against bronchoconstriction, and prostaglandin E2 reduces mucus secretion. Leukotriene B4 is a potent chemotactic agent and activator for neutrophils. Leukotrienes C4 and D4, formerly referred to as the slow-reacting substance of anaphylaxis, are very potent bronchoconstrictors with potency one thousand times greater than histamine. These leukotrienes stimulate mucus secretion and increase vascular permeability, producing edema. Leukotriene antagonists have been shown to reduce symptoms of asthma and seasonal allergic rhinitis, indicating the importance of these mediators in the pathogenesis of these disorders.

Complement plays an important role in protecting the host from infection. Individuals with inherited deficiencies of complement components are susceptible to bacterial infections. Complement also mediates inflammation. As previously described, anaphylatoxins (C3a and C5a) generated during complement activation react with basophils and mast cells, resulting in histamine release. C5a is also a chemotactic factor and activator for neutrophils. The binding of C3b to the surface of bacteria enhances phagocytosis. Another clinical manifestation of complement is recurrent episodes of submucosal and subcutaneous angioedema observed in patients with inherited deficiency of C1 inhibitor. The pathogenesis of angioedema in this disorder is not allergenic but is due to the lack of an inhibitor that prevents activation of both the complement and kinin systems. The uncontrolled production of bradykinin and a kinin-like fragment of C2 leads to angioedema that is not responsive to glucocorticoids as would be expected in allergic angioedema.

The immune system is a highly complex and integrated system, which, for the most part, protects us from the world of microorganisms and provides tolerance to self-antigens. In most instances, immunization from prior exposure to antigens is protective. Unfortunately, the immune response in allergic individuals is inappropriate and exaggerated. As our knowledge of the immune system expands, it is hoped that prevention and better treatment of allergic diseases will be achieved.

Antibodies

Brian Alan Smart

Antibodies are proteins with specificity for individual antigens. They are produced by B lymphocytes. The type and amount of antibody produced in response to an individual antigen challenge is determined, in large part, by the stage of differentiation that had been attained by the B lymphocyte that is producing the antibody. B lymphocyte differentiation is a complex process involving gene rearrangement, somatic mutation, and clone growth in response to antigen recognition. The antibody that is produced by B lymphocytes may be one of a variety of isotypes, all of which have slightly different structures and functions. Antibodies are the primary element of the humoral immune system and, because of the remarkable variety of antibody specificity and type, this system can respond to a virtually unlimited number of antigens.

Antibody production is closely linked to B lymphocyte differentiation. B lymphocytes originate from stem cells in the bone marrow. At this early point in development, these cells are called pro-B lymphocytes and do not produce or secrete antibody. These cells eventually pass through the pre-B lymphocyte developmental stage on the way to becoming immature B lymphocytes. These immature B lymphocytes are able to produce the μ heavy chain, which is linked to light chains to produce IgM, the first type of antibody produced. Soon thereafter, these cells become mature B lymphocytes and are capable of producing a small amount of IgD. When these mature B lymphocytes are activated by an antigen stimulus, they secrete specific IgM and IgD, undergo clonal expansion to produce large numbers of specific antibody-producing B lymphocytes, and undergo isotype switching to produce other types of antibodies: IgG, IgA, and IgE. On further exposure to antigen, the clonally expanded B lymphocyte population, now termed plasma cells, can produce a large amount of specific antibody.

One of the most remarkable characteristics of antibodies is their incredible variety of specificity. This variety is made possible by the organization of the immunoglobulin gene and its capacity for somatic mutation. Immunoglobulins are composed of tetramers of two heavy and two light chains. These heavy and light chains can combine in a variety of combinations, but, because of the process of allelic exclusion, the product of only one set of antibody genes is expressed by an individual cell. Heavy chains themselves are created by the combination of three gene products, named variable (V), diversity (D), and joining (J).

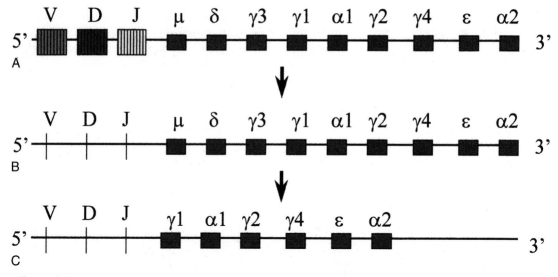

Figure 1–1. *A*, Organization and rearrangement of the heavy chain gene. The human heavy chain gene is composed of multiple, different copies of V, D, and J segments as well as the sequentially arranged constant region segments, μ to α2. *B*, The initial production of the μ heavy chain involves the random selection of single copies of V, D, and J segments. *C*, Isotype switching involves "cutting out" earlier constant region segments and "pasting" the remaining group of sequentially arranged constant region segments to the V, D, and J segments. In this example, the γ1 heavy chain is being produced.

There are many different copies of the V, D, and J gene segments (Fig. 1–1*A*), and they randomly combine to form heavy chains in a process called VDJ recombination (Fig. 1–1*B*). Similarly, light chains are composed of V and J segments, which are also present in a variety of different copies. Additional diversity is created by deletions and additions at the junctions between V, D, and J segments in heavy chains and between V and J segments in light chains. Most of the diversity of antibody specificity, however, comes from somatic mutation of the V gene segments. After B lymphocytes are exposed to antigens, a hypermutation mechanism is stimulated that introduces point mutations into these segments. In this manner, in the course of an immune response, B lymphocytes produce antibodies of progressively greater affinity. Furthermore, through gene rearrangement, the antigen-specific regions of these increasingly specific antibodies are "pasted" onto different heavy chain constant regions, leading to isotype switching, as described below (Fig. 1–1*C*). The wide variety among different antibodies afforded by the grouping of heavy and light chains, the gene segments used in formation of the heavy and light chains, the later modification of these gene segments, the somatic mutation of the variable regions, and the creation of different

isotypes of antibodies with the same specificity allow the humoral immune system to respond to an enormous variety of antigen challenges in a number of different ways.

After antibody specificity has been determined, an individual B lymphocyte or plasma cell can produce any of a number of antibody isotypes, the production of which is, in large part, determined by the stage of development the B lymphocyte has achieved. There are nine immunoglobulin isotypes which all appear to have slightly different functions (Table 1–1). The most prevalent group of isotypes in serum is IgG, with the subclasses IgG1, IgG2, IgG3, and IgG4. The four subclasses are very similar, with about 90% homology among them. They all exist as globular monomers and, because of their size and shape, are the only isotype group that passes through the placenta, conferring passive immunity to newborns. The subtypes do have some differences in function, however. For example, IgG1 and IgG3 are chiefly responsible for interacting with protein (generally, viral) antigens, whereas IgG2 is chiefly responsible for recognizing bacterial polysaccharide antigens. Unlike IgG, IgM is present only as a single isotype, which exists in serum as a pentamer. IgM is the earliest antibody produced and, because of its pentameric organization, is well suited, even in low con-

Table 1–1. **Antibody Isotype Characteristics**

Isotype	MW*	Common Form	Placental Transfer	Distinguishing Functions
IgM	970	Pentamer	No	Primary immune response, antigen receptor
IgD	184	Monomer	No	Antigen receptor
IgG1	146	Monomer	Yes	Secondary immune response, protein antigens
IgG2	146	Monomer	Yes	Secondary immune response, polysaccharide antigens
IgG3	170	Monomer	Yes	Secondary immune response, protein antigens
IgG4	146	Monomer	Yes	Secondary immune response
IgA1	160	Monomer/dimer	No	Mucosal immunity
IgA2	160	Monomer/dimer	No	Mucosal immunity
IgE	188	Monomer	No	Allergy, parasites

*Molecular weight in kilodaltons (kD).

centrations, to bind antigen. IgM also acts as a membrane-bound antigen receptor. IgA exists in both monomeric and polymeric (usually dimeric) forms and has two subclasses, IgA1 and IgA2. Remarkably, IgA production exceeds the production of all other immunoglobulin subtypes, including IgG. IgA appears to be very important in mucosal immunity, because a large amount of IgA is found in exocrine secretions. IgD is present in very small quantities and its particular function, aside from its role as a membrane-bound antigen receptor, remains unclear. IgE exists as monomer of a single isotype and is the antibody that is most important in mediating the allergic response and is also important in the immune response to parasites.

Whereas antibodies are produced exclusively by B lymphocytes, the control of antibody production is a complex process involving a variety of interactions with cells and cytokines. For example, the maturation of mature B lymphocytes into plasma cells involves B lymphocyte interaction with antigen-presenting cells in lymphoid tissues, such as lymph nodes, the spleen, and Peyer's patches. Another essential interaction is required for antibody switching. This occurs when CD40 on the B lymphocyte surface interacts with the CD40 ligand on T lymphocytes and other cell types. If this interaction does not occur, such as in the case of hyper-IgM syndrome, in which there is a deficiency of the CD40 ligand, the B lymphocytes are unable to mature fully and only produce IgM and IgD. Cytokines are stim-

ulatory proteins produced by a variety of cell types, including B lymphocytes, T lymphocytes, and monocytes. Some cytokines, such as interleukin 4 (IL-4), IL-5, and IL-7, for example, are essential, along with cell–cell interactions, for B lymphocyte growth and differentiation.

In summary, antibodies are proteins, produced by B lymphocytes, with specificity for individual antigens. Antibody production is a complex process that results in the production of a wide variety of highly specific antibodies of nine different isotypes. The control of antibody production is an essential process that involves B lymphocyte stimulation by other cells and by cytokines.

Suggested Reading

Alt FW, Oltz FM, Young F, et al: VDJ recombination. Immunol Today 13:306, 1992

Banchereau J, Rousset F: Human B lymphocytes: Phenotype, proliferation, and differentiation. Adv Immunol 52:125, 1992

Greenspan NA: Immunoglobulin function. *In* Rich RR, Fleisher TA, Schwartz BD, et al (eds): Clinical Immunology: Principles and Practice. St. Louis, Mosby, 1996, p 250

Harriman W, Volk H, Defranoux N, Wabl M: Immunoglobulin class switch recombination. Annu Rev Immunol 11:361, 1993

Noelle RJ, Snow BC: B cell differentiation. *In* Rich RR, Fleisher TA, Schwartz BD, et al (eds): Clinical Immunology: Principles and Practice. St. Louis, Mosby, 1996, p 149

Potter KN, Capra JD: Immunoglobulin genes and proteins. *In* Rich RR, Fleisher TA, Schwartz BD, et al (eds): Clinical Immunology: Principles and Practice. St. Louis, Mosby, 1996, p 50

Lymphocytes

Brian Alan Smart

Lymphocytes are a diverse group of mono-nuclear cells that play central roles in both humoral and cell-mediated immunity. All lymphocytes arise from the pluripotential hematopoietic stem cells in the bone marrow (Fig. 1–2). Through a complex and tightly regulated series of steps, including stimulation with cytokines (chemical messengers that influence the actions of other cells), stem cells differentiate first into lymphoid precursor cells and then into a number of cell types, including B lymphocytes, natural killer (NK) cells, and T lymphocytes. T lymphocytes further differentiate into cytotoxic and T helper lymphocytes. The T helper lymphocytes further differentiate into subtypes that are critical in regulating the allergic and inflammatory response.

LYMPHOCYTE DEVELOPMENT

B Lymphocyte Development

After differentiation from the common lymphoid precursor into B lymphocyte precursors, the B lymphocytes go through a number of developmental steps, most of which occur in the bone marrow. During these developmental steps, there is extensive gene rearrangement and somatic mutation, which allows B lymphocytes to fulfill their primary function, antibody production. Initially, B lymphocytes are capable of producing IgM and, soon thereafter, IgD; after further stimulation with antigen, receptor-mediated cell-to-cell contact, and cytokines, these cells mature into plasma cells that are capable of producing all antibody isotypes, including IgG, IgA, IgM, IgD, and IgE. Remarkably, not only are more immunoglobulin isotypes produced during differentiation (by gene rearrangement), but antibodies of increasing avidity are produced as well (by

somatic mutation). In addition, there is a selection process during B lymphocyte development in which self-reactive cells are removed and cells capable of producing specific, needed antibodies are stimulated to develop. The elegant process of B lymphocyte differentiation and antibody production is described in more detail in the section on Antibodies.

Natural Killer Cell Development

Natural killer cells are a small subgroup of lymphocytes. It is believed that these cells arise from T lymphocyte precursors because, in the absence of a thymus, T lymphocyte precursors develop into NK cells, whereas the same cells develop into mature T lymphocytes in the presence of a thymus.

T Lymphocyte Development

After differentiation from the common lymphoid precursors, T lymphocyte precursors further differentiate into cells that have the cell surface marker CD4 (helper cells), CD8 (cytotoxic cells), or neither CD4 or CD8 (the so-called $\gamma\delta$ cells). The development of CD4 and CD8 cells from T lymphocyte precursors occurs in the thymus in a series of stages that are characterized by the degree of cell surface expression of CD4, CD8, and the T-cell receptor that has α and β chains ($\alpha\beta$-TCR). For example, one of the earliest stages of development is the triple-negative precursor that does not express any of the previously mentioned molecules. Expression of CD4 and CD8 is then gained, to create the double-positive T-cell precursor. Eventually, expression of either CD4 or CD8 is lost, creating a single-positive cell. TCR expression is first measurable on the surface

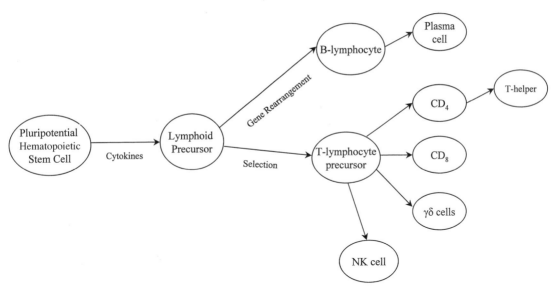

Figure 1–2. Lymphocyte development. Lymphocyte development starts with the pluripotential hematopoietic stem cell which, after specific cytokine stimulation, develops into the lymphoid precursor cell. This precursor cell may develop into B-lymphocytes in a process that involves, among other required steps, gene rearrangement. Upon further stimulation, B-lymphocytes may develop into plasma cells. The lymphoid precursor cells also may develop into T-lymphocyte precursor cells in a process that involves, among other steps, cell selection. Depending on the stimulus, these precursor cells may develop into CD4, CD8, γδ, or natural killer (NK) cells. CD4 cells further differentiate into subsets that are identified by differences in cytokine secretion.

of T-cell precursors that are committed to becoming double-positive. As the T-cell precursor matures, expression of the TCR increases, as well. During this maturation process, there is both negative selection (removal) of self-reactive T lymphocytes and positive selection (further development) of antigen-reactive T lymphocytes. The development of the γδ T lymphocytes (T lymphocytes with TCR composed of γ and δ chains) is slightly different from the development of αβ T lymphocytes in that there is not as much positive and negative selection and the CD4 and CD8 molecules are not expressed.

LYMPHOCYTE FUNCTIONS

B Lymphocytes

B lymphocytes are the group of cells responsible for humoral immunity. They fulfill this role by being the only type of cell that produces antibodies. Characteristics of the different antibody subtypes are further discussed in the section on Antibodies. B lymphocytes do, however, have other important roles besides antibody production, such as antigen presenta-

tion. For example, B lymphocytes, similar to other cell types, can process both intracellular and extracellular antigens and present them on their cell surfaces in the context of major histocompatibility complex (MHC) type I and II, respectively, to stimulate CD8 and CD4 T lymphocytes. B lymphocytes also secrete cytokines such as interleukin 12 (IL-12).

Natural Killer Cells

Natural killer cells are a subgroup of lymphocytes that are named for their ability to non-specifically (independent of MHC restriction) kill tumor cells and cells infected with virus. They also have other functions. For example, with antibody present, NK cells can provide some specific cytotoxicity, in a process called antibody-dependent cell cytotoxicity. NK cells also produce cytokines, such as interferon-γ (IFN-γ) and tumor necrosis factor alpha (TNF-α), that play roles in the regulation of other cells.

T Lymphocytes

T lymphocytes have the greatest variety of functions. For example, CD8 cells function in cytotoxic roles, whereas CD4 cells have many different roles as helper cells. The critical importance of normal T lymphocyte function, relative to other types of cells that have immunologic functions, is illustrated by the universal early fatality experienced by patients lacking functional T lymphocytes (severe combined immunodeficiency [SCID] patients); patients lacking any of the other elements of the immune system usually have much longer survival.

CD8 T Lymphocytes

T lymphocytes expressing CD8 function as cytotoxic cells. The cytotoxic function of a CD8 cell depends on the presentation of antigen by the MHC type I complex on the surface of another cell. All nucleated cells are capable of processing antigen and expressing it on the cell surface with MHC type I molecules. After antigen recognition, CD8 cells kill those cells that express the antigen. It is in this manner that cells infected with virus or intracellular parasites, as well as tumor cells, are destroyed. In addition to their directly cytotoxic effects, CD8 cells can release cytokines.

CD4 T Lymphocytes

T lymphocytes that express CD4 function as helper cells. These cells respond to antigen

presented by the MHC type II complex on the surface of another cell. The group of cells that present MHC type II is largely restricted to B lymphocytes, activated T lymphocytes, monocytes, macrophages, dendritic cells, and endothelial cells. Unlike the case with MHC type I, the antigen that is presented by MHC type II is obtained from outside the cell. Instead of inducing a cytotoxic response, MHC type II antigen presentation activates CD4 cells to regulate and stimulate other cells by cell-surface receptor interactions and by the production of cytokines. Cell-surface receptor interactions include the interaction of CD40 (expressed on B lymphocytes) with CD40 ligand (expressed on CD4 cells) to help induce isotype switching of immunoglobulins. The production of cytokines is of key importance to the function of CD4 cells. There are subgroups of CD4 cells that are, in fact, characterized by differences in their cytokine production.

CD4 Lymphocyte Subsets

Several different subsets of CD4 cells have been identified by differences in cytokine production. The best understood of these subsets include the Th1 (T helper 1) and Th2 cells (Fig. 1–3A). Th1 cells are characterized by production of the cytokines IL-2, IL-12, and IFN-γ (but not IL-4 or IL-5), which stimulate cell-mediated cytotoxicity (such as the activity of CD8 cells) and delayed hypersensitivity

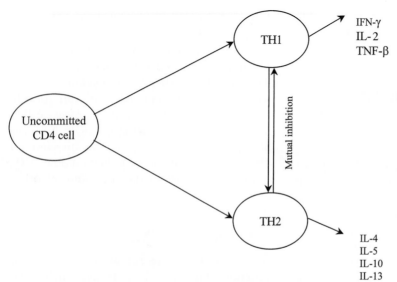

Figure 1–3. T-helper lymphocyte subsets. The uncommitted CD4 cell may differentiate into any of a number of cytokine-secreting cells. The best understood types are the T-helper 1 (TH1) and T-helper 2 (TH2) cells. TH1 cells secrete interferon-γ (IFN-γ), interleukin-2 (IL-2), and tumor necrosis factor-β (TNF-β), among other cytokines. TH2 cells secrete interleukins-4, -5, -10, -13 (IL-4, IL-5, IL-10, and IL-13), among other cytokines. The cytokines secreted by TH1 and TH2 cells have mutually antagonistic qualities and mutually inhibit the development of the other cell type.

(such as transplant rejection). In contrast, Th2 cells are characterized by production of IL-4 and IL-5, but not IL-2, IL-12, or IFN-γ. Th2 cytokines stimulate antibody production and are believed to be central players in the allergic response. Th1 and Th2 cytokines have mutually antagonistic qualities that lead to the development of CD4 cell populations that exclusively produce either Th1 or Th2 cytokines. There is, however, a newly characterized group of CD4 cells, called Th0 cells, that secrete both Th1 and Th2 cytokines. These Th0 cells may be precursors of Th1 and Th2 cells.

γδ T Lymphocytes

The function of γδ T lymphocytes is unclear. It is likely that these cells have a more primitive, less specific function than T lymphocytes with αβ T-cell receptors. There is evidence that γδ T lymphocytes secrete Th2 cytokines and may be essential to the development of allergic asthma. There is also some evidence that γδ T lymphocytes may play a role in autoimmune responses.

SUMMARY

Lymphocytes are an essential part of the immune system that arise from pluripotential progenitor cells in the bone marrow to provide a wide variety of functions. Lymphocyte development is a complex process that results in the production of B lymphocytes, NK cells, and T lymphocyte subsets. B lymphocytes primarily function as antibody-producing cells. NK cells have cytotoxic functions, and can function both specifically and nonspecifically. CD8 T lymphocytes primarily have cytotoxic functions and require specific antigen recognition to function. CD4 T lymphocytes stimulate activities of other cell types through cell-surface receptor contact and cytokine production. CD4 cells are further divided into T helper subsets that produce different types of cytokines, leading to different responses, such as allergy.

Suggested Reading

Abbas AK, Singer GG: Regulatory and effector functions of CD4+ T lymphocytes. *In* Rich RR, Fleisher TA, Schwartz BD, et al. (eds): Clinical Immunology: Principles and Practice. St. Louis, Mosby, 1996, p 264

Banchereau J, Rousset F: Human B lymphocytes: Phenotype, proliferation, and differentiation. Adv Immunol 52:125, 1992

Mosmann TR, Sad S: The expanding universe of T-cell subsets: Th1, Th2 and more. Immunol Today 19:138, 1996

Punt JA, Singer A: T cell development. *In* Rich RR, Fleisher TA, Schwartz BD, et al. (eds): Clinical Immunology: Principles and Practice. St. Louis, Mosby, 1996, p 157

Stevens CD: The lymphoid system. *In* Clinical Immunology and Serology: A Laboratory Perspective. Philadelphia, F.A. Davis, 1996, p 25

Zuany-Amorim C, Ruffle C, Haile S, et al: Requirement for γδ T cells in allergic airway inflammation. Science 280:1265, 1998

Cytokines

Lanny Rosenwasser

Cytokines are secreted proteins that have significant growth, differentiation, and activation functions on contiguous or distant cells and tissues. In other words, cytokines may have autocrine, paracrine, or endocrine functions.

Autocrine, or self-stimulatory, function is best illustrated by the cytokine interleukin 2 (IL-2). This cytokine, produced by T lymphocytes, is the major growth factor that drives T lymphocyte proliferation. Paracrine effects are common in situations in which cytokines produced by one cell type affect adjacent cells; for example, the bronchial epithelium in producing IL-8 can attract and activate neutrophils and eosinophils into the airway to mediate the inflammation associated with bronchial asthma. Finally, endocrine effects also occur with cytokines. Local production of IL-1 and TNF in the lung may have profound distant effects on tissues such as muscles, the liver, and even the brain to induce acute phase reactions, myalgias, and fever associated with inflammation and immune reactions. Cytokines have been categorized into six major families. These are interferons (IFN), interleukins (IL), growth and differentiation factors, colony stimulating factors, chemokines, and tumor necrosis factors (Table 1–2).

Cytokines are generally small proteins or glycoproteins with molecular weights in the range of 5 to 40 kD. Cytokines have unique receptors with specific cellular distribution patterns that mediate the responses to these factors as autocrine, paracrine, or endocrine mediators. Also, cytokines can produce a cascade of responses that modify inflammation, immunity, host defense, or other body functions; often three or four cytokines are required to synergize their activities to get the optimal function expressed. Hence, the production of red cells from precursors in the bone marrow requires the interaction of erythropoietin, IL-3, IL-1, and IL-11. These overlapping or redundant functions clearly identify the importance of many of the cytokine activities on body economy, because elimination or lack of function of one cytokine would not then prove to be detrimental to mounting a regulatory response. This section reviews the major cytokine families including the interferons, interleukins, chemokines, colony stimulating factors, differentiative and growth factors, and tumor necrosis factors (see Table 1–2). Each of these families are made up of multiple

proteins; however, because cytokines from different families may have overlapping functions, there are colony stimulating factors that may behave like interleukins, interleukins that behave like colony stimulating factors, and other examples of overlap.

INTERFERONS

The interferons were the first cytokine family to be described and defined by molecular characterization in the late 1970s and early 1980s. There are three members in the interferon family, IFN-α, -β, and -γ. The initial biologic activity recognized for this mediator was antiviral action as measured in a wide variety of assays that measure viral growth or killing (Table 1–3).

Interferon-α and IFN-β are both strong antiviral proteins and play a major role in host defense against viral infections. Interferon-γ has not only antiviral function but also has significant immunoregulatory functions in terms of activating other cells within the immune system. Interferon-γ, otherwise known as immune interferon, is the most important cytokine responsible for macrophage activation and cell-mediated immunity and has regulatory effects on T helper cells, cytotoxic T cells, γδ T cells, and NK cells. Interferon-γ stimulates expression of type I and type II MHC and multiple other receptors on the membranes of activated macrophages, T cells and NK cells. Interferon-γ can enhance killing mediated by a number of these immune effector cells.

INTERLEUKINS

The next family of cytokines to be described were the interleukins. These also have been

Table 1–3. **Interferons**

Cytokine	Abbreviation	Cellular Source
Interferon α	IFN-α	B cells NK cells Monocytes/macrophages
Interferon β	IFN-β	Fibroblasts Epithelial cells Macrophages
Interferon γ	IFN-γ	T cells NK cells Macrophages

molecularly identified and represent a very diverse and heterogeneous group of proteins that have various effects on immune responses and other important effects on host defense and inflammation. They are summarized in Table 1–4.

Interleukins are a diverse group of cytokines; they are really multiple families that have overlapping and redundant functions. For example, the interleukins that are most involved in T cell activation include IL-2, IL-4, IL-9, IL-15 and IL-17. These cytokines affect T-cell proliferation and activation through effects on distinct and different receptors, but they all have overlapping and redundant functions in this regard. In the same way, IL-1, IL-6, IL-8, IL-12, and IL-18 are cytokines synthesized predominantly by monocytes and macrophages that have proinflammatory and im-

mune modulatory effects unrelated to their activities on T and B cells. A further example involves the effect of IL-3, IL-7, and IL-11, which all stimulate the differentiation of precursor cells into mature hematopoietic, lymphoid, and myeloid cells.

CHEMOKINES

The chemokines are a family of structurally and functionally related proteins that include at least 14 distinct members (Table 1–5). They are produced by mononuclear phagocytic cells, T lymphocytes, NK cells, neutrophils, keratinocytes, hepatocytes, fibroblasts, and endothelial and epithelial cells. The peptides are small (8–10 kD), secreted, proinflammatory cytokines that exhibit between 20% and 50%

Table 1–4. **Interleukins**

Cytokine	Major Functions	Cellular Source
Interleukin 1	Immune reactivity, inflammation, fever	Macrophages
Interleukin 2	T cell growth and proliferation	T cells
Interleukin 3	Stimulation of bone marrow precursors	T cells
		Thymic epithelial cells
Interleukin 4	IgE isotype switch	T cells
	Allergic inflammation	Basophils
		Mast cells
		Eosinophils
Interleukin 5	Eosinophil activation	T cells
		Mast cells
		Eosinophils
Interleukin 6	Terminal differentiation	T cells
		Monocytes/macrophages
		Fibroblasts
		Endothelial cells
		Mast cells
		Hepatocytes
Interleukin 7	B and T cell development	Bone marrow stromal cells
Interleukin 8	Chemotaxis and activation of neutrophils	T cells
		Monocytes/macrophages
		Epithelial cells
		Fibroblasts
Interleukin 9	T cell and mast cell activity	T cells
		Mast cells
Interleukin 10	Cytokine synthesis and inhibition	Monocytes/macrophages
		T cells
Interleukin 11	B and T cell development	Bone marrow stromal cells
Interleukin 12	Interferon induction	Macrophages
		B cells
Interleukin 13	Similar to IL-4	T cells
		Mast cells
		Basophils
Interleukin 14	B cell proliferation	T cells
Interleukin 15	T cell proliferation	Monocytes/macrophages
		T cells
Interleukin 16	T cell chemotaxis	T cells
Interleukin 17	T cell proliferation	Monocytes/macrophages
Interleukin 18	Interferon inducer similar to IL-1 and IL-12	Monocytes/macrophages

Table 1–5. **Chemokines**

Cytokine	Cell Source	Predominantly Activates
C–X–C Subfamily		
IL-8 (NAP-1)	T cells/monocytes, endothelial cells	Neutrophils
		Lymphocytes
GRO α, β, γ	T cells/monocytes	Neutrophils
NAP-2	Platelets	Neutrophils
CTAP-III	Platelets	Neutrophils
BTG	Platelets	Neutrophils
γIP-10	T cells/monocytes	Neutrophils
ENA-78 (MIP-2)	T cells/monocytes	Neutrophils
C–C Subfamily		
MIP-1α	T cells/monocytes	Neutrophils
		Eosinophils
		Basophils
MIP-1β	T cells/monocytes	Neutrophils
MCP-1, MCP-2, MCP-3,	T cells/monocytes	Eosinophils
MCP-4		Basophils
RANTES	T cells/monocytes	Eosinophils
		Basophils
Eotaxin	T cells/monocytes	Eosinophils

homology in their amino acid sequences. The chemokines are characterized by the presence of four conserved cysteine residues and are subdivided into two families based on the positioning of these cysteines. The genes for the C–X–C subfamily are located on chromosome 4q, and its members are characterized by the separation of the first two cysteines by a variable amino acid. The C–C subfamily has the first two cysteine residues adjacent to each other, and its genes are located on chromosome 17q. These two subfamilies also may be distinguished by their primary target cell; the C–X–C subfamily primarily acts on neutrophils and the C–C family on eosinophils, monocytes, and T cells. Recently, a new subfamily of chemokines has been identified. Members of this group lack the first and third C and are referred to as the C subfamily.

COLONY STIMULATING FACTORS

The most clinically efficacious of any of the cytokines is a member of the colony stimulating factor family known as erythropoietin (EPO). It is produced by peritubular cells of the kidney and Kupffer cells of the liver and is involved in the stimulation, differentiation, and growth of erythroid progenitor cells. There is a synergy of erythropoietin with IL-1β, IL-3, and IL-11 in producing mature erythroid cells. In chronic diseases there is a defect in erythropoietin related to reduced renal EPO production. In affected patients, EPO replacement is a significant adjunct to treatment.

Other colony stimulating factors also have a wide variety of activities. The stem cell factor or c-kit ligand steel factor is an important stromal cell and fibroblast factor that is critical for the differentiation of mast cells and basophils into high-affinity IgE Fc receptor-bearing mature effector cells. This hematopoietic growth factor is involved in myeloid and lymphoid progenitor cell activation and is also important in the viability of germ cells and, hence, may be important for reproductive biology as well.

GROWTH AND DIFFERENTIATION FACTORS

Platelet-derived growth factor, whose cellular source is macrophages and whose targets include smooth muscle and endothelial cells, is important as a proliferative factor for endothelial cells and smooth muscle cells. It is therefore very important in vascular biology and in wound healing. Endothelial cell growth factor is also made by a variety of cells including stromal cells. It is involved in enhancing the

Table 1–6. **Role of Cytokines in Allergic Responses**

Allergic Response	Cytokine	Activity
IgE Regulation	IL-4, IL-13	ϵ isotype switch
	IL-4	Generation of IL-4–producing T lymphocytes
	IL-2, IL-5, IL-6	Synergize with IL-4, IL-13
	IFN-γ, TGF-β	Inhibit IL-4, IL-13
	IL-12	Stimulates IFN-γ production by NK cells and T cells
		Inhibits differentiation of IL-4–producing T lymphocytes
Eosinophilia	IL-5, IL-3, GM-CSF	Eosinophilopoietins
	RANTES, MIP-1α, eotaxin, MCP-3	Eosinophil chemotaxis and activation
	IL-1, TNF	Eosinophil activation
Mast cell development	IL-3, IL-9, IL-10, nerve growth factor, hematopoietic stem cell factor	Mast cell growth factors
	GM-CSF	Inhibits mast cell proliferation, basophil chemotaxis, and histamine release
	MIP-1α, MCP-1, MCP-3	Inhibition of histamine release
	RANTES	
	IL-8	

proliferation, growth, and differentiation of endothelial cells.

Transforming growth factor β (TGF-β) is made by chondrocytes, osteoclasts, osteoblasts, fibroblasts and monocytes, and some T cells. It stimulates osteoblast and osteoclast formation of extracellular matrix, wound healing, and scar formation; it inhibits NK cells and proliferation and activation of B and T lymphocytes. In the gut, it promotes IgA isotype switch by B lymphocytes and can, under some circumstances, inhibit macrophage killing. In allergic inflammation, the expression of TGF-β may be associated with the fibrosis observed in long-standing asthma and the subendocardial fibrosis associated with the hypereosinophilic syndrome. TGF-β may lessen allergic inflammation through a capacity to inhibit epsilon germ line transcription and IgE synthesis in IL-4–treated human B cells and through inhibition of mast cell proliferation.

TUMOR NECROSIS FACTORS

TNF-α is made primarily by macrophages. It is also known as keratan. It is involved in activation of a wide variety of cells including inflammatory cells. TNF-α works on diverse cell types and causes modulation of gene expression for growth factors, cytokines, transcription factors, cell surface receptors, and acute phase proteins, and it plays an important role in host defense. It is also an endogenous pyrogen and can stimulate catabolism as well.

The same activities have been attributed to lymphotoxin or TNF-β, which is made by T and B lymphocytes as well as macrophages.

ROLE OF CYTOKINES IN THE REGULATION OF ALLERGIC IMMUNITY AND INFLAMMATION

There are three major ways in which cytokines play a role in allergic inflammation and immunity. These are the activities of cytokines in the regulation of IgE; the contribution of cytokines to eosinophil activation and function; and the role cytokines play in mast cell development and activation. Such responses are summarized in Table 1–6.

Suggested Reading

Borish L, Rosenwasser LJ: CME: Update on cytokines. Journal of Allergy and Clinical Immunology 97:719, 1996
Borish L, Rosenwasser LJ: Cytokines in allergic inflammation. *In* Middleton Jr E, Reed CE, Ellis EF, Adkinson NF Jr, Yunginger JW, Busse WW (eds): Allergy: Principles and Practice, 5th ed. St. Louis, Mosby, 1998, pp. 108–123

Mosmann TR, Coffman RL: TH1 and TH2 cells: Different patterns of lymphokine secretion lead to different functional properties. Annual Reviews of Immunology 7:145, 1989

Oppenheim J, Zachariae COC, Mukaida N, Matsushima K: Properties of the novel proinflammatory supergene "intercrine" cytokine family. Annual Reviews of Immunology 9:617, 1991

Rosenwasser LJ, Borish L: Cytokines, interleukins, and growth factors. *In* Kaplan AP (ed): Allergy, 2nd ed. Philadelphia, W.B. Saunders, 1997, pp. 53–70

Eosinophils

Rafeul Alam

The eosinophil is a leukocyte of granulocytic lineage. The majority of eosinophils are in the tissue. The blood pool represents the cells that are in transit. It has been estimated that for every circulating eosinophil, there are 100 to 200 eosinophils in the tissue. Eosinophils develop, differentiate, and function in a distinct manner. Eosinophils play an important role in allergic and parasitic diseases. The goal of this section is to highlight some of the important aspects of eosinophil cell biology and functions.

ONTOGENY

Eosinophils differentiate from the pluripotent CD34+ stem cells. The exact mechanism of myeloid lineage commitment of stem cells is unknown, but most studies indicate that the early stages of commitment are independent of any known growth factors (stochastic stage). Cells beyond this stage begin to express receptors for some of the hematopoietic growth factors including those for IL-3, IL-5, G-CSF, and GM-CSF (deterministic stage). IL-5 plays a critical role in the final maturation of eosinophils. Mice transgenic for the IL-5 gene have increased eosinophilia. Targeted disruption of the IL-5 gene abrogates the ability of mice to mount an eosinophilic inflammatory response. Some of the transcription factors that favor eosinophilic differentiation in the stochastic stage inlude GATA1 and C/EBP-β. In the later stage, eosinophil differentiation is stimulated by IL-5, GM-CSF, and IL-6. Th2 cells produce most of these cytokines and critically regulate eosinophil production; however, IL-12 and IFN-γ, the two cytokines that promote Th1 response, block eosinophil differentiation. The life span of an eosinophil is relatively short. The maturation time of eosinophils in the bone marrow is 2 to 6 days, the circulating half-life is 8 to 12 hours, and the tissue survival time is only a few days. Eosinophils die of programmed cell death, so-called apoptosis. Growth factors and inflammatory cytokines such as IL-3, IL-5, IL-13, GM-CSF, and IFN-γ significantly delay eosinophil apoptosis. TGF-β and corticosteroids facilitate eosinophil apoptosis.

EOSINOPHIL STRUCTURE

Eosinophils are 12–17 μm in diameter. The mature eosinophil has a bilobed nucleus and numerous granules. The granules stain red with the acidic dye eosin (hence the name eosinophilic granulocyte). The reason for this staining pattern is that the granules contain very positively charged proteins such as major basic protein (MBP), eosinophil cationic protein (ECP), eosinophil-derived neurotoxin (EDN) and eosinophil peroxidase. The granules have an electron-dense crystalloid core, which is solely formed by MBP. The other granular proteins form the less electron-dense matrix. The granular content is released into the tissue upon activation of eosinophils.

EOSINOPHIL MEDIATORS

Activated eosinophils release their granular content—MBP, ECP, EDN, and eosinophil peroxidase. By virtue of their strong positive charge, MBP, ECP, and EDN induce intense tissue damage. MBP causes airway epithelial desquamation and destruction of basement membrane. It induces mast cell and basophil degranulation. Acting upon the muscarinic receptor-2 (M2), MBP augments acetylcholine release at the nerve ends and is implicated in the pathogenesis of bronchial hyperreactivity. MBP also has direct cytotoxic effects on parasites. ECP induces the formation of ion-nonselective pores in the membranes of target cells and thereby promotes cell death. Both ECP and EDN have ribonuclease activity. Eosinophil peroxidase induces damage to the tissue by generating hydrogen peroxide and halide acids.

Eosinophils are the major source of leukotrienes in an allergic reaction. Eosinophils metabolize arachidonic acid mainly into the cysteinyl-peptide leukotriene C4 (LTC4), which is then metabolized into LTD4 and LTE4. In addition, eosinophils produce another potent lipid mediator, platelet-activating factor (PAF). Most of these mediators are preferentially produced in the lipid bodies. The number of these lipid bodies increases on activation of eosinophils. The cysteinyl-leukotrienes and PAF are extremely potent bronchoconstrictors and play an important role in the pathogenesis of asthma. Further, they increase vascular permeability and mucus production.

Eosinophils produce many different cytokines. The amount of the cytokines produced by eosinophils is usually very low. In many eosinophil-rich inflammatory conditions, the concentration of the cytokines may exceed the biologic threshold. Some of the cytokines produced by eosinophils include IL-1, IL-3, IL-4, IL-5, IL-6, IL-8, IL-12, RANTES, MIP-1, and eotaxin. The production of eosinophil growth factors such as IL-5 and chemotactic factors such as eotaxin may have autocrine-like effects and may represent a self-perpetuating mechanism of inflammation.

EOSINOPHIL ADHESION AND MIGRATION

Eosinophils express a wide variety of adhesion molecules that facilitate their adhesion and subsequent migration from the bloodstream into the tissue. Like most leukocytes they express β2 integrins (e.g., CD11b/CD18). Unlike neutrophils, however, they express two α4 integrins, α4β1 and α4β7. Both of these integrins are also expressed on lymphocytes and basophils, which may explain the frequent colocalization of eosinophils and lymphocytes in certain inflammatory conditions. Eosinophil adhesion and chemotaxis are stimulated by cytokines (e.g, IL-16), C–C chemokines and inflammatory mediators such as C5a, PAF, and LTC4. Eosinophils predominantly express the C–C chemokine receptor 3 (CCR3) and, to a lesser extent, CCR1. The ligands for CCR3 are eotaxin, RANTES, MCP-2, MCP-3, and MCP-4. In addition to inducing chemotaxis, C–C chemokines also cause eosinophil degranulation. The stimulation of eosinophils with IL-5 causes *de novo* expression of C–C chemdune receptor 1 (CXCR1), and the cells become responsive to IL-8. IL-5 and GM-CSF, in addition to their growth factor activity, exert modest chemokinetic activity on eosinophils. The mechanism of chemotaxis of eosinophils involves the activation of MAP kinases (extracellular signal-regulated kinase [ERK] and p38 kinases) and phosphatidyl-inositol-3 kinase. The inhibition of these kinases completely abrogates chemotaxis.

EOSINOPHIL ACTIVATION

A number of endogenous molecules are known to activate eosinophils. IL-5 and GM-CSF activate eosinophils in a multifaceted manner. They stimulate their maturation, metabolism, mediator synthesis, and expression of adhesion molecules. Finally, they prime eosinophils for degranulation and cytotoxic activity. Primed eosinophils undergo degranulation in the presence of many factors including PAF, CCR3 ligands (e.g., RANTES, eotaxin, MCP-2, MCP-3, and MCP-4), multimeric and polymeric IgA, and IgG, and C5a. Eosinophils also express the α and γ subunits of the high-affinity IgE receptor complex, but not the β subunit. Under certain circumstances, these cells may be activated in an IgE-dependent manner. Eosinophils release their granular content (i.e., MBP, ECP, EDN, and EPO) and secrete PAF, LTC4, and reactive oxygen radicals in an immediate fashion. The synthesis and secretion of cytokines require longer times, usually 4 to 12 hours.

FUNCTION OF EOSINOPHILS

The physiologic function of eosinophils remains unclear. The general consensus has been that these cells play a critical role in host defense against parasitic infections. Recent studies indicate that the presence of eosinophils is not absolutely necessary for an immune response against parasites. Mice treated with anti-IL-5 antibody show unimpaired immune response. Eosinophils play an important role in the pathogenesis of allergic reactions. The activation of mast cells in immediate hypersensitivity reactions results in the elaboration of many eosinophil-active chemotactic factors including C–C chemokines, LTB4, LTC4, and PAF. These molecules are likely to attract eosinophils into the site of an allergic reaction. The influx of eosinophils along with lymphocytes and basophils typically manifests as the late-phase allergic reaction and is associated with the recrudescence of allergic symptoms 4 to 8 hours after the initial allergic insult. The importance of eosinophils in allergic diseases is underscored by the efficacy of corticosteroids. The latter agents inhibit eosinophil growth and survival. Further, they inhibit the production of many cytokines and chemokines that play an essential role in the chemotaxis and activation of eosinophils.

Suggested Reading

Alam R, Stafford S, Forsythe P, et al: RANTES is a chemotactic and activating factor for eosinophils. J Immunol 150:3442, 1993

Bochner BS, Schleimer RP: The role of adhesion molecules in human eosinophil and basophil recruitment. J Allergy Clin Immunol 94:427, 1994

Gleich GJ, Adolphson CR: The eosinophilic leukocyte: Structure and function. Adv Immunol 39:177, 1986

Heath H, Qin SX, Rao P, et al: Chemokine receptor usage by human eosinophils: The importance of CCR3 demonstrated using an antagonistic monoclonal antibody. J Clin Invest 99:178, 1997

Rothenberg ME: Eosinophilia. N Eng J Med 338:1592, 1998

Sanderson CJ: Interleukin-5, eosinophils and disease. Blood 79:3101, 1992

Schleimer RP, Bochner BS: The effects of glucocorticosteroids on human eosinophils. J Allergy Clin Immunol 94:1183, 1994

Weller PF: Human eosinophils. J Allergy Clin Immunol 100:283, 1997

Young JD, Peterson CG, Venge P, Cohn ZA: Mechanism of membrane damage mediated by human eosinophil cationic protein. Nature 321:613, 1986

Basophils and Mast Cells

Hitoshi Okazaki and Reuben P. Siraganian

Basophils and mast cells are the critical effector cells in allergic diseases. Despite their distinct lineage, they are usually discussed together because of their structural and functional similarities. They both have prominent

cytoplasmic granules that contain histamine and other mediators. On their surface they have high-affinity receptors for the Fc portion of IgE (FcεRI). These receptors were formerly believed to be specific for basophils and mast cells, but recently were found to be expressed also on eosinophils, Langerhans cells, and activated monocytes. Exposure to multivalent allergens (antigens) induces the degranulation and production of mediators from both basophils and mast cells that have antigen-specific IgE bound to the receptors on their surface.

Although basophils and mast cells have such similar features, there are differences between these two cell types. First, although they both originate from pluripotential hematopoietic stem cells in bone marrow, basophils are usually present only in the circulation, although they can move into tissues in certain types of allergic inflammation. On the other hand, mast cells normally reside in connective tissues, often located beneath epithelial surfaces, such as in the skin and the respiratory and gastrointestinal systems. Second, basophils are probably end cells that do not proliferate, and they have a short life span (i.e., several days' duration). In contrast, mast cells originate from bone marrow, with precursors that migrate and then mature in tissues, and they have the potential to proliferate and live longer (weeks to months) than the usual hematopoietic end cells. Table 1–7 offers a comparison of the characteristics of basophils and mast cells.

The roles of basophils and mast cells are usually discussed in the context of the allergic response, which is often harmful; therefore, their favorable functions have often been overlooked. Basophils and mast cells play an important role in host defense mechanisms against parasites and microorganisms. They are involved in the mechanisms for eliminating parasites through IgE-dependent or independent pathways. In addition, they have a role in defense against bacterial infections because they recruit circulating leukocytes by the release of TNF-α at sites of infection.

MEDIATORS FROM BASOPHILS AND MAST CELLS

Histamine is a major biogenic amine in human basophils and mast cells. It is formed from the amino acid histidine by histidine decarboxylase, and it is stored in granules where it is associated with proteoglycans. When cells are stimulated, histamine is released and dissociates from proteoglycans resulting in local effects such as vasodilation and the contraction of smooth muscle cells, for example, in bronchi or the gastrointestinal tract. Once histamine is released from cells, it is rapidly metabolized.

Neutral proteases also are a major component of the granules. They cleave peptide bonds, resulting in the degradation of proteins. Tryptase is one protease present in mast cells but not in basophils. The precise role of proteases is not clearly identified, but they may contribute to the airway hyper-responsiveness in asthma.

Lipid mediators are generated after stimulation of these cells. Arachidonic acid is released from cellular stores and is metabolized either by the cyclooxygenase pathway to generate prostaglandin (PG) D_2, or by the lipoxygenase pathway to generate leukotriene (LT) C_4 (LTD_4, LTE_4). Mast cells produce much more PGD_2 than LTC_4, whereas basophils produce LTC_4 but not PGD_2. These lipid mediators have potential inflammatory activities. Details about the lipid mediators in mast cells and basophils are discussed elsewhere in this text.

Table 1–7. **Basophils and Mast Cells**

Characteristics	Basophils	Mast Cells
Origin of precursor cells	Bone marrow	Bone marrow
Site of maturation	Bone marrow	Connective tissue
Localization	Circulation	Connective tissue
Life span	Days	Weeks to months
Ig receptors	FcεRI, FcγR	FcεRI
Mediators in granules	Histamine (<1 pg/cell), Chondroitin sulfate A	Histamine, Chondroitin sulfate A, Heparin, Proteases (Tryptase, Chymase, Cathepsin G, Carboxypeptidase)
Lipid mediators	LTC4	PGD2 > LTC4,
Cytokines	TNF-α, IL-4	TNF-α

Cytokines are newly generated mediators that are released slowly after stimulation of basophils and mast cells. There are several cytokines produced by basophils and mast cells. They have different bioactivities, such as induction and enhancement of inflammation, chemotactic activity for other cells, or modulation of the functions of other cells. Some cytokines such as tumor necrosis factor alpha (TNF-α) are prestored in basophils and mast cells, whereas other cytokines are only newly synthesized after stimulation. Cytokines produced by stimulated mast cells and basophils that are detected either at the mRNA or protein level are the following; IL-1, IL-3, IL-4, IL-5, IL-6, IL-8, IL-9, IL-10, IL-13, IL-16, TNF-α, TGF-β, granulocyte/macrophage colony stimulating factor (GM-CSF), INF-γ, macrophage inflammatory protein (MIP)-1α, MIP-1β, basic fibroblast growth factor, and other chemokines. Among these cytokines, IL-4, IL-10 and IL-13 are responsible for the regulation of IgE production from B cells as well as the surface expression of CD40L in mast cells and basophils. IL-5 is related to the recruitment and survival of eosinophils, whereas IL-8 is responsible for the recruitment of neutrophils. Thus, cytokine production from mast cells and basophils may modulate allergic inflammation, especially in the late phase, but the relative contribution of the cytokines produced by mast cells and basophils to the late allergic response remains to be elucidated.

MECHANISM OF SIGNALING BY FCεRI

The high-affinity receptor for IgE on the surface of the mast cells and basophils consists of three different subunits, α, β, and a dimer of the γ subunit. The α subunit of the receptor has a large extracellular domain, which is responsible for the binding to the Fc portion of the IgE molecules, and a relatively short intracellular tail. The β subunit has four transmembrane domains with both carboxy terminal and amino terminal ends in the cytoplasm. The γ subunit is a dimer, each subunit of which has a single transmembrane domain with a very short extracellular domain and relatively longer cytoplasmic tail. The cytoplasmic tails of the β and γ subunits are responsible for propagating the signals when the receptor is aggregated. These cytoplasmic tails contain the immunoreceptor tyrosine–based activation motif (ITAM), which can bind the Src homology (SH) 2 domain of proteins when the tyrosine residues of the ITAM are phosphorylated.

Table 1–8. **Proteins Involved in FcεRI Signaling**

Protein	Description
Syk	Member of Syk/ZAP-70 family of protein tyrosine kinases; binds to phosphorylated ITAMs and is activated
Lyn	Member of Src family of protein tyrosine kinases; associated with the plasma membrane and with FcεRI; probably phosphorylates β and γ subunits of FcεRI
PLCγ	Phospholipase; tyrosine phosphorylated after cell activation; hydrolyzes inositol phospholipids (PIP2) to inositol 1,4,5-trisphosphate (IP3) and diacylglycerol (DAG)
PI-3K	Lipid kinase; phosphorylates phosphatidyl inositol 4,5-bisphosphate to produce phosphatidyl inositol 3,4,5-trisphosphate; which recruits pleckstrin homology (PH) domain–containing proteins such as PLCγ and Btk to the proximity of the membrane
Btk	Bruton's tyrosine kinase; cytosolic molecule; translocates to the membrane; probably affects Ca^{2+} influx and the JNK pathway
FAK/Pyk2	Members of focal adhesion tyrosine kinase family; tyrosine phosphorylated by FcεRI and by integrin; interacts with other signaling molecules
Shc	Adaptor molecule; tyrosine phosphorylated after stimulation
Grb2	Adaptor molecule; binds Sos
Sos	Guanine nucleotide exchange factor of Ras
Vav	Guanine nucleotide exchange factor of Rac
Ras	Small GTP binding protein; activation leads to Erk pathway
Rac	Small GTP binding protein; activation leads to JNK pathway and changes in cytoskeleton
Erk	Ser/Thr kinase; phospholipase A2 and transcription factors are downstream
JNK	Ser/Thr kinase; probably related to the transcription of TNF-α
PLA₂	Phospholipase; phosphorylated by Erk; releases arachidonic acid
PKC	Protein kinase C; Ser/Thr kinase; β and δ isoforms are critical for secretion

JNK = c-Jun N-amino-terminal kinase.

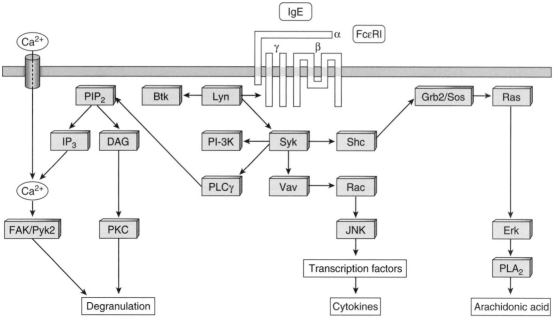

Figure 1–4. Signaling pathway initiated by aggregation of FcεRI in basophils or mast cells. The summary of the function of these proteins is in Table 1–8.

The phosphorylation of the tyrosine residues of cytoplasmic proteins is an early step in the signaling in FcεRI, suggesting the involvement of several tyrosine kinases in signaling. Among these kinases, Syk is the main tyrosine kinase propagating intracellular signals by binding to the ITAMs of the γ subunits, which are probably tyrosine-phosphorylated by Lyn or other Src family tyrosine kinases. Downstream of Syk is the tyrosine phosphorylation of the phospholipase C_γ (PLC$_\gamma$) that results in the increase in the catalytic activity of this enzyme. PLC$_\gamma$ catalyzes the hydrolysis of phosphatidylinositol 4,5-bisphosphate, resulting in the generation of inositol 1,4,5-trisphosphate and diacylglycerol, which are essential for the Ca^{2+} release from internal stores and protein kinase C activation respectively. The release of Ca^{2+} from the internal store is followed by the influx of Ca^{2+} from outside the cell. Downstream of Syk are other pathways that lead to the release of lipid mediators and cytokines. These intracellular proteins and pathways involved in FcεRI mediated secretion and production of mediators are shown in Table 1–8 and Figure 1–4. Some adaptor proteins such as Shc, Grb2, and Vav, and small G proteins such as Ras and Rac are also downstream of Syk. The Shc/Grb2/Sos→Ras→Erk pathway leads to the activation of phopholipase A_2 that results in the release of the lipid mediators. In contrast the Vav→Rac→JNK pathway is related to the production of cytokines.

SUMMARY

Basophils and mast cells are thought to be involved not only in allergic diseases such as asthma, allergic rhinitis, urticaria, and systemic anaphylaxis, but also in fibrotic disorders such as progressive systemic sclerosis and fibrotic lung disease. This finding suggests a role for mast cells and basophils not only in acute allergic response but also in chronic inflammation. Furthermore, these cells contribute to host defense against parasite infestations and bacterial infections. Therefore, the role of mast cells and basophils in human diseases might be much more extensive than previously thought.

Suggested Reading

Costa JJ, Weller PF, Galli SJ: The cells of the allergic response. JAMA 278:1815, 1997
Siraganian RP: *In* Middleton EJ, Reed CE, Ellis EF, et al (eds): *Allergy: Principles and Practice.* 5th ed. St. Louis, Mosby–Year Book, pp. 204–227

Lipid Mediators: Prostaglandins and Leukotrienes

Esther L. Langmack and Sally E. Wenzel

EICOSANOIDS

Prostaglandins, leukotrienes, lipoxins, and thromboxanes comprise a group of lipid-derived mediators known as eicosanoids. Unlike other biologically active molecules that are stored as preformed agents, eicosanoids are synthesized *de novo* from membrane phospholipids in response to cell stimulation by allergen, infection, inflammation, or trauma. Of the family of eicosanoids, the prostaglandins (PGs) and leukotrienes (LTs) have emerged as important mediators of inflammation in asthma and allergic reactions.

ARACHIDONIC ACID METABOLISM

Arachidonic acid is the substrate from which all eicosanoids are synthesized. The first step in eicosanoid synthesis is the liberation of arachidonic acid from cell membrane phospholipids by phospholipase A_2 (PLA_2) enzymes. PLA_2 enzymes hydrolyze the *sn*-2 fatty acid acyl ester bond of phosphoglycerides to release free arachidonic acid. Arachidonic acid release is believed to be the rate-limiting event in eicosanoid biosynthesis.

Phospholipase A_2 enzymes have been identified in many cells, including mast cells, neutrophils, eosinophils, and macrophages. PLA_2s are activated by receptor-mediated influx of calcium ions into the cell. Two of the best characterized mammalian PLA_2s are secretory PLA_2 and cytosolic PLA_2. Secretory PLA_2 is a 14-kD enzyme that is secreted from the cell and hydrolyzes phospholipids on the outer leaflet of the plasma membrane. In contrast, cytosolic PLA_2 is an 85-kD intracellular enzyme that, once it is phosphorylated, translocates from the cytosol to the nucleus, where it hydrolyzes phospholipids on the outer nuclear membrane.

Free arachidonic acid can then enter the arachidonic acid cascade (Fig. 1–5), where it serves as a substrate for one of several different enzymes, including cyclooxygenases and lipoxygenases. The final product derived from arachidonic acid depends on the type of cell, the nature of the stimulus driving lipid-mediator production, and a complex set of regulatory processes. Cyclooxygenase pathway products are the thromboxanes and the prostaglandins, PGD_2, PGE_2, PGI_2 (prostacyclin), and $PGF_2\alpha$. The products of 12-lipoxygenase and 15-lipoxygenase pathways include the lipoxins, 12-hydroxyeicosatetraenoic acid (12-HETE) and 15-hydroxyeicosatetraenoic acid (15-HETE). The contribution of 12- and 15-lipoxygenase pathways products to inflammation is just beginning to be understood. The products of the 5-lipoxygenase pathway are leukotriene B_4 (LTB_4) and the cysteinyl leukotrienes (cLTs), LTC_4, LTD_4, and LTE_4.

PROSTAGLANDINS

Prostaglandin biosynthesis begins with the conversion of arachidonic acid to an endoperoxide, PGH_2, by the enzyme cyclooxygenase (COX). Two isoforms of COX, have been identified, COX-1 and COX-2. COX-1 controls constitutive PG production under basal conditions and has a wide cellular distribution. In contrast, COX-2, an inducible enzyme expressed in a smaller number of cell types, appears to be responsible for PG biosynthesis at sites of active inflammation. PGH_2 is converted into PGD_2, PGE_2, PGI_2, $PGF_{2\alpha}$, or thromboxane A_2 (TXA_2) by individual synthases.

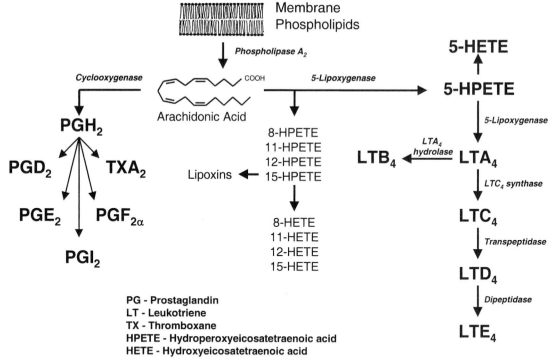

Figure 1–5. Phospholipase A_2 acts on stimulated cell membrane phospholipids to release arachidonic acid, the precursor of the prostaglandins and leukotrienes. Leukotrienes are synthesized via the 5-lipoxygenase pathway. LTA_4 is metabolized by LTA_4 hydrolase to generate leukotriene B_4 (LTB_4) or by leukotrine C_4 (LTC_4) synthase to form the cysteinyl leukotrienes. Prostanoids are synthesized by way of the cyclooxygenase pathway.

PGD_2, TXA_2, and $PGF_{2\alpha}$ cause broncho-constriction and vasospasm. In the lung, macrophages produce TXA_2 and $PGF_{2\alpha}$. TXA_2 is also synthesized by platelets. Pulmonary mast cells release PGD_2 after allergen stimulation. PGD_2 is the most powerful bronchoconstricting prostanoid, with an estimated potency one thousand times that of histamine. PGD_2 is metabolized to $9\alpha,11\beta$-PGF_2, another potent bronchoconstrictor. PGD_2 and $PGF_{2\alpha}$ are elevated in bronchoalveolar lavage (BAL) fluid of asthmatics at baseline, compared with normal controls. PGD_2 and TXA_2 increase in BAL fluid after endobronchial allergen challenge in atopic asthmatics patients.

Prostacyclin and PGE_2 have bronchoprotective action. Prostacyclin is elaborated by vascular endothelial cells and vascular and nonvascular smooth muscle cells. Prostacyclin is a potent pulmonary vasodilator that also protects against certain bronchoconstrictive stimuli. PGE_2 is generated by airway epithelial cells and alveolar macrophages. PGE_2 reduces mucus secretion and is a weak bronchodilator *in vitro*. In *in vivo* studies, inhaled PGE_2 has been shown to attenuate bronchoconstriction induced by exercise and allergen. Topical PGE_2 blocks inflammation associated with cutaneous allergen injection in atopic individuals. Unfortunately, the potential for use of PGE_2 as a therapeutic agent in asthma and allergy has been limited by its short half-life and gastrointestinal side effects.

Nonsteroidal antiinflammatory drugs (NSAIDs), such as aspirin and indomethacin, are COX inhibitors that reduce PG biosynthesis. In the lung, COX inhibition decreases production of both bronchoconstrictor and bronchoprotective PGs, such that these drugs have little overall effect on airway tone or inflammation, in most situations. The notable exception to this is the syndrome of aspirin-intolerant asthma, which affects 10% to 15% of all people with asthma. In these individuals, NSAIDs precipitate bronchospasm and rhinorrhea. In severe cases, this reaction progresses to an anaphylactoid reaction. Although the pathogenesis of the syndrome is incompletely understood, the reaction involves rapid release of large quantities of cLTs.

LEUKOTRIENES

Leukotriene production begins when 5-lipoxygenase translocates from the cell or nuclear cytosol to the nuclear envelope, where it associates with 5-lipoxygenase activating protein (FLAP). In the presence of calcium, adenosine triphosphate, and FLAP, 5-lipoxygenase then catalyzes both the oxygenation of arachidonic acid to form 5-hydroperoxyeicosatetraenoic acid (5-HPETE) and the conversion of 5-HPETE into LTA_4, an unstable epoxide. LTA_4 serves as the precursor for both LTB_4 and the cLTs. LTA_4 hydrolase transforms LTA_4 into LTB_4. LTC_4 synthase, a membrane-associated glutathione-S-transferase, converts LTA_4 into LTC_4, the first of the cLTs. LTC_4 is then further metabolized to LTD_4 and LTE_4 by the sequential enzymatic removal of γ-glutamate and glycine, respectively. LTE_4 is either excreted unchanged in the urine and bile or further metabolized to a number of biologically inactive molecules.

The type and amount of LT produced depend on the cell's expression of synthetic enzymes and the local inflammatory milieu. LTB_4 is produced by alveolar macrophages, monocytes, and neutrophils, whereas the cLTs are produced primarily by eosinophils, mast cells, and basophils. All of these cells play important roles in asthma and allergic inflammation. Cytokines, growth factors, and other lipid mediators released at the site of inflammation can modulate LT production. For example, neutrophils incubated in granulocyte-macrophage colony stimulating factor (GM-CSF) or platelet-activating factor increase LT synthesis in response to a second stimulus. This priming effect is also observed in eosinophils, which increase production of cLTs after exposure to IL-3, IL-5, and GM-CSF and a subsequent triggering stimulus. Exposure of eosinophils to IL-3, IL-5, and GM-CSF also increases eosinophil survival in tissues.

LTB_4 is an important proinflammatory lipid mediator. LTB_4 exerts its biologic effects through interaction with the BLT receptor. LTB_4 can amplify the inflammatory response in several ways. LTB_4 is a very potent chemotactic agent for neutrophils and eosinophils, and it promotes neutrophil adherence to vascular endothelial cells, thereby facilitating the influx of granulocytes into the site of inflam-

mation. LTB_4 stimulates neutrophil degranulation and superoxide generation, as well as production of cytokines, such as IL-6 from human monocytes.

Formerly known as the slow-reacting substance of anaphylaxis, the cLTs were first recognized for their capacity to induce sustained contraction of airway, gastrointestinal, and mesangial smooth muscle. LTC_4 and LTD_4 are among the most potent bronchoconstrictors identified to date, with a potency one thousand times that of histamine and a longer duration of action than histamine. cLTs act on a single airway smooth muscle receptor, designated the cys-LT_1 receptor. In addition to their actions as bronchoconstrictors, cLTs enhance and perpetuate inflammation through their effects on blood vessels, mucous glands, and cell migration. cLTs increase the permeability of vascular endothelium, leading to edema formation and facilitating cell migration into sites of inflammation. cLTs also stimulate bronchial mucus secretion and inhibit mucus clearance, thereby worsening airflow obstruction in asthma. In addition, cLTs may directly modulate influx of eosinophils into asthmatic airways. LTD_4 is a potent chemoattractant for human eosinophils *in vitro*. Inhalation of LTE_4 by patients with asthma dramatically increased the number of eosinophils in the lamina propria of airway mucosa.

The cLTs are released during allergen-mediated and other responses in asthmatic patients and individuals with allergic rhinitis. During the acute reaction to an allergen, activation of the high-affinity IgE receptor on mast cells and basophils stimulates rapid production and release of cLTs. Increased concentrations of cLTs have been found in BAL fluid of atopic asthmatics 5 minutes after endobronchial allergen challenge. Similarly, cLTs increase in nasal lavage fluid after nasal allergen challenge in subjects with allergic rhinitis. Pretreatment with the LT receptor antagonist zafirlukast attenuated both the early and late decreases in forced expiratory volume in one second (FEV_1) after allergen challenge, confirming the importance of the cLTs in allergen-induced bronchospasm. Zafirlukast likewise decreased allergic symptoms in patients with seasonal allergic rhinitis. The release of cLTs has also been demonstrated in patients with spontaneous exacerbations of asthma, in aspirin-intolerant asthmatic patients challenged with aspirin, and after exercise in children with exercise-induced asthma.

Advances in the understanding of the biosynthesis of the LTs and their role in inflammation has led to the development of several classes of pharmacologic agents for treatment of asthma: LT receptor antagonists (LTRAs), 5-LO inhibitors, FLAP inhibitors, and LTC_4 synthase inhibitors. LTRAs, including zafirlukast and montelukast, block the cys-LT_1 receptor. 5-LO inhibitors, such as zileuton, inhibit the activity of 5-lipoxygenase, thus decreasing production of LTB_4 as well as the cLTs. Both LTRAs and zileuton have been shown to improve asthma symptoms and relieve bronchospasm in laboratory challenges and clinical trials, thereby confirming the importance of these molecules in asthma and allergic diseases. FLAP and LTC_4 synthase inhibitors are still in development, and their effectiveness in the treatment of asthma has yet to be conclusively demonstrated.

Suggested Reading

Alam R, Dejarnatt A, Stafford S, et al: Selective inhibition of the cutaneous late but not immediate allergic response to antigens by misoprostol, a PGE analog. Results of a double-blind, placebo-controlled randomized study. Am Rev Respir Dis 148:1066, 1993

Bass DA, Thomas MJ, Goetzl EJ, et al: Lipoxygenase-derived products of arachidonic acid mediate stimulation of hexose uptake in human polymorphonuclear lymphocytes. Biochem Biophys Res Commun 100:1, 1981

Coleman RA, Eglen RM, Jones RL, et al: Prostanoid and leukotriene receptors: A progress report from the IUPHAR working parties on classification and nomenclature. Adv Prost Throm Leuko Res 23:283, 1995

Christie PE, Tagari P, Ford-Hutchinson AW, et al; Urinary leukotriene E_4 concentrations increase after aspirin challenge in aspirin-sensitive asthmatic subjects. Am Rev Respir Dis 143:1025, 1991

Churchill L, Chilton FH, Resau JH, et al: Cyclooxygenase metabolism of endogenous arachidonic acid by cultured human tracheal epithelial cells. Am Rev Respir Dis 140:449, 1989

Dahinden CA: Regulation of leukotriene production by cytokines. Adv Prost Throm Leuko Res 22:327, 1994

Dahlen SE, Hedqvist P, Hammarstrom S, et al: Leukotrienes are potent constrictors of human bronchi. Nature 288:484, 1980

Donnelly AL, Glass M, Minkwitz MC, et al: The leukotriene receptor antagonist, ICI 204,219, relieves the symptoms of acute seasonal allergic rhinitis. Am J Respir Crit Care Med 151:1734, 1995

Drazen JM, O'Brien J, Sparrow D, et al: Recovery of leuko-

triene E_4 from the urine of patients with airway obstruction. Am Rev Respir Dis 146:104, 1992

Ford-Hutchinson AW, Bray MA, Doig MV, et al: Leukotriene B_4, a potent chemokinetic and aggregating substance released from polymorphonuclear leukocytes. Nature 286:264, 1980

Hardy CC, Bradding P, Robinson C, et al: Bronchoconstrictor and anti-bronchoconstrictor properties of inhaled prostacyclin in asthma. J Appl Physiol 63:1567, 1988

Henderson WR: Eicosanoids and lung inflammation. Am Rev Respir Dis 135:1176, 1987

Henderson WR: The role of leukotrienes in inflammation. Ann Intern Med 121:684, 1994

Holgate ST, Bradding P, Sampson AP: Leukotriene antagonists and synthesis inhibitors: New directions in asthma therapy. J Allergy Clin Immunol 98:1, 1996

Hoover RL, Karnovsky ML, Austen KF, et al: Leukotriene B_4 action on endothelium mediates augmented neutrophil endothelial adhesion. Proc Natl Acad Sci USA 81:2191, 1984

Hyman AL, Spannhake EW, Kadowitz PJ: Prostaglandins and the lung. Am Rev Respir Dis 117:111, 1978

Kikawa Y, Miyanomae T, Inoue Y, et al: Urinary leukotriene E_4 after exercise challenge in children with asthma. J Allergy Clin Immunol 89:1111, 1992

Kudo I, Murakami M, Hara S, et al: Mammmalian nonpancreatic phospholipases A_2. Biochim Biophys Acta 117:217, 1993

Laitinen LA, Laitinen A, Haahtela T, et al: Leukotriene E_4 and granulocytic infiltration into asthmatic airways. Lancet 341:989, 1993

Leslie CC: Properties and regulation of cytosolic phospholipase A_2. J Biol Chem 272:16709, 1997

Liu MC, Bleecker ER, Lichtenstein LM, et al: Evidence for elevated levels of histamine, prostaglandin D_2, and other bronchoconstricting prostaglandins in the airways of subjects with mild asthma. Am Rev Respir Dis 142:126, 1990

MacDermot J, Kelsey CR, Waddell KA, et al: Synthesis of leukotriene B_4 and prostaglandins by human alveolar macrophages: Analysis by gas chromatography/mass spectrometry. Prostaglandins 27:163, 1984

Marom Z, Shelhamer JH, Bach MK, et al: The effects of arachinoids and leukotrienes on the release of mucus from human airways. Chest 81:365, 1982

Marom Z, Shelhamer JH, Kaliner M: Effects of arachidonic acid, monohydroxyeicosatetraenoic acid and prostaglandins on the release of mucous glycoproteins from human airways in vitro. J Clin Invest 67:1695, 1981

Melillo B, Woolley KL, Manning PJ, et al: Effect of inhaled PGE_2 on exercise bronchoconstriction in asthmatic subjects. Am J Respir Crit Care Med 149:1138, 1994

Naclerio RM, Baroody FM, Togias AG: The role of leukotrienes in allergic rhinitis: Review. Am Rev Respir Dis 143:S91, 1991

Nagy L, Lee TH, Goetzl EJ, et al: Complement receptor enhancement and chemotaxis of human neutrophils and eosinophils by leukotrienes and other lipoxygenase products. Clin Exp Immunol 47:541, 1982

Pavord ID, Wong CS, Williams J, et al: Effect of inhaled prostaglandin E_2 on allergen-induced asthma. Am Rev Respir Dis 148:87, 1993

Rola-Pleszczynski M, Stankova J: Leukotriene B_4 enhances interleukin-6 (IL-6) production and IL-6 messenger RNA accumulation in human monocytes in vitro: translational, and posttranscriptional mechanisms. Blood 80:1004, 1992

Seibert K, Masferrer J, Zhang Y, et al: Mediation of inflammation by cyclooxygenase-2. Agents Actions 46(suppl):41, 1995

Spada CS, Nieves AL, Krauss AH, et al: Comparison of leukotriene B$_4$ and D$_4$ effects on human eosinophil and neutrophil motility in vitro. J Leukocyte Biol 55:183, 1994

Sweatman WJ, Collier HO: Effects of prostaglandins on human bronchial muscle. Nature 217:69, 1968

Szczeklik A: Mechanism of aspirin-induced asthma. Allergy 52:613, 1997

Taylor IK, O'Shaughnessy KM, Fuller RW et al: Effect of cysteinyl-leukotriene receptor antagonist ICI 204,219 on allergen-induced bronchoconstriction and airway

hyperreactivity in atopic subjects. Lancet 337:690, 1991

Tischfield JA: A reassessment of the low molecular weight phospholipase A$_2$ gene family in mammals. J Biol Chem 272:17247, 1997

Wenzel SE, Larsen GL, Johnston K, et al: Elevated levels of leukotriene C$_4$ in bronchoalveolar lavage fluid from atopic asthmatics after endobronchial allergen challenge. Am Rev Respir Dis 142:112, 1990

Wenzel SE, Westcott JY, Smith HR, et al: Spectrum of prostanoid release after bronchoalveolar allergen challenge in atopic asthmatics and in control groups. Am Rev Respir Dis 139:450, 1989

Complement and Kinin Systems

Bruce C. Gilliland

The complement and kinin systems play important roles in normal physiologic processes as well as in autoimmune and allergic disorders. Both systems are composed of specific plasma proteins that interact in a cascade sequence to mediate a variety of biologic effects including inflammation and host defense.

COMPLEMENT SYSTEM

The complement system is comprised of plasma proteins that interact in a coordinated cascade and other plasma and cell membrane proteins that regulate these events (Table 1–9). The plasma complement proteins are mostly synthesized in the liver. Synthesis also occurs in monocytes or macrophages; fibroblasts; and in epithelial cells of the pulmonary, gastrointestinal, and genitourinary tracts. In addition to its important role in protecting the host from infection, complement also mediates tissue damage in a variety of immunologically mediated disorders including systemic lupus erythematosus, cryoglobulinemia, and hypersensitivity vasculitis.

Complement is activated through two major pathways: the classical pathway and the alternative pathway. Each pathway has its characteristic activators that initiate a series of steps resulting in the formation of a structurally different but functionally identical enzyme complex, C3 convertase, which cleaves and activates complement protein 3 (C3). Subse-

Table 1–9. **Components of the Complement Cascade**

Pathway	Approximate Molecular Weight (kD)	Serum Concentration (~µg/ml)
Classical Pathway		
C1q	410	80
C1r	83	50
C1s	83	50
C2	117	25
C3	185	1200
C4	205	600
Alternative Pathway		
C3	185	1200
Factor B	83	180
Factor D	25	—
Properdin	160	25
Terminal Pathway		
C5	190	75
C6	120	60
C7	110	55
C8	150	80
C9	71	60

quently, both pathways lead to cleavage of C5 by their respective C5 convertases, followed by the assembly and insertion of the terminal complement components known as the membrane attack complex into the membrane of a cell or microorganism resulting in cell damage or lysis.

Classical Complement Pathway

The classical complement pathway is typically activated by immune complexes containing antibodies of IgM or IgG subclasses 1 and 3 or by the binding of these antibodies to antigens on the membranes of cells or microorganisms. C1 can be directly activated in the absence of antibody by substances such as C-reactive protein, pneumococcal polysaccharides, gram-negative bacteria, and various viruses.

Activation of the classical pathway starts with the binding of C1 to antibody or other activators (Fig. 1–6). C1 is a calcium-dependent molecular complex composed of one molecule of C1q and two molecules each of C1r and C1s. C1q has six globular heads that recognize sites on IgG, IgM, or other activators such as C-reactive protein. The binding of two or more globular recognition heads of C1q to an activator alters C1r, converting it to an active protease enzyme. C1r in turn activates C1s, making C1s the active protease that acts on C4 and C2. C1s cleaves many molecules of C4 and C2, releasing two small peptides, C4a and C2a, into plasma. The remaining larger fragments C4b and C2b form a magnesium-dependent complex, C4b2b, which is the classical pathway C3 convertase. C4b attaches covalently to the surface of the activator, allowing the C3 convertase to be assembled at this site. Each C1s generates several thousand molecules of C3 convertase. The pathway is further amplified as each C3 convertase generates many thousand molecules of activated C3 (C3b) that covalently bind to the activating surface around the initiating C3 convertase. The high density of C3b on the surface of the activator is important for opsonization of microorganisms and the clearance of circulating complexes (see Biological Activities of Complement Components and their Fragments).

Activation of C4 and C2 can occur inde-pendent of C1 through mannose binding protein (MBP), the lectin pathway. MBP is a naturally occurring plasma protein that increases during acute phase reactions. MBP is structurally similar to C1q and circulates in a complex with a serine protease that is similar to C1r and C1s. The MBP–serine protease complex recognizes and binds to bacteria expressing terminal mannose or N-acetylglucosamine on their surface, leading to activation of the serine protease. C4 and C2 are subsequently cleaved as in the classical pathway to form C4b2b, the C3 convertase. The active serine protease can also directly act as a C3 convertase.

Regulation of complement activation is critical in allowing the complement system to appropriately destroy invading microorganisms and remove harmful circulating immune complexes while at the same time protecting host cells and tissues from complement-mediated damage (Table 1–10). The initiation of classical pathway activation is controlled by the C1 inhibitor, which binds to activated C1r and C1s, removing them from the antibody–C1qrs complex. C1 inhibitor reduces fluid phase activation and excessive activation on the surface of the activating target. The mannose binding protein–serine protease is also blocked by the C1 inhibitor. Other regulatory proteins prevent excessive activation and consumption of C3 convertase. Decay accelerating factor (CD55), which is attached to host cells, functions by dissociating C3 convertase deposited on these cells. C4b-binding protein also accelerates dissociation of C3 convertase, but acts primarily on the fluid phase C3 convertase. Some regulatory proteins facilitate the proteolytic cleavage of C3b and C4b by serving as a cofactor for the serine protease, factor I. On the host cells, membrane cofactor protein (CD46) is the cofactor for factor I, which degrades C3b and C4b and protects host cells from complement-induced damage. In the fluid phase, C4b-binding protein serves as a cofactor for factor I, which cleaves C4b into C4c and C4d (Fig. 1–7).

Alternative Complement Pathway

The alternative pathway does not require antibody for activation but instead is activated by

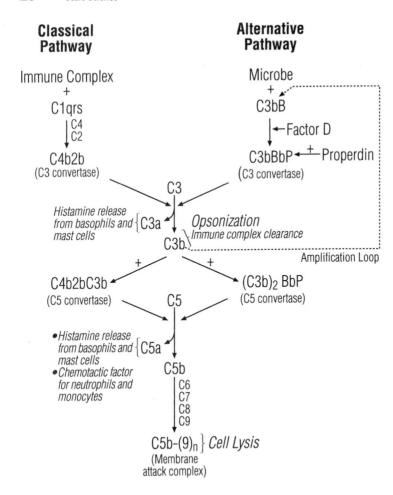

Classical Pathway

Alternative Pathway

Figure 1–6. The complement system. The two major pathways of complement activation are the classical and alternative pathways. Each pathway forms separate but functionally identical C3 and C5 convertases that cleave C3 and C5 respectively, leading to the formation of C3b and C5b and the release into the plasma of biologically active fragments C3a and C5a. The formation of C5b initiates the assembly and insertion of the terminal components into the cell membrane, resulting in cell lysis.

polysaccharides present in cell membranes of various pathogenic bacteria, parasites, viruses, and fungi (see Fig. 1–6). The first step is the covalent binding of C3b to the surface of an activator, which permits the attachment of factor B to form a magnesium-dependent complex, C3bB. Factor B in the C3bB complex is cleaved by factor D, present as an active en-

Table 1–10. **Regulatory Proteins of the Complement System**

Protein	Function
Control of initiation of the classical pathway	
C1 inhibitor (C1-INH)	Inactivates C1r and C1s
Regulation of C3 convertase	
Decay accelerating factor (CD55)	Accelerates dissociation of C3 and C5 convertases on host cells
C4b-binding protein	Accelerates dissociation of fluid phase C3 and C5 convertases of classical pathway and cofactor for factor I cleavage of C4b
Factor I	Degrades C3b and C4b in presence of cofactor protein
Membrane cofactor protein (CD46)	Membrane-bound cofactor for factor I cleavage of C4b
Factor H	Accelerates the dissociation of alternative pathway C3 and C5 convertases and cofactor for factor I cleavage of C3b
Properdin	Stabilizes alternative pathway C3 convertase
Terminal Pathway	
Membrane inhibitor of reactive lysis (CD59)	Blocks assembly and insertion of terminal components on host cells by binding C8 and preventing polymerization of C9
S-protein	Binds to C5b-7 complex and prevents its insertion into the cell membrane

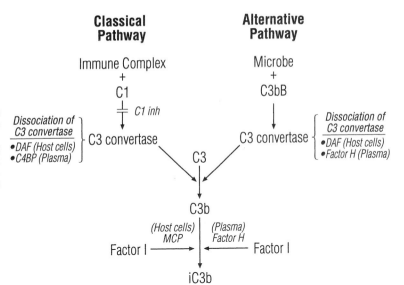

Figure 1–7. Regulatory proteins of the classical and alternative complement pathways. *C1inh,* C1 inhibitor; *DAF,* decay accelerating factor; *C4BP,* C4b binding protein; *MCP,* membrane cofactor protein. MCP and factor H are cofactors for the serine protease, factor I.

zyme, to form C3bBb, which is unstable and rapidly destroyed. The complex, however, is stabilized by the addition of properdin (P) to form C3bBbP, the alternative complement pathway convertase. The C3 convertase cleaves C3 to form C3b, which complexes with additional factor B to form C3bB. The latter is cleaved by factor D to generate additional C3bBb. The availability of C3b to create more C3 convertase provides amplification or a positive feedback loop for the alternative pathway.

The regulation of the alternative pathway is directed at controlling C3 convertase formation in the fluid phase or on the target cell. The alternative pathway does not have an inhibitor similar to C1 inhibitor to block its initiation. This pathway instead is regulated by either dissocation of C3 convertase or prevention of its formation. Decay accelerating factor (CD55) accelerates the dissociation of alternative pathway C3 convertase that forms on the host cell and protects host tissues from complement induced damage. Factor H, a plasma protein, accelerates the decay of fluid phase C3 convertase. Factor H and membrane cofactor protein each serve as cofactors for the proteolytic cleavage of C3b into inactive C3b (iC3b). Membrane cofactor protein only functions in this role on the host cell to which it is attached.

For activation of the alternative pathway to occur, C3b must be available in the plasma so that it can bind to an activating substance such as a pathogenic bacteria. Small amounts of C3b are normally found in plasma as a result of low-grade C3 convertase activity. The formation of the initial C3 convertase requires the presence of a metastable form of C3. C3 continually undergoes spontaneous hydrolysis of its thioester bond to form C3 (H_2O), which is capable of forming a complex with factor B in the presence of magnesium. Factor B in the complex is then cleaved by factor D to form C3(H_2O)Bb, an initiator of C3 convertase that cleaves C3 to C3b and C3a. This C3 convertase has a very short half-life.

Terminal Complement Pathway

Activation and assembly of the terminal complement components (C5b-9), referred to as the membrane attack complex, results in cell membrane damage (see Fig. 1–6). The initial step is the cleavage of C5 by either the classical or alternative pathway C5 convertase. Each C5 convertase is created by the addition of C3b to either the classical or alternative pathway C3 convertase, forming, respectively, C4b2bC3b or C3bBbC3b. Cleavage of C5 yields a large fragment C5b and a small fragment C5a. The latter is released into plasma and has important biologic functions (Table 1–11). C5b binds a single molecule of C6 followed by a single C7 molecule to form a C5b67 complex

Table 1–11. **Biologic Functions of Complement**

Complement Protein	Function
C2 fragment	Kinin-like activity: venular permeability and vasodilatation; contributes to the swelling in hereditary angioedema
C3a, C5a	Anaphylatoxins: release of histamine from mast cells and basophils; C3a inhibits antibody production; C5a stimulates antibody production
C5a	Chemotactic factor for neutrophils and monocytes; increases adhesiveness and is a potent activator of inflammatory mediators from these cells; stimulates oxidative burst in neutrophils
C3b	Enhances phagocytosis and clearance of immune complexes
C5b-9	Membrane attack complex: produces cell injury and lysis

that inserts into the cell membrane. With the addition of a single C8 molecule to the C5b67 complex, some cell damage occurs. Multiple molecules of C9, ranging from 6 to 12, react with the C5b-8 complex to create a stable transmembrane channel. The C5b-9n complex is inserted through the cell membrane with the hydrophobic residue on the outside in contact with the lipid bilayer. The transmembrane channel formed permits the influx of water and sodium, leading to osmotic lysis of the cell or microorganism. A single C5b-9n transmembrane channel will lead to osmotic lysis. Under normal circumstances, many transmembrane channels are present in an affected cell.

The terminal complement pathway or membrane attack complex is regulated at several steps (see Table 1–10). Membrane inhibitor of reactive lysis (CD59) prevents insertion of the terminal complement components into the membrane of host cells by binding C8 and C9, thereby protecting the host cells from lysis as innocent bystanders. This regulatory protein as well as decay accelerating factor, a regulator of C3 convertase, are attached to the cell surface by a phosphoinositide glycosidic linkage. Another inhibitor, S-protein, also called vitronectin, binds to the C5b67 complex preventing insertion of this complex into the cell membrane. The SC5b67 fluid-phase complex can still incorporate C8 and C9 but is unable to lyse cells. The importance of the two regulatory proteins is exemplified by the disorder paroxysmal nocturnal hemoglobinuria (PNH) in which these two proteins are lacking. The absence of these two regulatory proteins from cells of affected patients makes their red blood cells extremely sensitive to complement lysis.

Biologic Activities of Complement Components and their Fragments

Complement activation leads to release of fragments that have important biologic activities (see Table 1–11). The fragments C3a and C5a, referred to as anaphylatoxins, induce degranulation of mast cells and basophils and release of histamine causing venular permeability, vasodilatation, and increased contractility of gastrointestinal and bronchial smooth muscles. These fragments cause smooth muscle contractility independent of histamine release. In addition, C5a is a chemotactic factor for neutrophils and monocytes. C5a also increases the adhesiveness of these cells and stimulates the production of oxygen-free radicals. C5a is believed to play a role in the adult respiratory syndrome in patients undergoing renal hemodialysis. The dialysis membrane activates the alternative complement pathway, leading to the generation of C5a, which causes aggregation and activation of neutrophils in the pulmonary circulation and results in lung injury. Both C3a and C5a affect antibody production with C3a inhibiting and C5a stimulating production. The activity of C3a and C5a is regulated by a serum carboxypeptidase that cleaves the C-terminal arginine from these proteins and reduces their functions.

A fragment of C2 released following C2 activation has kinin-like properties that cause vascular permeability and edema. This fragment may contribute to the development of edema in patients with hereditary angioedema (see Kinin System). The activation and assembly of the terminal complement components

(C5b-9) results in cell damage and destruction.

Biologic Activities of Complement Receptors

The interaction of cell surface complement receptors (CR) with C3b and its degradation products provides mechanisms for facilitating phagocytosis, clearance of circulatory immune complexes, and regulation of the immune system (Table 1–12). CR1, the receptor for C3b, is present on neutrophils, monocytes and macrophages, erythrocytes, follicular dendritic cells, and B lymphocytes. The binding of C3b-coated cells or microorganisms to CR1 on neutrophils and macrophages enhances their phagocytosis. Attachment of CR1 on phagocytic cells to C3b-containing immune complexes deposited on vascular endothelium or other sites causes vasculitis and tissue damage. CR1 on erythrocytes also plays an important role in the clearance of circulating immune complexes. CR1 on erythrocytes binds C3b-containing immune complexes, which are carried by the erythrocytes to the liver and spleen where they are removed and digested. The erythrocytes are released back into the circulation.

CR3 is the receptor for iC3b, a degradation product of C3b. CR3, present on neutrophils and macrophages, binds iC3b-coated cells or microorganisms enhancing their phagocytosis.

CR4 is also a receptor for iC3b and is present on neutrophils, monocytes, macrophages, dendritic cells, and NK cells. It has been shown to mediate adhesion of neutrophils to endothelium.

CR2 is the receptor for C3d and C3dg, which are subsequent degradation products of C3b. CR2 is present on the membrane of B lymphocytes and forms a complex with several other proteins. Interaction of C3dg with this complex lowers the threshold of B lymphocytes for activation by T lymphocyte-dependent antigens. CR2 is also found on follicular dendritic cells. Of interest is that Epstein-Barr virus binds to the same complex receptor, permitting its entry into B lymphocytes.

C1q receptors (C1qR) are found on neutrophils, monocytes, and most B lymphocytes. The binding of C1q to the C1qR on neutrophils or monocytes leads to enhanced phagocytosis of C1q-containing immune complexes. The C1q receptor reacts only with C1q that has been dissociated from C1r and C1s by C1 inhibitor.

Hereditary Deficiencies of Complement Proteins

Inherited deficiencies of individual complement components are recognized for most of the proteins in the complement system (Table 1–13). Complete absence of a complement protein occurs infrequently, but may be associated with increased susceptibility to serious bacterial infections or to the development of autoimmune disorders similar to systemic lupus erythematosus. Complement proteins are encoded by genes on autosomal chromosomes except for the properdin gene, which is on the X chromosome. Complement deficiencies are inherited as an autosomal recessive trait. Complete deficiency of a complement protein results from inheritance of a null (nonsynthesis) gene from each parent. An individual with

Table 1–12. **Complement Receptors**

Receptor Protein	Specificity	Expressed on These Cells	Function
C1qR	C1q	Neutrophils, monocytes, B lymphocytes	Enhances phagocytosis
CR1	C3b/C4b	Erythrocytes, neutrophils, monocytes/ macrophages, follicular dendritic cells, B lymphocytes	Clearance of immune complexes, enhances phagocytosis
CR2	C3d, C3dg	B lymphocytes, follicular dendritic cells	Lowers threshold of B lymphocyte activation
CR3	iC3b	Neutrophils, monocytes/macrophages, natural killer cells	Mediates adhesion of leukocytes to endothelium, enhances phagocytosis
CR4	iC3b	Neutrophils, monocytes/macrophages, dendritic cells and natural killer cells	Mediates adhesion of leukocytes to endothelium

Table 1–13. **Hereditary Deficiencies of Complement Proteins**

Protein	Pattern of Inheritance	Clinical Features
C1q, C1r, or C1s	Autosomal recessive	Lupus-like illness, susceptibility to bacterial infections
C4 or C2	Autosomal recessive	SLE and lupus-like illness, dermatomyositis, glomerulonephritis, vasculitis
C3	Autosomal recessive	Recurrent, pyogenic infections, lupus-like illness
C5, C6, C7, or C8	Autosomal recessive	Lupus-like illness, recurrent *Neisseria* infections
Properdin	X-linked	Recurrent *Neisseria* infections, recurrent pyogenic infections
Factor D	Autosomal recessive	*Neisseria* infections
Factor H or I	Autosomal recessive	Recurrent pyogenic infections
C1 inhibitor	Autosomal dominant	Hereditary angioedema

only one normal gene (heterozygote) will have one-half of the normal amount of the protein.

Complete deficiency of a component of the classical pathway—C1q, C1r, C1s, C4, or C2—may be associated with a lupus-like disorder. Complete C2 deficiency is the most common deficiency, affecting 1 in 10,000 individuals. Dermatomyositis, glomerulonephritis, and vasculitis have been observed in C4- or C2-deficient patients. Individuals who are C4-deficient are also more likely to develop systemic lupus erythematosus. C4 differs from other complement components by being encoded by two distinct genes, designated C4A and C4B. Null alleles at these two gene loci are common. Individuals with a null allele at one of the two C4 loci will have serum levels 75% of normal, those with two null alleles will have levels 50% of normal, those with three null alleles will have serum levels 25% of normal, and those with all four null alleles will have no C4 protein. C4A homozygous deficiency (two null alleles at C4A) is 10 to 15 times more common in patients with systemic lupus erythematosus than in the unaffected population. The development of lupus-like disorders in individuals with deficiencies of classical pathway complement proteins is believed to be caused by inadequate clearance of circulating immune complexes. The absence of an early acting complement protein prevents formation of C3b, which normally would bind to immune complexes leading to their removal by the spleen and liver. Persistence of circulating immune complexes increases their likelihood of being deposited in the kidney and other tissue sites, resulting in tissue damage.

Individuals with classical pathway complement protein deficiencies are more susceptible to infection with encapsulated bacteria. These infections are usually not serious unless other host defense defects are present. Complement deficiencies in the alternative pathway predispose individuals to serious recurrent bacterial infections, because this pathway is the first line of host defense before the development of antibodies. Factor D deficiency has been described in a few patients, and all had recurrent meningococcal disease. Properdin-deficient individuals are usually teenage boys with systemic meningococcal disease. The meningococci often belong to uncommon serogroups.

Individuals with complete absence of C3 protein have increased susceptibility to encapsulated bacteria such as meningococcus, pneumococcus, and *Haemophilus influenzae*. Lupus-like disorders also occur in C3-deficient patients. Low levels of C3 may also be caused by hypercatabolism of C3. In the absence of C3 inactivator (factor I), C3b is not degraded to C3bi, resulting in additional production of C3 convertase. The positive feedback provided by C3b eventually results in depletion of C3 levels. Affected individuals are susceptible to infections with encapsulated bacteria.

Individuals with a hereditary deficiency of a terminal complement protein may present in their teenage years with systemic gonococcal infections or recurrent meningococcal meningitis. About 50% of individuals with a homozygous deficiency of a terminal complement component, however, are healthy. Complete deficiency of C5, C7, or C8 may rarely be associated with systemic lupus erythematosus or a lupus-like disorder. The strongest correlation between a complement component deficiency and an autoimmune disease is seen when early acting components are absent.

Inherited deficiency of C1 inhibitor (INH) is associated with hereditary angioedema (HAE). HAE is characterized by recurrent episodes of subcutaneous and submucosal tissue edema that last up to 72 hours. Episodes may involve the throat, compromising breathing, or cause acute abdominal pain and obstruction when involving the intestine. The mechanisms for angioedema are believed to be excessive formation of bradykinin and C2 kinin because of low levels of C1 inhibitor. Diagnosis is made by the demonstration of low levels of C1 inhibitor protein or low or absent C1 inhibitor function. Approximately 15% of HAE-affected individuals make a nonfunctional C1 inhibitor protein. Complement measurements show low C4 and C2 serum levels. C4 levels are usually low between attacks. C3 levels and CH50 activity are normal.

Acquired angioedema is clinically similar to HAE and is also caused by low levels of C1 inhibitor. In acquired angioedema, low levels of C1 inhibitor are caused by autoantibodies to the inhibitor or by excessive utilization of C1 inhibitor because of increased activation of C1 by immune complexes. Excessive activation of C1 with increased utilization of C1 inhibitor is seen in systemic lupus erythematosus and malignancies. It should be remembered, however, that most patients with angioedema, especially with associated urticaria, do not have an inherited or acquired deficiency of C1 inhibitor.

Clinical Significance

Complement measurements may be helpful in the diagnosis and assessment of immunologically mediated disorders (Table 1–14). The tests that are most generally available are analysis of hemolytic complement activity and determination of protein levels of C3 and C4. Hemolytic complement activity is usually expressed in CH_{50} units. A CH_{50} unit is determined by the amount of serum that will lyse 50% of a known amount of sheep erythrocytes optimally sensitized with rabbit antisheep erythrocyte antibodies. Immunoassay techniques are used to quantitate C3 and C4 protein levels. The normal range of serum levels for CH_{50}, C3, and C4 are quite broad, making it difficult to know whether the complement system is activated unless the levels fall below the established normal range. Even then, low levels of complement may be caused by decreased synthesis; for example, C3 synthesis may be reduced in systemic lupus erythematosus. Complement is also an acute phase reactant, and complement levels are usually increased in patients with infectious diseases and connective tissue disorders. The increase is usually no greater than two-fold over the baseline level and occurs within a week of the onset of inflammation. In comparison, C-reactive protein increases 100- to 1000-fold within hours. In the setting of inflammation, levels of C3, C4, or CH_{50} at the lower limit of normal may signify activation of complement.

The detection of cleavage products of complement components is a sensitive method for determining complement activation. The measurement of cleavage products has the advantage of not being influenced by alterations in the rate of synthesis. Cleavage products most commonly measured include anaphyla-

Table 1–14. **Measurement of Complement**

Condition	C1 INH	C1	C4	C3	CH$_{50}$
Classical pathway activation (e.g., SLE*, SBE†, mixed cryoglobulinemia)	NA	NA	↓	↓	↓
Alternative pathway activation (e.g., membranoproliferative glomerulonephritis type II and partial lipodystrophy associated with the C3 nephritic factor)	NA	NA	N‡	↓	N
Deficiency of a complement component (e.g., C2). May be associated with lupus-like disorder or recurrent bacterial infections depending on the absent complement component	NA	N	N	N	Absent
Hereditary angioedema	↓ §	N	↓	N	N or sl ↓
Acquired angioedema	↓	↓	↓	N	N or sl ↓

*Systemic lupus erythematosus
†Subacute bacterial endocarditis
‡Normal
§Protein measurement of C1 INH may be normal but protein is nonfunctional. Functional assay of C1 INH is required.
NA = Not applicable. Measurement is not of clinical value in these disorders.

toxins (C3a and C5a), C4d, C3d, and Bb. An increased level of Bb and not C4d indicates predominantly activation of the alternative pathway. Detection of increased amounts of membrane attack complex C5b-9 in serum also provides evidence of complement activation. The binding of S-protein to C5b-9 prevents insertion of this complex into cell membranes, allowing it to be measured in the serum or other body fluids (e.g., synovial fluid). Assays for cleavage products are not widely available in clinical laboratories.

The CH_{50} assay is the best screening test for a homozygous deficiency of a complement protein, because an affected individual will have no detectable serum complement hemolytic activity. The absence of any one complement protein blocks the subsequent activation of complement components required for hemolysis of the sheep erythrocytes. Some hemolysis will occur with complete deficiency of C9 (see *Terminal Complement Pathway*). In individuals with no detectable hemolytic complement, the missing component is identified by assays for individual complement components available in specialty laboratories.

Reduced levels of C3, C4, and CH_{50} may be present in patients with circulating immune complexes, for example, those with systemic lupus erythematosus, mixed cryoglobulinemia, hypersensitivity vasculitis, poststreptococcal glomerulonephritis, subacute bacterial endocarditis, infected atrioventricular shunts, pneumococcal sepsis, and the prodromal phase of hepatitis B infection. Low levels of C3 with normal levels of C4 and CH_{50} are observed in membranoproliferative glomerulonephritis and partial lipodystrophy. These disorders are associated with the C3 nephritic factor. This nephritic factor has been shown to be an IgG autoantibody directed to the activated factor B present in the alternative pathway C3 convertase, C3bBb. The autoantibody decreases the natural decay of the convertase and also interferes with its dissociation by factor H. The cell-bound C3 convertase stabilized by the nephritic factor has a significantly longer half-life, which results in an increased turnover of the C3b amplification loop without activation of the terminal complement components. The increased activation of C3 results in depressed serum levels of this protein. Low complement values also occur in severe hepatic failure and malnutrition because of decreased synthesis. Some patients with systemic lupus erythematosus have low levels of C3 owing to decreased synthesis of C3 as well as increased consumption.

Summary

The complement system is a highly integrated and remarkably regulated system consisting of plasma and cell membrane proteins and cell receptors. Its primary function is to protect the host from infection by mediating inflammation. Biologic activities of complement are chemotaxis, phagocytosis, cell adhesion, cell injury and lysis, and B cell differentiation. The importance of complement in host defense is underscored by the increased susceptibility to recurrent bacterial infection in those rare individuals who have an inherited deficiency of a single complement component. Complement plays an adverse role in a variety of immunologic disorders by mediating inflammation and tissue damage. An unusual form of angioedema occurs in individuals with an inherited deficiency of C1 inhibitor. Measurement of complement is of value in several clinical disorders.

KININ SYSTEM

The kinin system consists of a group of plasma proteins that, once activated, interact in a sequential manner to generate bradykinin, a biologically active nonapeptide. These biologic activities include the ability to induce vasodilatation, vascular permeability, pain, contraction of smooth muscle at many sites, and bronchoconstriction and the activation of phospholipase A2 resulting in the formation of arachidonic acid and production of prostaglandins and leukotrienes. Many of these activities are proinflammatory. Kinins are responsible, in part, for some of the clinical features of asthma and allergic rhinitis. Bradykinin is also involved in maintaining normal vascular homeostasis by regulating systemic blood pressure and cardiovascular circulation. Another kinin referred to as kallidin (lysl-bradykinin) is formed locally in tissue and has similar biologic activities (Table 1–15).

Table 1–15. Functions of Bradykinin

Vasodilatation
Vascular permeability
Bronchoconstriction
Contraction of gastrointestinal and uterine
    smooth muscle
Mediation of pain
Facilitation of arachidonic acid metabolism
Blood pressure homeostasis and
    cardioprotection

Components of the Kinin System

The major plasma proteins are Factor XII [Hageman factor], prekallikrein, and high-molecular weight [HMW] kininogen. Most HMW kininogen circulates as a complex with prekallikrein in a 1:1 molar ratio and with Factor XI in a 2:1 molar ratio. Factor XI does not play a role in bradykinin formation. The activation and interaction of these plasma proteins depend on their binding to a suitable negatively charged surface such as lipid A, a component of endotoxin located in the outer membrane of all gram-negative bacteria, or other naturally occurring polysaccharides. Endothelial cells have receptors on their surface for HMW kininogen or Factor XII permitting activation of Factor XII along this surface and initiation of bradykinin production. Kallikrein can also be activated by tissue injury and by plasmin.

Steps in the Generation of Bradykinin

The initial step in the generation of bradykinin is autoactivation of Factor XII once it binds to a negatively charged surface (Fig. 1–8). Bound Factor XII is cleaved by activated Factor XII (Factor XIIa) to form additional Factor XIIa and fragments of Factor XII [XIIf]. Trace amounts of Factor XIIa are believed to be present in normal plasma to account for the initial cleavage of Factor XII. Factor XIIa rapidly converts prekallikrein to the active enzyme kallikrein and also activates Factor XI to Factor XIa, which can initiate the intrinsic coagulation pathway. Kallikrein cleaves surface-bound HMW kininogen to generate bradykinin. Plasma kallikrein is very specific in using HMW kininogen as a substrate and is unable to cleave low-molecular weight kininogen. Factor XIIf is not bound to the contact surface and can activate prekallikrein to kallikrein at distant sites.

The complex of prekallikrein and HMW kininogen binds to the activating contact surface through HMW kininogen allowing this complex to be in juxtaposition to Factors XII and XIIa. Kallikrein, in addition to generating bradykinin, activates Factor XII to form more Factor XIIa and Factor XIIf, which in turn activates prekallikrein to kallikrein providing a positive feedback loop. The activation of Factor XII by kallikrein is many-fold more rapid than the autoactivation of Factor XII and accounts for most of the activation of Factor XII.

Bradykinin Function and Degradation

The functions of bradykinin arc mediated through its interaction with either B1 or B2 receptors, which are present on the membrane surface of many cell types including vascular endothelial, smooth muscle, and synovial lining cells. B1 receptors are thought to be induced during inflammation.

Figure 1–8. The kinin system. Activation of the kinin cascade is initiated by the binding of factor XII to a negatively charged surface. The complex of prekallikrein and high molecular weight (HMW) kininogen also binds to the activating surface through HMW kininogen, allowing the components of the kinin system to be in close proximity. (Kallikrein provides a positive feedback loop by activating factor XII.) C1 inhibitor (C1inh) inhibits factor XIIa, factor XIIf (not shown), and prekallikrein.

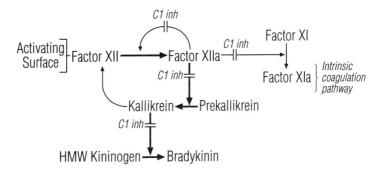

Bradykinin is rapidly digested by carboxypeptidase N (also referred to as anaphylatoxin inactivator or kininase 1). The degraded bradykinin is still able to react with bradykinin receptors in the vasculature to produce hypotension. Further cleavage of this protein by angiotensin converting enzyme (ACE) produces inactive peptides. In the pulmonary vasculature, bradykinin is inactivated by ACE (also referred to as kininase II). The cough and angioedema associated with the administration of ACE inhibitors for treatment of hypertension and diabetes mellitus may be caused by the inhibition of bradykinin degradation leading to increased tissue levels of bradykinin.

Regulation of the Kinin System

Low-grade activation of Factor XII and prekallikrein may be continously ongoing but held in check by plasma inhibitors. The introduction of a negatively charged activating surface changes the balance in favor of increased activation of the kinin-generating system. The fact that plasma inhibitors are not bound to the contact surface further favors activation. Plasma inhibitors, however, do play a role in controlling the degree of activation. C1 inhibitor is the major inhibitor of Factors XIIa and XIIf. C1 inhibitor and alpha 2 macroglobulin are the main inhibitors of kallikrein.

Tissue Kallikrein Pathway

Tissue kallikrein is a low-molecular weight kallikrein that is distinct from plasma kallikrein. Large amounts of this protein are produced by salivary glands, the pancreas, and the kidney. It is also found in other tissues including the brain, pituitary gland, colon, and prostate. Tissue kallikrein preferentially cleaves low-molecular weight kininogen but also can cleave HMW kininogen to form kallidin (lysl-bradykinin). The lysine is removed by a plasma aminopeptidase to form bradykinin. Kallidin and bradykinin have the same biologic activities.

Clinical Significance

Activation of the kinin system has been observed in allergic rhinitis and asthma. Bradykinin has been found in nasal secretions and bronchoalveolar lavage fluid and may contribute to nasal stuffiness and discharge in allergic rhinitis and bronchoconstriction and bronchial mucosal edema in asthma. Bradykinin acts directly on the smooth muscle of the bronchi to cause bronchoconstriction but also may react with receptors on sensory nerves in the airways to produce reflex bronchospasm and cough. Bradykinin may also stimulate bronchial epithelial cells to release neutrophil and mononuclear chemotactic factors. The kinin system is activated in endotoxic shock, resulting in hypotension. In patients with acute hemorrhagic pancreatitis, release of tissue kallikrein with activation of bradykinin is believed to be partially responsible for the formation of ascites and subsequent hypotension. Both sodium urate and calcium pyrophosphate crystals act as activating contact surfaces for the generation of bradykinin, which may contribute to the inflammatory response and pain observed in gout and pseudogout. Plasma kallikrein has been found in the synovial fluid of patients with rheumatoid arthritis and may be a factor in joint inflammation. Excessive kinin occurs in many other acute and chronic inflammatory disorders, including inflammatory bowel disease, connective tissue diseases, and inflammatory skin diseases.

The kinin system is also involved in the pathogenesis of hereditary angioedema. In this disorder, C1 inhibitor is present in very low concentrations or is dysfunctional, resulting in decreased inhibition of activated Factor XII, kallikrein, and C1r and C1s of the complement system. Kallikrein has been found in induced blister fluid of patients with HAE. Furthermore, an amount of contact activator insufficient to activate the kinin system in normal plasma produces rapid activation in plasma of HAE-affected patients. Once the kinin system is triggered in these patients, angioedema can develop very quickly. The complement system is also activated in HAE and may play a role in the development of angioedema, as a fragment of C2 reportedly has kinin-like properties.

The kinin system is important in the homeostasis of the cardiovascular system. Brady-kinin exerts vasodilatory effects by stimulating endothelial cells to release nitric oxide and prostacyclin. The beneficial effects of ACE inhibition in patients with myocardial ischemia and heart failure are believed to be due to the increased levels of bradykinin resulting in vasodilatation and improved blood flow. The kinin system also plays a role in the regulation of blood pressure and renal blood flow.

Summary

Bradykinin is the major product of the kinin system and has several important biologic activities. These include vasodilatation and vascular permeability, contraction of smooth muscle, mediation of pain, and activation of phospholipase A2 leading to the eventual formation of prostaglandins and leukotrienes. Bradykinin causes bronchoconstriction in asthma and nasal stuffiness and discharge in allergic rhinitis. It acts as a proinflammatory mediator in many acute and chronic inflammatory diseases. Bradykinin also plays an important role in the regulation of the cardiovascular system, providing cardioprotection and blood pressure homeostasis.

Acknowledgment

The author would like to thank Robert Sherwood for his assistance in preparing this section.

Suggested Reading

Complement System

Ahearn JM, Rosengard AM: Complement receptors. *In* Volanakis JE, Frank MM (eds): The Human Complement System in Health and Disease. New York, Marcel Dekker, 1998, p 167

Ahmed AE, Peter JB: Clinical utility of complement assessment. Clin Diagn Lab Immunol 2: 509, 1995

Denson P: Complement deficiencies and infections. *In* Volanakis JE, Frank MM (eds): The Human Complement System in Health and Disease. New York, Marcel Dekker, 1998, p 409

Fearon DT: The complement system and adaptive immunity. Semin Immunol 10:355, 1998

Frank MM: The complement system. *In* Frank MM, Austen KF, Claman HN, Unanue ER (eds): Samter's Immunologic Diseases, 5th ed. Boston, Little, Brown, 1994, p 489

Ghebrehiwet B: The complement, system: Mechanisms of activation, regulation, and biologic functions. *In* Kaplan AP (ed): Allergy, 2nd ed. Philadelphia, WB Saunders 1997, p 219

Holers VM: Complement. *In* Rich RR (ed): Clinical Immunology: Principles and Practice. St. Louis, Mosby-Year Book, 1996, p 363

Liszewski MK, Farries TC, Lublin DM, et al: Control of the complement system. Adv Immunol 61:201, 1996

Moxley G, Ruddy S: Immune complexes and complement. *In* Kelley WN, Harris ED Jr., Ruddy S, Sledge CB (eds): Textbook of Rheumatology, 5th ed. Vol. 1, Philadelphia, WB Saunders Co, 1997, p 228

Ruddy S: Complement deficiencies and Rheumatic Deseases. *In* Kelley WN, Harris ED, Jr., Ruddy S, Sledge CB (eds): Textbook of Rheumatology, 5th ed. Vol 2. Philadelphia, WB Saunders 1997, p 1305

Volanakis JE: Overview of the complement system. *In* Volanakis JE, Frank MM (eds): The Human Complement System in Health and Disease, New York, Marcel Dekker, 1998, p 9

Whaley K, Schwaeble W: Complement and complement deficiencies. Semin Liver Dis 17:297, 1997

Kinin System

Atkins PC, Miragliotta G, Talbot SF, et al: Activation of plasma Hageman factor and kalllikrein in ongoing allergic reaction in the skin. J Immunol 139:2744, 1987

Baumgarten CR, Togias AG, Naclerio RM, et al: Influx of kininogens into nasal secretions after antigen challenge of allergic individuals. J Clin Invest 76:191, 1985

Berkenboom G: Bradykinin and the therapeutic actions of angiotensin-converting enzyme inhibitors. Am J Cardiol 82:11S, 1998

Christiansen SC, Proud D, Cochrane CG: Detection of tissue kallikrein in the bronchoalveolar lavage fluids of asthmatic subjects. J Clin Invest 79:188, 1987

Curd JG, Prograis LF, Cochrane CG: Detection of active kallikrein in induced blister fluids of hereditary angiooedema patients. J Exp Med 152:742, 1980

Kaplan AP, Shibayama Y, Reddigari S, et al: The intrinsic coagulation/kinin-forming cascade: Assembly in plasma and cell surfaces in inflammation. Adv Immunol 66:225, 1997

Mombouli JV: ACE inhibition, endothelial function and coronary artery lesions. Role of kinins and nitric oxide. Drugs 54 (Suppl 5):12, 1997

Morrison DC, Cochrane CG: Direct evidence for Hageman factor (factor XII) activation by bacterial lipopolysaccharides (endotoxins). J Exp Med 140:797, 1974

Pang L, Knox AJ: Bradykinin stimulates IL-8 production in cultured human airway smooth muscle cells: Role of cyclooxygenase products. J Immunol 161:2509, 1998

Reddigari SR, Silverberg M, Kaplan AP: Bradykinin formation: plasma and pathways. *In* Kaplan AP (ed): Allergy, 2nd ed. Philadelphia, WB Saunders, 1997, p 235

Riccio MM, Proud D: Evidence that enhanced nasal reactivity to bradykinin in patients with symptomatic allergy is mediated by neural reflexes. J Allergy Clin Immunol 97:1252, 1996

Sato E, Koyama S, Nomura H, et al: Bradykinin stimulates alveolar macrophages to release neutrophil, monocyte, and eosinophil chemotactic activity. J Immunol 157:3122, 1996

Chapter 2

Skin Tests, *In Vitro* Tests

Laurie A. Myers

Although many allergic diseases can be diagnosed with a comprehensive history and physical examination, *in vivo* allergy tests are of value to confirm clinical suspicions and to identify specific allergens. Skin tests are immediate and reproducible, making this technique ideal for diagnosing allergic diseases. *In vitro* allergy tests are usually reserved for the rare patient who cannot undergo skin testing.

IN VIVO ALLERGY TESTING

Background

Blackley described the first skin test in 1865 when he scratched his forearm, placed ryegrass pollen on it, and developed itching, erythema, and swelling. In 1907 Von Pirquet developed a scratch test for tuberculosis. Smith, in 1909, and Schloss, in 1912, then recognized the usefulness of scratch testing for diagnosing food allergy; Walker employed scratch testing for diagnosing allergy to animal dander in 1917. Lewis and Grant studied dermatographia and vascular reactions of the skin to histamine or injury. They recognized that the scratch itself could induce a wheal in normal skin and that it was difficult to introduce a constant dose of test solution into the scarified area. To overcome these difficulties, they developed the prick test in 1924. Skin testing has stood the test of time; details of the procedure are now more standardized but its rationale has not changed. Skin testing remains the preferred method of diagnosing IgE-mediated diseases.

Pathophysiology of Skin Testing

In vivo skin testing is a useful technique that demonstrates the presence of allergen-specific IgE by introducing an extract of a relevant antigen or allergen into the skin. If the allergen successfully crosslinks specific IgE on the surface of sensitized cutaneous mast cells, a characteristic wheal-and-flare reaction develops (Fig. 2–1). The wheal-and-flare response to allergen is identical to that induced directly

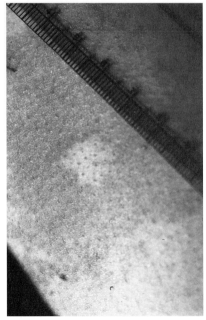

Figure 2–1. Cutaneous wheal-and-flare response to histamine.

by histamine and is the product of both inflammatory and neurogenic cellular interactions. This immediate hypersensitivity response results from mast cell degranulation with the release of pre-formed mediators and the generation of newly synthesized ones. Of the multitude of physicochemically discrete compounds released from mast cells, histamine primarily mediates the wheal-and-flare response because it can be detected 5 minutes after allergen challenge and peaks at 30 minutes. Biologic effects of histamine include arteriolar vasodilatation, extravasation of plasma fluid, and axonal stimulation. The immediate effect is assessed grossly as the triple response of Lewis: localized erythema, edema, and widespread flare.

Studies have shown that the histamine flare can be reduced with topical anesthetics and is reduced in patients with spinal cord injuries, suggesting that the flare depends on sympathetic nervous system interactions with the skin and higher centers. Substance P may be one of several critical neuropeptides that links the sympathetic nervous system to the cutaneous response. It is located in afferent sensory fibers that mainly form neuroeffector junctions with those mast cells close to blood vessels. Antidromic stimulation of these nerves or histamine itself can release substance P. This neuropeptide acts in a positive feedback manner to induce mast cell degranulation, vasodilation, and the consequent flare. Overall, the wheal-and-flare reaction is mainly due to mast cell–derived histamine; the neurogenic interactions seem to intensify the vascular response.

The immediate wheal-and-flare response may be followed by a late phase reaction (LPR). This is a diffusely edematous, only slightly indurated lesion at the same site as the wheal-and-flare. The incidence of isolated LPRs is 6% to 14% but up to 85% of LPRs are preceded by an immediate reaction. The intensity of the LPR correlates directly with that of the immediate reaction. The LPR starts 1 to 2 hours after antigen challenge, peaks at 6 to 12 hours, and resolves in 24 to 48 hours. Like the immediate response, the LPR also requires allergen and specific IgE interactions but the pathophysiology of the LPR is less well understood. Mediators from degranulated mast cells likely cause the influx of inflammatory cells such as CD4+ lymphocytes, neutrophils, and eosinophils that not only initiate but also sustain the LPR. Histamine, kallikrein, thromboxane B_2, interleukin 4, interleukin 5, RANTES, leukotriene C_4, prostaglandin D_2, and platelet activating factor have all been implicated in producing the LPR. Why the LPR does not always follow the immediate response is not known. More importantly, its clinical significance and role in diagnosing IgE-mediated disease has not been proved.

Methods of Skin Testing

In vivo allergy testing includes two general methods, epicutaneous and intracutaneous skin tests. With epicutaneous testing the allergen is placed on the skin before introducing it into the epidermis; with intracutaneous skin tests, the allergen is injected directly into the dermis. Epicutaneous techniques include scratch, prick, or puncture methods. With scratch testing, the superficial layers of the skin are abraded with a blunt instrument and the allergen is applied to a 0.3- to 0.6-mm site. This method lacks precision, yields false-positive and inconsistent results, and is no longer used as a diagnostic tool to detect allergy. Prick and puncture testing are the preferred methods to screen for IgE-mediated diseases. Intracutaneous tests may be used for low potency extracts or to detect low-grade sensitization. Skin testing is not without risks; therefore, the precautions listed in Table 2–1

Table 2–1. **Skin Testing Precautions**

- *Never* perform skin testing unless a physician is available immediately to treat systemic reactions
- Have emergency equipment readily available
- Perform intracutaneous tests only in those patients who have negative prick or puncture test results
- Do not test the patient if allergic symptoms, particularly wheezing, are present
- Use extracts of known potency and stability
- Be certain that the test concentrations are appropriate
- Include a positive and negative control solution
- Perform tests in normal skin
- Determine and record medications taken by the patient and time of last dose
- Record the reactions at the proper time

Adapted from Middleton E Jr, Ellis EF, Reed CE, eds: *Allergy: Principles and Practice*, 4th ed. St Louis, Mosby, 1993; with permission.

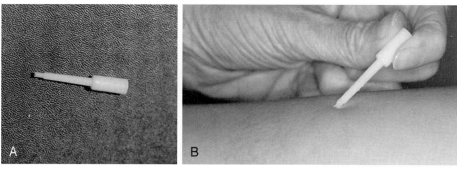

Figure 2–2. *A,* Prick method using Greer DermaPIK (Greer Laboratories, Lenoir, NC). *B,* The device is held at a 45° angle to pass through the extract and prick the epidermis.

should be taken before performing allergy skin testing.

Prick and Puncture Tests

Prick or puncture tests are widely used in the initial evaluation of an atopic patient. Prick testing is mainly performed by the Pepys method, which is a modification of the test originally described by Lewis and Grant. In this method, a drop of the allergen extract (1:10–1:20 weight/volume) is applied directly to the patient's skin. Allergens should be placed at least 2 cm apart on the patient's back, volar surface of the arm, or forearm. An appropriate device is used to pass through the extract at a 45° to 60° angle. The epidermis is then gently pricked and lifted ever so slightly before withdrawing the device (Fig. 2–2). This technique should not induce bleeding; it simply disrupts the epidermis enough to allow the extract to penetrate. Appropriate devices for prick testing include a 25- to 27-gauge hypo-

dermic needle, blood lancet, bifurcated needle, or one of several proprietary devices. The puncture test differs from the prick test in that the device is held at a 90° angle to the skin and pushed through the extract into the superficial layers of the skin without lifting the epidermis (Fig. 2–3). Separate instruments should be used for each allergen to avoid contaminating different sites. No differences in the presence of skin reactions are observed if the allergen extract is removed immediately after pricking or if it remains on the skin for 15 minutes.

Because prick tests do not reproducibly inject an exact amount of allergen into the skin, cutaneous responses vary with seemingly minor differences in technique such as force, duration, depth, or angle of the prick. For these reasons, commercially available, standardized devices have been engineered to ensure more uniform technique and allergen injection. These should increase the reproducibility of skin tests among different users. Most of these devices are designed for the puncture

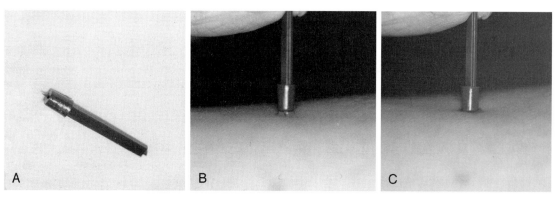

Figure 2–3. *A,* Puncture method using a Morrow-Brown disposable needle. *B,* The needle is held perpendicular to the skin. *C,* The needle is pushed through the extract and into the epidermis.

method. A skilled operator performing the puncture test with a commercial device and modified prick test with a hypodermic needle can produce results with coefficients of variation of 8.4% and 13.4%, respectively. Desirable devices are ones with similar precision and little interpatient variation. In general, metallic devices produce larger wheals but induce more bleeding and the smallest wheals are produced by pricking with a hypodermic needle, intradermal needle, or a plastic device. The accuracy of these devices is measured by the rate of false-positive or false-negative reactions and should also be considered when choosing an appropriate device. Alternative devices may also have the allergen preloaded, have multiple points on each head, or allow the simultaneous placement of multiple allergens. Cost and ease of use often dictate which device investigators choose for skin testing. Regardless of the actual device chosen for skin testing, the reliability and reproducibility of prick test results still greatly depend on the skill of the operator.

Intracutaneous Tests

Intracutaneous skin tests are often performed in the patient with a convincing history of IgE-mediated illness whose screening prick test results are negative. Prick testing should precede intracutaneous testing to detect highly sensitive patients who may be at risk for a systemic reaction from the testing procedure. A tuberculin syringe and 26- or 27-gauge needle is used to inject 0.01 to 0.05 ml of extract intracutaneously. The needle is held at a shallow angle to the skin with the bevel facing down and advanced into the superficial dermis before the extract is injected (Fig. 2–4). The test sites are placed 5 cm apart on the upper arm or volar surface of the forearm so that a tourniquet can be applied to attenuate a systemic reaction. A small wheal or bleb should form at the injection sites. It is important to expel any air from the syringe to avoid false-positive reactions and to penetrate only superficial layers of the skin to avoid false-negative ones.

The size of the skin reaction depends more on the concentration of the extract than the volume of injected extract. In general, ex-

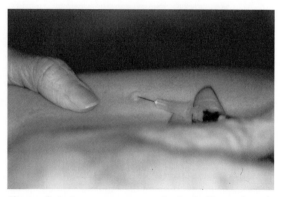

Figure 2–4. Intracutaneous method of skin testing. A small-gauge needle is held at a shallow angle to the skin; extract is injected, and a bleb forms at the injection site.

tracts used for intracutaneous skin testing are 100 to 1000 times more dilute than prick test reagents. Recently, extracts have been more precisely standardized using a definition of bioequivalency units (BAU). With potent extracts of 100,000 BAU, the range of intracutaneous test solutions is 100 to 1000 BAU. With less potent extracts of 10,000 BAU, the range is 10 to 100 BAU. A single concentration of allergen is generally used to determine the presence or absence of allergen-specific antibodies but more information about the degree of sensitivity may be obtained by performing threshold dilution titration tests with threefold or tenfold serial dilutions.

Negative and positive controls are always placed and are used to interpret reactions to the specific allergens. Allergen extracts may contain preservatives that induce false-positive reactions so an appropriate negative control is often the diluent used to stabilize the allergen such as 50% glycerin. Negative control solutions generally detect nonspecific skin reactivity; they may cause a positive wheal-and-flare reaction in a dermatographic patient. False-positive reactions may also occur with excessive trauma to the skin. The positive control solution is histamine or a mast cell secretagogue such as codeine phosphate. Commercially prepared histamine used for prick testing comes as 5.43 mmol/L and for intradermal testing as 0.0543 mmol/L. Positive control solutions are placed to ensure that the patient is physiologically capable of producing a wheal-and-flare response, has not taken an antihistamine, and that the operator's technique is adequate.

Comparison of Prick and Intradermal Skin Testing

Both the U.S. Joint Council of Allergy, Asthma, and Immunology and the European Academy of Allergology and Clinical Immunology recommend prick and puncture tests as the primary test for the diagnosis of IgE-mediated allergic diseases. When performed by an experienced technician, prick tests are relatively simple, inexpensive, safe, and painless. These factors make them ideal for evaluating the pediatric patient. In general, prick tests are less sensitive, especially with low-potency extracts, more specific, and correlate better with clinical symptoms than intradermal tests. Intradermal tests are more sensitive and have more reproducible results than prick tests, perhaps by virtue of the larger quantity of allergen that is consistently injected. Intradermal testing can be painful, difficult to perform in children, and can also induce more false-positive reactions than prick tests. They also carry a higher risk for systemic reactions. See Table 2–2 for a summary of these comparisons.

The correlation between a positive prick test response to aeroallergens and inhalation challenges ranges from 60% to 90% and is only 30% to 40% for intracutaneous tests. Correlations vary according to the allergen, test dose, and grading system. The correlation of

Table 2–2. **Relative Advantages of Prick and Intradermal Skin Testing**

Characteristic	Prick Test	Intradermal Test
Simplicity	+ + +	+ +
Speed	+ + + +	+ +
Interpretation of positive and negative reactions	+ + + +	+ +
Discomfort	+	+ + +
False-positive reactions	Rare	Possible
False-negative reactions	Possible	Rare
Reproducibility	+ + +	+ + + +
Sensitivity	+ + +	+ + + +
Specificity	+ + + +	+ + +
Detection of IgE antibodies	Yes	Yes
Safety	+ + + +	+ +
Testing of infants	Yes	Difficult

Adapted from Middleton E Jr, Ellis EF, Reed CE, eds: *Allergy: Principles and Practice,* 4th ed. St Louis, Mosby, 1993; with permission.

positive prick test responses to foods with food challenges in patients with atopic dermatitis ranges from 25% to 75%. This depends on the food being tested and the characteristics of the reported allergic reaction to the food in question. It is not accepted practice to perform intracutaneous testing for foods because of the high rate of false-positive reactions that cannot be confirmed with food challenges. If a prick test response is negative to a food, there really is no reason to pursue intracutaneous testing because the negative predictive value of the prick test is 82% to 100%, meaning that these patients rarely have positive responses to food challenges. The higher degree of sensitivity achieved with intracutaneous testing is desirable for diagnosing venom or penicillin allergy. For these allergens, intracutaneous testing is a better predictor of clinical allergy.

Interpretation of Skin Test Results

A positive skin test result to an aeroallergen is defined as a wheal of 3 mm or greater in the context of no reaction at the negative control site. However, a positive skin test reaction only implies the presence of allergen-specific IgE on cutaneous mast cells that have degranulated in response to a specific allergen. It is possible for people to have allergen-specific IgE in the absence of clinical symptoms. Further interpretation of a positive skin test result relies on the patient's history that clinical symptoms are provoked by exposure to that allergen. This may be difficult to elicit in patients with perennial symptoms or in those who are not aware of low levels of exposure. As a general rule, all skin test results should be interpreted in the context of the patient's history and physical examination.

Measurement

Responses to immediate hypersensitivity skin tests reach a peak response in 8 to 10 minutes for histamine, 10 to 12 minutes for mast cell secretagogues, and 12 to 17 minutes for allergens. For very precise measurements, the size of both the peak wheal and the flare response are then determined in the following manner: the largest diameter of the response and the diameter of the response midway and perpendicular to this are averaged to determine the size of wheal and flare independently. Often, in routine practice, allergy tests are simply read at 15 minutes using only the single largest wheal's diameter.

Grading Systems

Graded systems are useful because a reading of only positive or negative ignores the relationship between increasing wheal size and the likelihood of clinical sensitivity. Grading systems for prick tests usually consider only the size of the wheal, not the flare. One system from Scandinavia grades the skin prick test result by comparing the size of the wheal induced by the allergen to the size of the wheal induced by the histamine (Table 2–3). Generally, only wheals ≥3 mm are considered positive. A useful grading system for intradermal skin tests employs measurements of both the wheal and the flare and the presence of pseudopods (Table 2–4). These grading systems assume that the negative control site has no measurable wheal or flare. In everyday practice, reactions are often graded from 0 to 4+, with only 3+ and 4+ reactions considered positive. A 3+ reaction is ≥3 mm and circular; a 4+ reaction is of the same size and pseudopodial (Table 2–5).

Table 2–3. Grading of Skin Prick Tests by Comparison to Histamine Positive Control

Grade	Percent of the Area of the Wheal Induced by Histamine Reference (5.43 mmol/L)
−	Same size as negative
+	25
+ +	50
+ + +	100
+ + + +	200

From Middleton E Jr, Ellis EF, Reed CE, eds: *Allergy: Principles and Practice,* 4th ed. St Louis, Mosby, 1993; with permission.

Table 2–4. Grading System to Measure Skin Reactions with Intradermal Tests

Grade	Erythema	Wheal
0	<5 mm	<5 mm
+ / −	5–10 mm	5–10 mm
1+	11–20 mm	5–10 mm
2+	21–30 mm	5–10 mm
3+	31–40 mm	5–10 mm or with pseudopods
or	>40 mm	
4+		>15 mm or with many pseudopods

From Middleton E Jr, Ellis EF, Reed CE, eds: *Allergy: Principles and Practice,* 4th ed. St Louis, Mosby, 1993; with permission.

Factors Affecting Skin Test Results

Medications

Atopic patients often use prescription or over-the-counter medications for symptomatic relief prior to skin testing and may be taking medications for concomitant illnesses. Many of these will suppress *in vivo* allergy reactions. Histamine antagonists may inhibit the cutaneous reaction to allergens as well as to histamine and should be withheld prior to skin testing. The duration of this inhibition, particularly with first-generation H_1-receptor antagonists, varies with different products. Chlorpheniramine, diphenhydramine, and promethazine suppress skin test reactions for 1 to 3 days, whereas hydroxyzine, clemastine, and cyproheptadine may suppress reactions for up to 10 days. The second-generation H_1-receptor antagonists cetirizine, terfenadine, and loratadine can also suppress skin test reactions for up to 10 days, but astemizole may inhibit skin test reactions for 60 days. Fexofenadine ap-

Table 2–5. Grading System for Prick or Intradermal Skin Tests

Grade	Cutaneous Response
0	No response
1+	Erythema only
2+	Erythema with wheal <3 mm
3+	Erythema with circular wheal ≥3 mm
4+	Erythema with pseudopodial wheal ≥3 mm

pears to have a pharmacokinetic profile similar to its parent compound, terfenadine, and therefore may suppress skin test reactions for up to 10 days. Topical and intranasal antihistamines may also suppress skin test reactions.

Tachyphylaxis develops after days or weeks of treatment with first-generation antihistamines; this phenomenon may also reduce their inhibition of skin test reactions; however, this reduced sensitivity is not observed with the second-generation antihistamines. The maximal inhibition of skin test reactions with loratadine does not occur until day 28 of use. This may reflect a cumulative effect on the degree of skin test suppression which could also prolong the duration of suppression. In most pharmacologic studies investigating the efficacy of antihistamines, measured outcomes are onset of action, degree of suppression of wheal-and-flare, and duration of action. In these studies, however, the skin tests are often performed after administering the test medication for only a few days. In practice, patients referred for allergy testing have often taken antihistamines for weeks or months and it is not uncommon to see suppression of skin test reactions for several weeks after the last dose. But most authors report that accurate skin test results can often be obtained even if patients have failed to withhold H_1-blockers or after shorter periods of abstinence. These discrepant observations may reflect differences in potency of extracts, use of prick versus intracutaneous tests, or routine versus intermittent dosing. To account for this interpatient variability, it may be prudent to withhold diphenhydramine and chlorpheniramine for 3 to 5 days, hydroxyzine, cyproheptadine, and clemastine for 10 to 14 days; and all other H_1-receptor antagonists for 2 to 3 weeks prior to skin testing. Astemizole has a longer half-life and may need to be withheld for several months prior to skin testing. Patients taking H_2-receptor antagonists show only minimal and not clinically significant suppression of allergy skin test reactions.

Short- or long-term oral corticosteroid therapy does not inhibit histamine-induced cutaneous reactivity. Therefore, it is accepted that inhaled corticosteroids do not inhibit allergy skin test reactions, although this assumption has not been studied. Potent topical glucocorticosteroids have been shown to inhibit the immediate wheal-and-flare response. This inhibition occurs only at the site of steroid application and, in practice, would only preclude skin testing in the patient with extensive cutaneous disease.

Other medications that have been shown to inhibit *in vivo* allergy testing include tricyclic antidepressants, phenothiazines, dopamine, and clonidine. Theophylline, β-agonists, and cromolyn can be administered prior to skin testing. β-blockers and angiotensin-converting enzyme (ACE) inhibitors may potentiate cutaneous reactivity. Interpatient variability in responses to medications and conflicting data on the duration and degree of cutaneous inhibition underscore the importance of a positive control. In general, a positive histamine control provides good evidence that allergy testing can be pursued and accurately interpreted.

Age

Patient age affects skin testing. Infants have decreased histamine reactivity and may respond to skin testing by producing a large flare and small wheal. After infancy, cutaneous reactivity to histamine gradually increases until age 15 to 20 years, stabilizes, and then decreases after age 50. It has been shown that the cutaneous response to allergens also increases with age. These results suggest that allergy skin testing can be pursued at any age but the results should be interpreted by comparing the size of the wheal produced by the allergens to that produced by the histamine.

Other Variables

Cutaneous reactivity varies with location. The upper and middle portions of the back are more reactive than the lower portion, and the back is more reactive than the forearm. The antecubital fossa is more reactive than the wrist and the ulnar side of the arm is more reactive than the radial. Seasonal variations in skin test results have been observed with pollen allergy. Cutaneous reactivity may increase after a pollen season, perhaps because of a priming effect on the skin, and then decline in the off season. Patients with atopic dermatitis may have decreased responses to histamine. Cutaneous diseases in general may limit the ability to perform testing on intact skin. Patients with spinal cord injuries, peripheral neuropathies, cancer, and chronic renal failure may all exhibit decreased cutaneous reactivity.

Selection of Allergenic Extracts

Number of Tests to Perform

Hundreds of commercially prepared allergenic extracts are available for skin testing, and clinical considerations are necessary to determine which ones are relevant for the evaluation of each patient. A detailed clinical and environmental history can usually limit the need for extensive testing. Younger patients are most likely sensitized to foods or to perennial allergens such as dust mites, animal danders, indoor molds, or cockroach. The older child and adult with seasonal symptoms are likely to be sensitized to outdoor airborne pollens. For these patients, appropriate skin testing requires that the investigator be familiar with the prevalent pollens in the patient's geographical area. Pollens of the same class often cross-react (i.e., timothy and fescue grass, hickory and pecan tree); therefore, testing with a limited number of each of the prevalent tree, grass, and weed pollens is usually sufficient to determine sensitization, but a more comprehensive evaluation may be necessary for the patient considering immunotherapy. In screening the older child or adult for inhalant allergies, a representative panel of extracts may include indoor aeroallergens (dust mite, animal danders, cockroach), airborne pollens (grasses, trees, and weeds), and mold spores.

Standardization of Extracts

The value of *in vivo* skin testing may be limited by the quality of the extract. The potency of extracts has traditionally been labeled according to their weight per volume or protein nitrogen units (PNU). These are determined by *in vitro* methods and do not consistently correlate with their actual biologic activity. Furthermore, the biologic activity of extracts labeled with similar potency from the same manufacturer can still vary greatly from lot to lot. Experts around the world have now set standards for reference extracts. In this country, allergen standardization is regulated by the Food and Drug Administration, Center for Biologics Evaluation and Research. The new standard in the United States is bioequivalency allergy units per milliliter (BAU/ml). Standardized extracts are those that, as determined by skin testing, are bioequivalent. Their potency is also confirmed by *in vitro* assays. Extracts standardized with regard to biologic activity yield the most reproducible, accurate results and should be employed whenever possible. Because standardized extracts contain consistent allergen levels, their use may increase the safety and efficacy of immunotherapy. Standardized extracts are now available for dust mite, cat dander, short ragweed, *Hymenoptera* venoms, and grasses while many others await FDA approval or are candidates for standardization.

Preservation of Extracts

In order to preserve their quality, extracts are stabilized in 50% glycerin for epicutaneous testing and 2% glycerin or 0.03% human serum albumin for intracutaneous testing. Potency declines with time, method of storage, and dilution. When not in use, extracts should be stored at 4° to 8° C. Extracts, especially dilute ones, should be replaced at regular intervals.

Safety of Skin Testing

When performed by a skilled investigator following recommended precautions, *in vivo* skin testing is a safe procedure. The most common adverse event is a large, localized reaction that can occur immediately after testing or later. These occur less frequently with prick testing. The probability of inducing systemic allergic reactions by skin testing is less than 0.02%. However, deaths have been reported from skin testing. All occurred with intracutaneous testing and, except for one fatality, were not preceded by epicutaneous testing. Intracutaneous testing injects a larger amount of allergen deeper into the skin, which may increase the risk for a systemic reaction. Other contributing factors may be using an incorrect dose of allergen, intracutaneous testing with foods, testing a symptomatic patient, testing during the pollen season, testing a highly sensitive patient, especially one with a previous systemic reaction, or testing patients using a β-blocker, ACE-inhibitor, or monoamine oxidase inhibitor.

IN VITRO ALLERGY TESTING

Skin prick tests are the preferred method of diagnosing allergic diseases. Situations exist, however, in which this technique cannot be performed. Patients with extensive atopic dermatitis may not have enough disease-free skin to place the tests. Others may have such severe allergic symptoms that they cannot discontinue their antihistamines. Furthermore, the patient who experienced a life-threatening allergic reaction may be reluctant to undergo *in vivo* testing. *In vitro* methods of allergy testing permit further evaluation of IgE-mediated processes in these situations without the risk of a systemic reaction. A complete list of clinical indications for *in vitro* testing is given in Table 2–6. These are not absolute indications, and good clinical judgment should mandate which method of allergy testing is most appropriate for an individual.

Table 2–6. **Clinical Indications for *In Vitro* Allergy Testing**

- Generalized dermatologic conditions, including dermatographism
- Concomitant use of histamine antagonists, tricyclic antidepressants, potent topical corticosteroids, or other medications that suppress cutaneous responses
- Concomitant use of β-blockers, monoamine oxidase inhibitors, or ACE inhibitors which may increase the risk of a systemic reaction
- Poorly controlled asthma
- History of a life-threatening allergic reaction
- Pregnancy
- Postmortem evaluation (i.e., for possible insect venom, latex, or food-induced anaphylaxis)
- Allergic bronchopulmonary aspergillosis

Methods of Testing

The most common *in vitro* methods of allergy testing are modifications of noncompetitive, solid-phase immunoassays. The radioallergosorbent test (RAST) is such a test and a useful technique for detecting the presence of allergen-specific IgE. With this method, allergen is covalently bound to a solid-phase support such as nitrocellulose. The patient's serum is then incubated with the solid phase. If there is any allergen-specific IgE present, it binds to the protein, and any free antibodies are washed away. The solid phase is next incubated with I^{125}-labeled, purified antihuman IgE and washed again. This step detects any allergen-bound IgE. The amount of radioactivity measured from the solid phase then reflects the quantity of allergen-specific IgE present in the test serum.

The enzyme-linked immunosorbent assay (ELISA) method can also detect allergen-specific IgE. This method differs from the RAST in the ligand used to detect IgE bound to the solid phase. Instead of radiolabeled anti-IgE, the ELISA uses an enzyme covalently bound to antibody. This ligand is often peroxidase coupled with anti-human IgE. When the appropriate substrate is added, it produces color in the presence of the enzyme portion of the bound ligand. The optical density then reflects the amount of allergen-specific IgE present in the patient's serum (Fig. 2–5). RASTs that detect allergen-specific IgG have no role in the evaluation of the allergic patient.

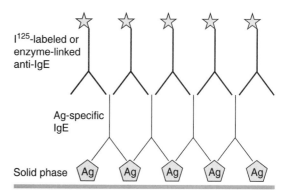

Figure 2–5. Radioallergosorbent test or enzyme-linked immunosorbent assay. Allergen (Ag) bound to the solid phase is incubated with test serum. Allergen-specific IgE binds. Anti-IgE labeled with I^{125} or linked to an enzyme binds, and radioactivity or optical density is measured.

Other Methods

Patients with allergic diseases often have elevated total serum IgE antibody or peripheral blood eosinophilia. Unfortunately, these measures are of little value in the evaluation of suspected allergic diseases, largely because of their variability among nonallergic individuals and lack of specificity. For example, an elevated serum IgE concentration is also seen with human immunodeficiency virus infection and in many primary immunodeficiencies such as Wiskott-Aldrich, DiGeorge, and Hyper-IgE syndromes. Eosinophilia can be seen with drug reactions, helminth infections, Churg-Strauss vasculitis, eosinophilic leukemia, and idiopathic hypereosinophilic syndrome. Both IgE and eosinophil levels may be elevated in graft-versus-host disease or allergic bronchopulmonary aspergillosis. These are, therefore, nonspecific markers of allergic and also other processes. Their presence may support the diagnosis of allergy and prompt a more thorough investigation for allergen-specific IgE.

Interpretation of *In Vitro* Results

A major problem with *in vitro* assays for allergen-specific IgE is deciding what constitutes a positive result. There is no general consensus on this matter, so results of assays are expressed in different ways. Some are expressed relative to that of nonallergic patients who have no allergen-specific IgE. For instance, a positive result may be one that is two to three standard deviations greater than the mean of the negative control. Or the test results can be expressed as a ratio of the mean of the negative control; a ratio greater than three is considered positive. RAST results also may be expressed relative to that of sera from highly allergic patients producing the same specific IgE. In this method, a standard curve derived from sera of allergic patients is divided into classes, ranging from 0 to 4, and the test serum is compared to the standard curve. In the modified RAST, 25 IU/ml of IgE is incubated with radiolabeled anti-IgE. The amount of time it takes to measure 25,000 counts of radioactivity determines how long the test serum

is counted. The total count obtained from the sample is then expressed in classes 0 to 5. This method increases sensitivity but lacks specificity. Proper interpretation of these tests requires that each assay be run with a positive and a negative control.

Besides the issue of defining a positive test result, other technical difficulties with *in vitro* assays exist: (1) standard curves are not always formulated for each allergen-specific IgE under question and may not be a valid representation of different allergens; (2) RASTs for unusual allergens may be limited by the unavailability of a positive control; (3) serum with high total IgE may produce nonspecific binding and weakly positive results for many allergens. In this situation, positive results can be verified by inhibition assays in which free allergen is incubated with the test serum. If the results are caused by allergen-specific IgE interactions, the addition of free allergen will inhibit binding by at least 80%; (4) binding allergen to the solid phase may alter the relevant epitope and not allow adequate recognition by IgE; (5) IgG antibodies in test serum may block the binding of IgE; and (6) IgE may cross-react with different allergens.

Accurate and precise assay results should correlate with clinical symptoms, skin tests, or provocation tests. Test quality often depends on the allergen being tested. Positive results with potent allergens, such as ragweed, dust mite, and cat dander, or purified epitopes correlate better than results with weaker allergens. *In vitro* assays with food proteins are especially problematic. They can be falsely negative if many allergenic epitopes are present and the clinically relevant one is not present in sufficient quantity to bind IgE. Also, food proteins may cross-react with inhalant allergens to produce false-positive results. Overall, the positive predictive value of *in vitro* allergen-specific IgE assays for clinical allergy is greatest for pollens, followed by dust mite, anaphylactogenic foods, animal danders, and fungi and is least predictive for nonanaphylactogenic foods. The interpretation of *in vitro* allergy test results is similar to that of *in vivo* test results in which the presence of allergen-specific IgE does not always indicate clinical allergy. The results still need to be interpreted with respect to the patient's history and physical examination.

COMPARISON OF *IN VIVO* AND *IN VITRO* ALLERGY TESTING

Confirming the presence of allergen-specific IgE is the most useful test in evaluating allergic diseases. Both *in vivo* and *in vitro* methods of allergy testing are able to do this. The availability of skilled specialists or qualified laboratories often dictates which method to pursue. The issue of quality control for allergy testing cannot be underestimated, because variations in technique may yield results invalid for clinical recommendations. In the current era of managed care, cost is another important factor in deciding which method to use. An individual RAST may cost three times that of a skin prick test. Table 2–7 summarizes the advantages of *in vivo* and *in vitro* methods of allergy testing.

CONCLUSIONS

The diagnosis of allergic diseases can be made on clinical grounds. Allergy testing is helpful to confirm clinical suspicions and to identify specific allergens. This information is necessary to make allergen avoidance recommendations (i.e., dust mite, animal dander) and to formulate a plan for immunotherapy. By de-

Table 2–7. **Advantages of *In Vivo* Versus *In Vitro* Allergy Testing**

In Vivo Testing	*In Vitro* Testing
Increased sensitivity	No need to stop medications
Increased specificity	
Better clinical correlation	No clinical contraindications
Less expensive	
Results immediately visible to patient	No risk of systemic reaction

tecting allergen-specific IgE, both *in vivo* and *in vitro* methods are valid techniques of diagnosing allergic diseases. (In this author's opinion, unconventional methods of allergy testing provide no useful information. These are discussed in Chapter 6.) When performed with quality extracts and standard techniques, *in vivo* allergy testing is a safe, accurate, and rapid diagnostic tool to identify IgE-mediated diseases. Only skilled operators should perform these procedures. Their experience and good judgment are necessary for proper interpretation of the results and to maintain the integrity of skin testing. Few clinical situations call for *in vitro* allergy tests. Regardless of the method used, clinical recommendations should not be based solely on the results of allergy tests. The physician's history, physical examination, and clinical expertise should determine the significance of allergy test results.

Chapter 3

Pulmonary Function Testing and Bronchial Provocation

Sandra D. Anderson

THE ETERNAL DILEMMA

The eternal dilemma is matching the respiratory symptoms of the patient with objective measurements. The reason for this is that the perception of severity of symptoms will be different for each patient and can change in the same patient over time. In an attempt to resolve this dilemma diary cards for recording asthma symptoms and daily home peak flow measurements were introduced for children in the early 1970s. This approach is now widely used in adults. Home monitoring and keeping diaries takes time and requires compliance. Also, the measurement of peak flow may not always reflect significant changes in lung function, particularly in children, and can be affected by medication use.

In addition to evaluation of patients who are known to have asthma, there is an increasing requirement to evaluate healthy subjects who have no current symptoms but give a past history consistent with asthma. These people are often seeking entry into the military or industry and have answered in the affirmative to a written question on past history of asthma. Another group of healthy subjects seeking objective evaluation for symptoms are elite athletes who complain of persistent cough, discomfort of breathing or both that could be asthma. Thus, there is a growing need, at the time of consultation, to establish whether a person with or without current symptoms does

have asthma and if the disease is severe enough to warrant treatment.

It is now accepted that pulmonary function tests (PFTs) and bronchial provocation tests (BPTs) can provide objective evidence of the existence of asthma. The results of such tests can also demonstrate that the same respiratory symptoms may result from widely differing physiology. For example, shortness of breath on exertion could reflect airway narrowing in one patient, obesity in another, or be an indication that maximal, but normal, flow limitation has been achieved, as might be expected in the elite athlete. Pulmonary function tests are used to determine if airway narrowing (airflow limitation) is present, whether it is acutely reversible in response to a bronchodilator, or exacerbated by a bronchoconstricting stimulus. When spirometry results are normal, BPTs are particularly useful to confirm the presence of airway hyper-responsiveness (AHR), the hallmark of asthma, and to determine its severity. Bronchial provocation tests are also useful for measuring changes in airway responsiveness following treatment with inhaled steroids and to identify drugs that prevent exercise-induced asthma. The information obtained from BPTs is a valuable addition to clinical assessment and past history and may be achieved more rapidly and reliably than home monitoring of peak flow variability and symptoms.

SPIROMETRY AND FLOW RATES

Measurement

The most important measurement of pulmonary function is spirometry, the documentation of forced expiratory volume to residual volume after maximal inspiration to total lung capacity. Spirometry refers to the two volumes measured during this maneuver. They are the forced expiratory volume in one second (FEV_1) and the forced vital capacity (FVC), and they are measured in liters or milliliters and expressed at body temperature and pressure fully saturated with water vapor (BTPS). The ratio of these two volumes (FEV_1/FVC %) is also documented. The forced expiratory volume in relation to time is illustrated in Figure 3–1.

The forced expiratory flow in relation to expired volume is given in Figure 3–2. There are many indices that can be obtained from the flow–volume curve. The most common is the peak expiratory flow (PEF). This is usually reached in the first 200 msec of a forced maneuver and reflects flow through the large airways. The PEF is measured as liters/sec or liters/min. The index most commonly used to describe flow through the medium to small airways is the forced expiratory flow in the middle half of the vital capacity, known as the FEF_{25-75} (also known as the maximum midexpiratory flow MMEF or MEF). Values for FEF_{25-75} are measured in liters/sec. The results of spirometry are effort dependent, particularly the measurement of PEF and FEV_1. Although much of the FEF_{25-75} is measured over the effort-independent part of the flow–volume curve, it is dependent on the full vital capacity being expired. The repeatability of FEV_1, FVC, and PEF is very good, and values are usually within 8% to 10% in patients; variation is less in healthy subjects. The FEF_{25-75} is less reproducible and for repeated blows there may be a 15% difference.

Traditionally spirometry has been measured with a water-sealed spirometer or bellows system with volume being recorded against

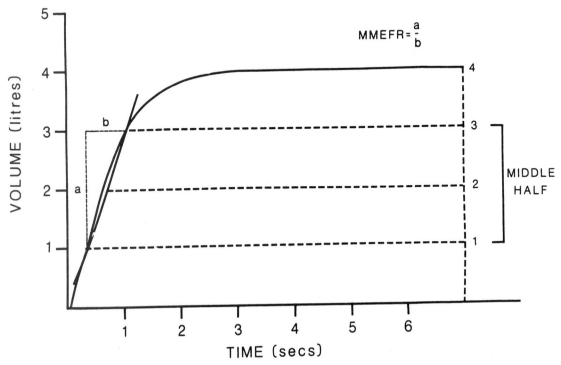

Figure 3–1. Forced expired vital capacity in relation to time. The maximum mid expiratory flow rate (MMEFR), also known as the forced expiratory flow rate, through the middle half of the vital capacity (FEF_{25-75}). It is calculated from a spirogram by measuring the time *(b)* taken to expire the middle portion of the vital capacity *(a)*. It is corrected to liters per second. (From Ellis E, Alison J: Key Issues in Physiotherapy. Oxford, Butterworth, Heineman, 1992, p 31. Used by permission.)

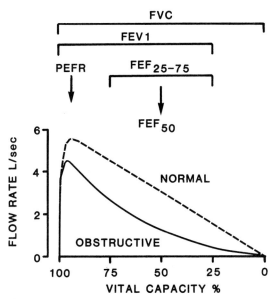

Figure 3–2. The forced expiratory flow in relation to volume during a forced vital capacity (FVC) maneuver as it would be seen before (normal) and after (obstructive) a provoking stimulus or before (obstructive) and after (normal) bronchodilator administration in a person with acutely reversible airflow limitation. The peak expiratory flow rate (PEFR), forced expiratory volume in one second (FEV$_1$), and flow rates through the middle portion of the vital capacity (FEF$_{25-75}$) are shown in relation to volume. In this example, the FVC remained the same; however, the FVC is normally reduced in exercise-induced asthma and is often increased after bronchodilator use. (From Anderson SD, Brannan J, Trevillon L, et al: Lung function and bronchial provocation tests for intending divers with a history of asthma. SPUMS Journal 25:233, 1995. Used by permission.)

time (see Fig. 3–1). The development of electronic spirometers allowed simultaneous plotting of expiratory flow against volume and this development has permitted easier examination of changes in response to acute intervention (e.g., bronchodilator, bronchoconstrictor) or chronic intervention (e.g., treatment with inhaled steroids or removal from a sensitizing agent).

Normal Values

To compare values for spirometry with normal, a set of predicted values is required. Predicted normal values vary according to gender, age, height, and ethnic origin and are usually chosen to suit the population being tested with many different sets being available. Commonly used ones include that described by Crapo and colleagues for North Americans and one

developed by Quanjer and coworkers for Europeans. A value greater than 80% or more of predicted normal is usually considered to be within the normal range, if all other volume values also are a similar percentage. The value of 80% usually represents the 95% confidence limit or the lower end of the normal range. Nonwhites usually have smaller lungs and 80% to 90% of the predicted value for white people is considered within normal limits by most laboratories. Because values for FEF$_{25-75}$ are more variable, the lower end of the 95% confidence interval is about 67% rather than 80%. The person measuring spirometry should be aware of the criteria for acceptability of the results.

Significance of Measurement of Spirometry and Flow–Volume Curves

The documentation of normal spirometry (FEV$_1$, FVC, and its ratio) and normal flow rates (FEF$_{25-75}$) excludes airway narrowing at rest. The documentation of a normal peak flow does not exclude airway narrowing as it only measures the peak of the flow and does not include airflow throughout the rest of the vital capacity (see Fig. 3–2). Normal spirometry does not preclude the possibility that airway narrowing may occur in response to a provoking stimulus. Many people with a past or a current history of asthma, but normal spirometry results and flow rates, can have airway narrowing provoked by a wide variety of stimuli including exercise. It is important to examine all indices of lung function. For example, a patient with life-long but well-treated asthma may have a PEF close to normal but abnormal FEV$_1$ and FEF$_{25-75}$ results. In Figure 3–2 two flow–volume curves are illustrated, an obstructive one that may be recorded at rest or after a stimulus such as exercise and a normal one that may be recorded before exercise or after use of a bronchodilator.

Response to Bronchodilator

The documentation (see Fig. 3–2) of abnormal spirometry or flow rates and reversal of these 15 to 20 min after the administration of a rapidly acting β_2-adrenoceptor agonist (e.g. terbutaline, albuterol) may be all that is needed to decide whether a person has asthma. Measuring response to an inhaled bronchodilator is an important test. For this reason, it is necessary to ensure that an adequate dose deposits in the airways by administering the bronchodilator by nebulizer or giving twice the standard dose of bronchodilator from a metered dose inhaler. An acute increase in FEV_1 to within the normal predicted range is, in a person with airflow limitation at rest, a consistent finding in a person with asthma. If the FEV_1 increases more than 15% (some suggest 12% or more) it is also considered consistent with a diagnosis of asthma. The response to a bronchodilator can confirm the presence of asthma but it does not give information about its severity. Referring a patient for a BPT is justified to assess asthma severity. A BPT can also help to determine the dose and type of medication required, particularly when exercise-induced asthma is being evaluated.

It is more difficult to assess airway responsiveness on the basis of changes in FEF_{25-75} and the result is valid only when the vital capacity remains the same (see Fig. 3–2). An increase of 25% in FEF_{25-75} after bronchodilator administration is considered a significant response. The importance of the FEF_{25-75} is appreciated when it is understood that it is this part of the flow–volume curve in which tidal breathing occurs during exercise. At rest, the flow generated during tidal breathing is low but flow increases with increasing intensity of exercise. The capacity for flow to increase is determined by the maximum flow–volume characteristics of the lung. If flow rates through the middle portion of the vital capacity are low, then the ability to increase flow is reduced. It is thought that breathlessness on exertion occurs when flow reaches the limit of the flow–volume curve. This could happen with similar propensity, but for different reasons, in both elite athletes and in patients with airflow limitation. Any increase in FEF_{25-75} in response to a bronchodilator may result in a patient reporting improved exercise tolerance. Likewise any decrease in FEF_{25-75} may result in a patient or athlete reporting poorer exercise performance.

STATIC LUNG VOLUMES

It would be common practice for a person referred for an asthma assessment to a pulmonary function laboratory to have a measurement of all lung volumes (Fig. 3–3). The reason for this is to determine if there is any hyperinflation (abnormally high total lung capacity and functional residual capacity in relation to other volumes) or gas trapping (an abnormally high residual volume in relation to other volumes). Hyperinflation results in muscular and mechanical inefficiency; a greater effort is required to breathe and the need for more effort can contribute to symptoms. These abnormalities are all reversible in persons with asthma. The techniques used to make the measurements are most commonly body plethysmography, helium dilution, or nitrogen washout and details for their use are given elsewhere. The advantage of measuring spirometry at the same time as lung volumes in body plethysmography is that the flow–volume curve can be accurately positioned in relation to total lung capacity and residual volume. Further, indirect measurements of airway caliber are made during body plethysmography that, unlike spirometry, are not dependent on expiratory effort. These include airway resistance (Raw) and conductance (Gaw). Normal values for Raw range from 0.6 to 2.4 L/sec/cm H_2O and Gaw from 0.42 to 1.67 L/sec/cm H_2O. These values can also be corrected for the absolute lung volume at which they are measured (FRC) and expressed as specific airways resistance (sRaw) and specific compliance (sGaw). Body plethysmography is measured in a box around 650 liters in size. For patients with physical disabilities or those who cannot tolerate enclosed spaces, lung volumes measured by gas dilution is a better option.

As with spirometry, values for total lung capacity (TLC), functional residual capacity (FRC), and residual volume (RV) are generally considered within the normal range if measured between 80% and 120% of the predicted value. To be considered normal, however, all the volumes would be expected to be a similar

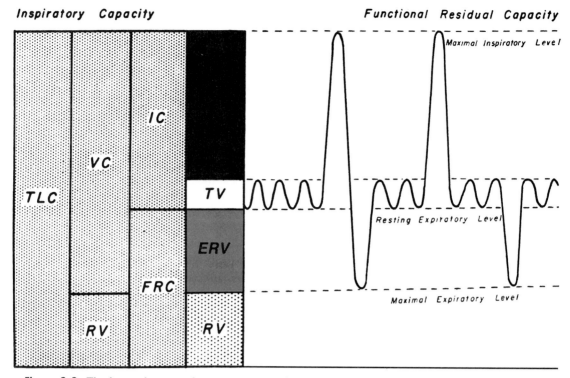

Figure 3–3. The lung volumes as they appear on a spirogram. Total lung capacity (TLC) is reached after one inhales to the maximal inspiratory capacity (IC). The residual volume (RV) is the volume of air left in the lung after a vital capacity maneuver (VC) is performed. When one is breathing with a normal tidal volume (TV), the functional residual capacity (FRC) is the volume in the lung. The thoracic gas volume measured during plethysmography is approximately equal to the FRC and TV. The inspiratory reserve volume (IRV) and expiratory reserve volume (ERV) are both used to increase tidal volume during exercise, but the IRV is used more frequently than the ERV. (From Comroe JH, Forster RE, Dubois AB, et al: The Lung, 2nd ed. Chicago, Year Book, 1962, p 8. Used by permission.)

percentage within that range. Thus, a vital capacity of 85% and a FRC of 120% is not normal and suggests that hyperinflation is occurring. Demonstration of the presence of hyperinflation or gas trapping and airflow limitation with a positive response to bronchodilator administration is in keeping with a diagnosis of asthma. The documentation of normal lung volumes at rest does not preclude the possibility that changes could occur acutely in response to a bronchoconstricting stimulus. [This is particularly important in the assessment of a person's suitability to self-contained underwater breathing apparatus (SCUBA) dive.] Acute airway narrowing provoked by exercise or hypertonic saline is frequently accompanied by hyperinflation and gas trapping. Indeed hyperinflation acts as a distending force to open narrowed airways and is thought of as nature's bronchodilator.

BRONCHIAL PROVOCATION TESTS

Background

Measurements of airway hyper-responsiveness (AHR) were first suggested to assess asthmatics by Tiffeneau, who also introduced the measurement of FEV_1. At that time acetylcholine was used as the provoking agent. Later Parker and coworkers introduced methacholine, a stable synthetic derivative of acetylcholine, into the laboratory. Since that time BPTs using methacholine and histamine have become widely used both in laboratories and in the field to identify AHR. Their safety, efficacy, and repeatability have been well established over many years. In the 1970s the physical challenge tests were introduced to overcome some of the limitations of the pharmacologic challenge tests. The osmotic challenges were introduced in the 1980s and 1990s. As a result, a wide range of BPTs is now available. These tests are both sensitive for identifying AHR and specific for recognizing currently active asthma. There are two types of BPTs, direct and indirect (Table 3–1).

Direct Provocation Tests

The stimuli used for direct BPTs include methacholine, histamine, leukotrienes, and prostaglandins. Methacholine or mecholyl is the most commonly used agent for pharmacologic challenge in North America and is tolerated better than histamine. Pharmacologic agents act directly by way of receptors (e.g., acetylcholine, histamine, prostaglandin, and leukotriene) to cause the airways to narrow. The receptors involved are all found on the bronchial smooth muscle but may also occur elsewhere (e.g., on vascular smooth muscle). The

precise reason that persons with asthma have AHR in response to agents like methacholine is not known. It may relate to the desquamation of the airway epithelium, which allows rapid passage of the stimulus to the smooth muscle. It may relate to the smooth muscle itself being more responsive in the presence of inflammation. It may simply relate to the amplifying effects of smooth muscle contraction in the presence of airway edema. Direct challenge tests give good information about end-organ responsiveness to the stimulus applied.

Strengths and Limitations of Direct Provocation Tests. The major perceived strengths in using methacholine or histamine in the clinical setting are the high sensitivity for detecting AHR and a high negative predictive value, the inexpensive nature and portability of the equipment, the ability to obtain a dose–response curve, the transient nature of the airway response elicited by them, and the safety record for their use.

Table 3–1. **Indications for the Use of Bronchial Provocation Tests**

Test	Indications for Use
Methacholine and histamine inhalation challenge	• to document bronchial responsiveness in a person with typical symptoms but no objective evidence of bronchial hyper-responsiveness • to document bronchial responsiveness in a person who may become exposed or has been exposed to sensitizing agents or has been withdrawn from exposure
Exercise challenge	• to make a diagnosis of exercise-induced asthma (EIA) in asthmatic patients with a history of breathlessness during or after exertion • to confirm that the drugs prescribed prevent exercise-induced asthma and permit normal exercise performance • to select the appropriate combination of drugs and determine dosage for patients whose exercise-induced asthma is not controlled by a single drug • to evaluate the effect of steroid therapy on severity of exercise-induced asthma and the type and amount of medication required to control exercise-induced asthma if it occurs
Isocapnic hyperventilation	• to make a diagnosis of exercise-induced asthma in a person who gives a history of breathlessness during or after exertion, particularly super-fit athletes • to assess the severity of exercise-induced asthma in a person already diagnosed with exercise-induced asthma • to exclude asthma as a cause of breathlessness on exertion • to exclude airway narrowing as the cause of postexercise cough • to assess EIA in a fit person and for whom dry air is a real challenge, i.e., breathing by SCUBA during exercise
Hyperosmolar aerosols (saline or mannitol)	• these challenge tests are most useful for identifying persons with currently active asthma and to assess its severity • to assess a person for suitability to dive with SCUBA • to assess indirectly the presence of endogenous mediators which cause the airways to narrow • to assess response to chronic treatment with corticosteroids • as an alternative test for exercise or isocapnic hyperventilation as a test to identify patients with exercise-induced asthma • to assess airway hyper-responsiveness consistent with asthma in patients with bronchiectasis and cystic fibrosis and to help clear secretions

The major limitations for the use of agents such as methacholine or histamine is that a positive airway response is neither specific for the diagnosis of asthma nor predictive of responsiveness to inhaled steroids. These agents do not identify people with exercise-induced asthma.

People with rhinitis, other lung diseases, obesity, sleep apnea, congestive heart failure, or with restricted movement of the chest wall may have AHR to histamine or methacholine. Abnormal baseline lung function is also associated with AHR to methacholine and histamine. Healthy subjects can also be responsive.

Although responsiveness to histamine and methacholine does decrease in response to treatment with inhaled steroids, as shown in drug trials in known asthmatics, these tests have not been widely advocated for assessing individual patients in a clinical setting. The reason for this may be because of some limitations of the methods. First, many subjects with responsiveness to pharmacologic agents will not necessarily respond to treatment with inhaled steroids; subjects with chronic airflow limitation are a good example of this. Second, the majority of subjects with asthma who take inhaled steroids remain responsive to pharmacologic agents. Even those who are symptom- and medication-free with normal lung function for long periods can remain very responsive. Thus, a clear end-point for treatment, i.e., the normal healthy range, is not always achievable or even identifiable. Third, changes in responsiveness to pharmacologic challenge tests may not be significantly different when different doses of steroids are used. Some authors have found no alteration in responsiveness when steroids were either given or withdrawn, and others have found that responsiveness returns to pretreatment levels within a few weeks after stopping treatment. The wide variation in the change in the responsiveness to histamine and methacholine reported in these studies suggests that these agents are not ideal for following response to treatment with steroids or withdrawal from steroid treatment. Finally, pharmacologic agents cannot be used to identify persons with exercise-induced asthma, to assess its severity, or to assess the benefit of drugs such as nedocromil sodium, sodium cromoglycate, or leukotriene antagonists used to treat it. These findings are important particularly for assessing persons for occupations in which exercise may be an important provoking stimulus (e.g., the military).

In the random population it is acknowledged that pharmacologic tests are less sensitive and have low specificity for identifying asthma and thus have a low positive predictive value. Thus people with symptoms of asthma can have airway responsiveness in the normal range, and a high proportion of persons (30% to 50%) with AHR to histamine or methacholine have no symptoms of asthma. These anomalies have been appreciated by epidemiologists for many years. Today we find increasing numbers of the so-called random population being referred to the laboratory for evaluation for employment so that these anomalies may well apply to them.

Indirect Provocation Tests

The indirect provocation tests usually refer to physical stimuli such as airway drying and cooling or changes in airway osmolarity, and they include exercise, hyperventilation, cold air, and nonisotonic aerosols (e.g., distilled water, hypertonic saline, and mannitol). These stimuli are thought to cause the release of endogenous mediators such as histamine, leukotrienes, prostaglandins, and possibly neuropeptides, which, in turn, cause the airways to narrow. Because the airway response is dependent on the presence of these mediators, it is considered that the indirect challenge tests reflect the cellular and neural pathways involved in airway inflammation, the underlying abnormality in asthma.

Strengths and Limitations of Indirect Provocation Tests. The perceived strengths of using exercise, hyperventilation, cold air, or nonisotonic aerosols are their high specificity and high positive predictive value for identifying currently active asthma. Challenge with hypertonic saline has the added advantage that sputum can be collected for analysis of inflammatory cells at the same time. The airway response to these challenge tests is markedly diminished or completely inhibited by treatment with inhaled corticosteroids. This suggests that the reason one becomes hyper-responsive to these stimuli must relate directly to airway inflammation. For this reason the use of indirect challenge tests to assess the effects of drug treatment is now being more widely appreciated. Further, these tests identify people with exercise-induced asthma, a factor important in the selection of employees for certain occupations or suitability to dive with SCUBA. Indirect tests can be used to investigate drugs used in the treatment of exercise-induced asthma such as sodium cromoglycate, nedocromil sodium, and leukotriene antagonists. Healthy persons are not responsive to these agents, and 99% of the healthy population have a fall in FEV_1 of less than 10% of baseline after the maximal dose of these stimuli.

The major limitation of indirect provocation tests is that they do not always identify persons with mild asthma and are thus regarded as less sensitive compared with pharmacologic challenge tests. Another limitation is the nature of the equipment involved. The need to condition the inspired air to be cold or just dry has limited the use of exercise, and the need for special gas mixtures has limited the use of hyperventilation to pulmonary function laboratories. In the last decade hypertonic saline (4.5%) has been used as a surrogate challenge for hyperpnea with dry air. This test requires an ultrasonic nebulizer that is portable and a balance is required for weighing. A new hyperosmolar challenge that involves the inhalation of a suitably dried powder preparation of mannitol has been developed as a simple disposable test kit.

Bronchial Provocation Tests for Specific Inhalation Challenge

Bronchial provocation tests can also be carried out with specific agents to which the patient has been exposed and may be sensitized. These tests are usually confined to research laboratories with an interest in occupational asthma. Special equipment is required so as not to expose the investigator. A late response, 6 to 9 hours after challenge, and an increase in nonspecific AHR often occur after such tests. Thus, they are not readily available. These tests are described in detail elsewhere.

Challenge Testing

The range of challenge tests offered by laboratories varies, but most should offer at least one direct and one indirect challenge test. The choice of test will depend on the question being asked and the strengths and limitations of the tests available. It is very important to tell laboratory staff the precise question you wish to have answered, for example, does the patient have exercise-induced asthma?

If you simply want to know whether the patient with normal spirometry results, with or without symptoms, has AHR to a pharmacologic agent, then a challenge with methacholine or histamine should be requested. This evaluation could be needed for a person entering an industry that is known to be associated with more respiratory symptoms in persons with existing AHR (e.g., aluminium, furniture, timber, western red cedar, wheat). It should be noted that if the same occupation requires the person to exercise, a diagnosis of exercise-induced asthma cannot be ruled out on the basis of a negative result to a pharmacologic challenge.

If you want to know if a patient has exercise-induced asthma, then you should request either a single level or multilevel hyperventilation test or a vigorous exercise test for 8 min using dry air at room temperature. This test can be repeated on a separate day to determine effectiveness of acute and chronic treatment for exercise-induced asthma. Hyperventilation at a rate equivalent to $30 \times FEV_1$ for 6 min is the protocol recommended for military recruits, elite athletes, and people without a clear history of asthma or taking medication. Hyperventilation is a very potent stimulus, so a multilevel test protocol, rather than a single level protocol, should be requested in those with known or suspected asthma. Cold air challenge should be requested only if that is the sole stimulus of which the subject complains, because sensitivity for detecting AHR with cold air is very low both in the field and in a clinical setting.

Consider the usefulness of an indirect challenge in a patient with a clear history of asthma and normal spirometry results who is not taking treatment. If that patient has a negative response to a properly performed indirect challenge test, it is most likely that airway inflammation is not present or sufficiently active for mediators to cause the airways to narrow. Such patients could include those who suffer transiently from asthma, for example following a viral infection or seasonal exposure to allergens. These same patients are likely to remain responsive to inhaled histamine or methacholine out of season at a time of no symptoms and normal lung function.

If you want to know if a patient has currently active asthma and is likely to respond to steroids, you may also request an indirect challenge test. In this respect, hypertonic saline, mannitol, distilled water, or hyperventilation would all be more sensitive for detecting AHR than exercise or cold air challenge. The challenge can be repeated 6 to 9 weeks after initiation of treatment with inhaled steroids to assess changes in responsiveness. The successful end-point of treatment is an airway response in the healthy range (Fig. 3–4). Fifty percent of subjects may be expected to achieve this response and be negative to these challenge tests in this period. Many of these persons will still have AHR to inhaled pharmacologic agents.

If you want to know if inflammation is under control in a patient who is being treated with steroids, you could similarly ask for an indirect challenge. Although a challenge with a nonisotonic aerosol would also be appropriate, the patient may identify better with an exercise or hyperventilation challenge. Most patients with asthma have exercise-induced asthma, and a positive test result would reinforce the need to continue or to increase treatment, or to adhere to prescribed treatment. By contrast, a negative result to an exercise challenge could encourage less treatment, i.e., a lower dose of steroids. Exercise-induced asthma is one of the first physiologic abnormalities to develop in asthma and is the last to disappear with steroid treatment. Exercise-induced asthma diminishes with increasing doses of steroids and is superior to symptom and peak flow scores in detecting differences in steroid dose.

In a patient who details symptoms of exercise-induced asthma it is best to have an objective measurement, because symptoms are a poor predictor of both the existence of exercise-induced asthma and its severity. Thus, the

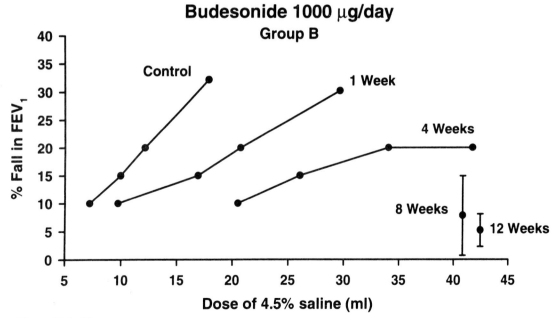

Figure 3–4. The mean response dose curves to hypertonic saline in 6 of 12 subjects before and for up to 12 weeks of treatment with budesonide given by way of Turbuhaler in a dose of 1000 μg per day. The data represent the 50% of subjects who achieved values for PD_{15} within the normal range of responsiveness to hypertonic saline after 12 weeks of treatment. The values at 8 and 12 weeks are shown as the mean percentage fall in forced expiratory volume in 1 second plus or minus 1 standard deviation ($FEV_1 \pm 1$ SD). (Data from du Toit JI, Anderson SD, Jenkins CR, et al: Airway responsiveness in asthma: Bronchial challenge with histamine and 4.5% sodium chloride before and after budesonide. Allergy and Asthma Proceedings 18:7, 1997. Used by permission.)

discomfort of breathlessness may not necessarily be related to a reduction in flow but rather an indication that maximal flow has been achieved. True exercise-induced asthma can often be distinguished from normal exercise limitation by eliciting a history of breathlessness that is worse 5 to 10 minutes after cessation of exercise compared with during exercise.

Baseline Lung Function

Bronchial provocation tests should be performed in the presence of the best lung function. They are not recommended for patients with a baseline FEV_1 less than 75% of the predicted value or the predicted value minus 3 standard deviations, because the results in these individuals are not really meaningful. For persons with baseline values less than 75% of predicted it is recommended to measure the airway response to a bronchodilator. Spirometry should always be repeated after chronic treatment with steroids.

Although the patient with abnormal baseline spirometry results is more likely to have AHR, patients with normal spirometry may also have AHR. This fact was made evident many years ago from studies in exercise-induced asthma. Patients can have severe AHR in response to exercise, hypertonic saline, or hyperventilation with normal spirometry and minimal or no symptoms.

The increasing use of inhaled steroids has led to a marked improvement in spirometry in most younger patients with asthma. Some may achieve flow rates throughout their vital capacity totally within the normal range while others may achieve a marked improvement in spirometry without all the values returning to normal. Performing a BPT within 1 to 2 weeks of starting inhaled steroids is preferable to having a BPT performed in the presence of significant airflow limitation. The baseline FEV_1 should improve sufficiently within 14 days of the beginning of steroid therapy to perform a BPT. The true responsiveness of the airways will be measured in response to the stimulus if the lung function is normal. This is particularly important for direct challenge tests which are more affected by baseline lung function.

Performing a Bronchial Provocation Test

The patient is required to perform many forced expiratory maneuvers after the inhalation of a substance, or after strenuous exercise, or after hyperventilating voluntarily at high flow rates. Thus, the patient needs to be cooperative and be willing to try hard with each maneuver. Some patients will experience wheezing, cough, mild dyspnea, and chest tightness during or after bronchial provocation; many patients do not experience symptoms at all.

An exercise challenge is best performed by a patient younger than 50 years with a normal electrocardiogram. Hyperventilation is performed best by those with an FEV_1 greater than 1.5L. Depending on the protocol used, pharmacologic agents and hyperosmolar agents are administered either during tidal breathing or with a single inspiration; single inspiration administration requires less effort and thus may be more attractive for assessing some patients. As provocation tests can lead to transient arterial hypoxemia, it is not advisable to perform these tests in some patients. The referring practitioner should be aware of or be informed by the laboratory of any contraindications for testing.

Medications

A person being referred to a laboratory should be advised to withhold medications that could affect their airway response to the bronchial provocation tests. For short-acting antihistamines such as diphenhydramine hydrochloride, the medication should be stopped 48 hours before the test. Long-acting antihistamines such as fexofenadine, astemizole, and loratadine should be stopped 1 week before the test. Ordinary preparations of oral bronchodilators should not be used for 12 hours, and sustained release oral bronchodilators for 24 hours. For the short-acting β_2-adrenoceptor agonists (albuterol, terbutaline) and for sodium cromoglycate and nedocromil sodium, a period of 6 hours is sufficient. The longer-acting β_2-adrenoceptor agonists, such as salmeterol, must be stopped for 48 hours. Inhaled corticosteroids (budesonide, beclomethasone, fluticasone) should not be taken on the day of the study. Caffeine-containing substances should also be avoided on the day of study.

Evaluation of the Results

Expression of the Sensitivity to a Provoking Stimulus.

Many indices of lung function have been used to assess AHR; however, the measurement of change in FEV_1 has become the international gold standard. The reduction in FEV_1 in response to the stimulus is expressed as a percentage of the baseline FEV_1 measured immediately before the challenge or after administration of a placebo and is known as the percent fall in FEV_1. Values for percent fall in FEV_1 are plotted against the log of the cumulative dose or the concentration of the substance administered. The dose or concentration required to induce a particular percent fall FEV_1 is derived by linear interpolation. The dose or concentration of the substance required to induce a 10%, 15%, or 20% fall in FEV_1 is

known as the PD_{10}, PD_{15}, or PD_{20}, and the concentration is indicated as PC_{10}, PC_{15}, or PC_{20} (Figs. 3–5 and 3–6). For the hyperventilation test, using a progressive protocol, the ventilation required to provoke a response is used and is quantified as the ventilation required to provoke either a 10% fall in FEV_1 (PVE_{10}) or a 15% fall in FEV_1 (PVE_{15}) (Fig. 3–7). For challenge by exercise or a single dose of hyperventilation, the maximum percent fall in FEV_1 documented in the 15 to 20 min after challenge is used. In order to express overall bronchial lability, the percent increase in FEV_1 after bronchodilator administration can be added to the percent fall in FEV_1 after a stimulus. If this value is greater than 23% it is indicative of airway hyper-responsiveness.

PROTOCOLS

Methacholine and Histamine

The most common protocols used are those described by Chai et al, Cockcroft et al, and Yan et al and have been recently summarized

PHARMACOLOGICAL CHALLENGE

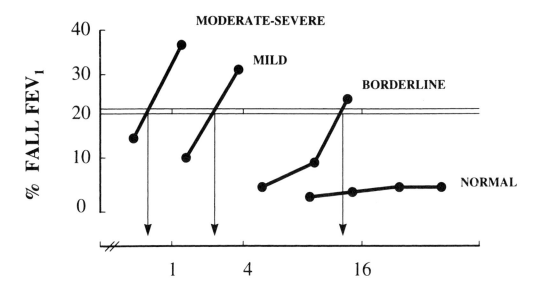

Figure 3–5. The percentage fall from baseline in forced expiratory volume in 1 second (FEV_1) in response to inhaling increasing concentrations of methacholine. The severity of the response is determined by the dose of methacholine required to provoke a 20% fall in FEV_1.

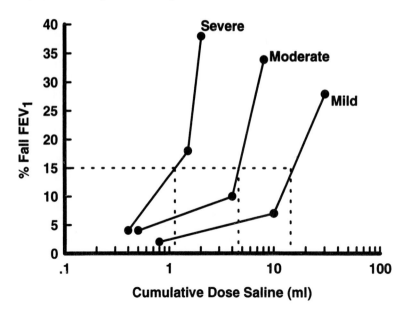

Figure 3–6. The percentage fall in forced expiratory volume in 1 second (FEV_1) in response to inhaling hypertonic (4.5%) saline. The severity of the response is determined by the dose of hypertonic saline required to provoke a 15% fall in FEV_1. The fall in healthy subjects is also shown. A similar illustration could be drawn for subjects inhaling distilled water.

by Sterk et al. Both the Chai technique, which uses an electrically controlled dosimeter, and the Yan technique, which uses a hand-held nebulizer, require multiple single-breath inhalations from FRC to TLC. The Cockcroft technique requires tidal breathing.

Commercial preparations of methacholine (acetyl-beta-methylcholine chloride) are available for use in humans and only require dilution. Otherwise solutions need to be prepared in the range of 0.03 to 16 mg/ml and delivered from appropriate nebulizers; further details for preparation are found elsewhere.

Significance of the Results

A positive test result occurs if the provoking concentration required to induce a 20% fall in FEV_1 (PC_{20}) is less than 8 mg/ml or, in some laboratories, 16 mg/ml, or when a provoking dose PD_{20} is less than 4 micromols or PD_{20} of less than 8 micromols (see Fig. 3–5). A value for a PC_{20} of less than 1.0 mg/ml or a PD_{20} less than 1.0 micromol is usually considered indicative of active asthma. Values for PC_{20} between 4 and 16 mg/ml are regarded as borderline, between 1 and 4 mg/ml as mild, and

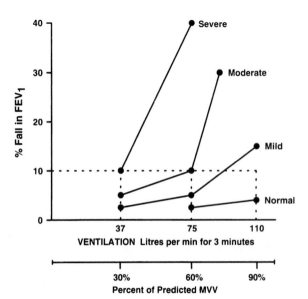

Figure 3–7. The percentage fall in forced expiratory volume in one second (% fall FEV_1) in response to eucapnic hyperventilaion with dry air containing 5% carbon dioxide (CO_2) for three asthmatic subjects. The severity of the response is determined by the level of ventilation required to provoke a 10% reduction in FEV_1. The fall for normal healthy subjects is also shown.

less than 1.0 mg/ml as moderate to severe AHR.

Indirect Challenge Tests

Exercise

Most laboratories work to a standard protocol that involves the subject exercising by cycling or running sufficiently hard to raise the ventilation rate per minute to approximately 20 times the FEV_1 (50% to 60% of maximum voluntary ventilation) and sustaining this rate for at least 4 and preferably 6 minutes. Compressed air is inspired by way of a demand valve, and only mouth breathing is used. It is not necessary to cool the inspired air, and increasing the duration of exercise while the patient is breathing dry air at room temperature at the target ventilation rate will induce a greater airway response. It is easier to inspire conditioned air and measure ventilation while cycling compared with running because the head is in a more stable position. The FEV_1 is measured before and at 3, 5, 7, 10, and 15 minutes after exercise. A bronchodilator is given after this time. Supplemental oxygen should be available at all times and, if needed, should be delivered with a bronchodilator. Some subjects find exercise difficult to perform. For further details of the laboratory protocol see Anderson et al for cycling, Woolley et al for running in adults and Haby et al for field studies.

Significance of the Results

If a reduction in FEV_1 of 10% or more is obtained using a standardized laboratory protocol, the person being tested is considered to have a positive test result. A value of 15% or more is usually taken as positive for exercise performed in the field. If the patient is not taking steroids, percent falls in FEV_1 between 10% to 25% are considered mild, 26% to 50% moderate, and greater than 50% severe exercise-induced asthma. If the person is taking steroids, the category is adjusted down so that moderate exercise-induced asthma would be represented by a 10% to 25% fall in FEV_1. If the test result is negative, the referring practitioner should be assured by the laboratory staff that the test was performed with the appropriate ventilation rate achieved and sustained and that the water content of the air was less than 10 mg/L of air inspired (e.g., temperature less than 23°C and relative humidity less than 50%). In the absence of a measure of ventilation, 90% to 95% of the maximum predicted heart rate should be obtained to confirm work intensity. It is particularly important that sufficient time has passed since the last medication dose or the last attack of asthma provoked by exercise.

Eucapnic or Isocapnic Hyperventilation

This test is an excellent surrogate for exercise and was developed and standardized by members of the U.S. Army to assess recruits for exercise-induced asthma. Hyperventilation with dry air is a more potent challenge than exercise because the inhibiting factors provided by the increased sympathetic drive of exercise are absent. As it requires a minimum FEV_1 of 1.5L, this test is not necessarily suitable for all children or for the elderly.

The patients voluntarily increase their ventilation while breathing dry air containing 4.9% CO_2, 21% O_2, and the balance N_2. The air is inspired from a reservoir and exhaled into a dry gas meter. The expired CO_2 levels remain the same (isocapnia) and within normal limits (eucapnia) for ventilation rates between 30 and 110 L/min. The test can be performed at progressively increasing levels of ventilation (e.g., 30%, 60%, and 90% of maximum voluntary ventilation), or at a single level for 6 minutes at a high ventilation rate (30 × FEV_1). The single level hyperventilation test is very potent and, for patients with known asthma, we use and recommend a test that comprises progressively increasing levels of ventilation for 3 minutes rather than a single high ventilation rate for 6 minutes. We recommend the 6 minute test in elite athletes who lack significant history of exercise-induced asthma and those with a history not requiring medication.

Significance of the results

A fall in FEV_1 of 10% or more is taken as abnormal (see Fig. 3–7).

Nonisotonic Aerosols

In 1980, Allegra and Bianco described the use of distilled water as a provocation test in patients with asthma. The importance of osmolarity was appreciated later when it was found that the airways of asthmatic, but not healthy, subjects were sensitive to both an increase and a decrease in osmolarity. This led to the development and standardization of distilled water and hyperosmolar saline (4.5%) as bronchial provocation tests. Since that time, these aerosols have been widely used in the field to study both adults and children, to assess the effects of drugs used in the treatment of asthma, and to assess airway inflammation in children. More recently, hypertonic saline has been used in the field to identify children with currently active asthma and in the workplace. A new hyperosmolar challenge has been developed recently in Australia. It uses a dry powder of mannitol as the provoking stimulus. As the mechanism whereby exercise and hyperventilation provoke airway narrowing is thought to be a transient hyperosmolarity of the airways, hyperosmolar challenges have been used as surrogates to identify exercise-induced asthma. In field studies it has been shown that a person who has a positive response to hypertonic saline is 4.3 times more likely to have exercise-induced asthma than one who does not.

Hypertonic (4.5%) Saline and Distilled Water

The protocol requires the subject to inhale an aerosol of 4.5% sodium chloride or distilled water for up to 16 minutes. The aerosol is generated by an ultrasonic nebulizer and the rate of delivery of the aerosol should be at least 1.2 ml/min, preferably 1.5 ml/min or more, delivered to the inspiratory port of a large, two-way valve. The FEV_1 is measured before challenge and 60 seconds after exposure to the aerosol. The time of inhalation is doubled for each exposure—30 seconds, 60 seconds, 2 minutes, 4 minutes, 8 minutes—until a 15% reduction in FEV_1 occurs and at least 18.6 ml of 4.5% saline has been delivered to the subject over 15.5 min. The dose of aerosol is measured by weighing the canister and tubing before and after challenge. If the total time of exposure and the total dose are known, the dose delivered per minute can be calculated and a dose–response curve drawn to calculate PD_{15}. Cough can occur during challenge with these aerosols. It is more of a problem with water, and for this reason challenge by hypertonic saline has become more popular. With hypertonic saline the patient may cough initially but cough subsides after 2 or 3 minutes.

Dry Powder Mannitol

The protocol requires the inhalation of progressively increasing doses of mannitol, which is suitably prepared for delivery, from a dry powder inhaler. The FEV_1 is measured on at least two occasions 60 sec after inhaling each dose of mannitol: the doses are 0, 5, 10, 20, 40, 80 (2×40), 160 (4×40), 160 (4×40), and 160 (4×40) mg. The test is stopped after a fall of 15% occurs in FEV_1 or a dose of 635 mg of mannitol has been given. Spontaneous recovery of FEV_1 occurs within 30 to 60 min or within 10 min after a standard dose of bronchodilator. The time to perform the test is 5 to 25 min and is much shorter than most other challenge tests. Because the mannitol is delivered as a powder, it has the advantage of not exposing the investigator to the provoking aerosol. The mannitol test may become more widely available in the future.

Significance of the Results

A fall in FEV_1 of 15% or more is considered as an asthmatic response but a fall greater than 10% is outside the normal range for healthy subjects. A person who has a positive test result to hypertonic (4.5%) saline, distilled water, or mannitol would be expected to have a positive response to challenge with hyperventilation or exercise. A person who has a positive response to a methacholine or histamine challenge would not necessarily have a positive response to a 4.5% saline, water, mannitol, or exercise challenge. Hyperosmolar aerosols are excellent testing agents for patients who are being evaluated for suitability for SCUBA diving, because these patients will be exposed to a similar stimulus during dives.

These challenge tests have been used to measure changes in AHR in response to chronic treatment with steroids and acute treatment with sodium cromoglycate, and nedocromil sodium. A negative test result in a patient taking inhaled steroids suggests that the inflammation is under control with therapy or the patient's condition is in remission at the time of the investigation.

CONCLUSION

The direct, or pharmacologic, challenges have their optimal diagnostic value (the highest combination of positive and negative predictive power) when the pretest probability is in the range of 30% to 70%. They are not helpful when the pretest likelihood of asthma is very low or very high. They are not useful when lung function is low. Even given a positive response, it is hard to interpret test results unless the PC_{20} is in the range of less than 1 mg per ml. Asthmatic patients whose disease is well controlled by inhaled steroids continue to have positive responses to testing for years, so that the end-point for treatment and back titration cannot be always identified as the normal healthy range. False-positive test results to methacholine and histamine can lead to unjustified treatment. For example, many elite athletes who complain of breathlessness on exertion and other respiratory symptoms can have positive responses to histamine or methacholine, but do not have exercise-induced asthma, or abnormal lung function, and do not require treatment for a physiologic abnormality. Perhaps more importantly, exercise-induced asthma may occur in those patients who have a negative result with inhaled histamine or methacholine challenge, and the person may need treatment. Both these situations would be of concern for people in some occupations and for sporting governing bodies whose administrators would not wish to incorrectly exclude or include (or have drugs used)

in otherwise fit persons. If the person is being assessed for an occupation such as the police or the military, it may be more relevant to measure responsiveness to the physical challenges such as exercise, hyperventilation, or hyperosmolar challenge. A positive response to histamine or methacholine in someone who has not had a symptom of asthma for years is hard to interpret if there is no response to an indirect challenge. In the hard-to-decide cases it may be beneficial to perform both types of challenge on separate days. This type of testing should not be viewed as an unattractive choice, because it is likely to give important outcomes particularly for those occupations that can potentially cause respiratory symptoms.

The indirect or physical challenges are used to identify currently active asthma and to assess its severity. Thus, a person with a positive result on indirect challenge is likely to require treatment with inhaled steroids, have exercise-induced asthma, and be unsuitable for a variety of activities. An additional value of the indirect challenge is that it can be used to monitor response to inhaled steroids into the healthy range and to back-titrate steroids. A negative test result to these challenges in a patient with known asthma suggests that the inflammation is under control with therapy or is in remission at the time of investigation. Although a negative test result in a person with symptoms does not necessarily exclude asthma, it does suggest that the disease is only mild and the patient does not require steroids.

Suggested Reading

American Thoracic Society: Lung function testing; selection of reference values and interpretive strategies. Am Rev Respir Dis 144:1202, 1991

Anderson SD, Brannan J, Spring J, et al: A new method for bronchial provocation testing in asthmatic subjects using a dry powder of mannitol. Am J Respir Crit Care Med 156:758, 1997

Anderson SD: Exercise-induced asthma. *In* Kay AB (ed): Allergy and Allergic Disease. Oxford, Blackwell Scientific, 1997, p 692

Anderson SD, Smith CM, Rodwell LT, et al: The use of nonisotonic aerosols for evaluating bronchial hyperresponsiveness. *In* Spector S (ed): Provocation Testing in Clinical Practice. New York, Marcel Dekker, 1995, p 249

Anderson SD, Gibson PG: Use of aerosols of hypertonic saline and distilled water (fog) for the patient with asthma. *In* Barnes PJ, Grunstein MM, Leff AR, Woolcock AJ (eds): Asthma. Philadelphia, Lippincot-Raven, 1997, p 1135

Anderson SD, Rodwell LT, Daviskas E, et al: The protective effect of nedocromil sodium and other drugs on airway narrowing provoked by hyperosmolar stimuli: A role for the airway epithelium. J Allergy Clin Immunol 98(No 5 Part 2):S124, 1996

du Toit JI, Anderson SD, Jenkins CR, et al: Airway responsiveness in asthma: Bronchial challenge with histamine and 4.5% sodium chloride before and after budesonide. Allergy and Asthma Proceedings 18:7, 1997

Juniper EF, Kline PA, Vanzieleghem MA, et al: Long term effects of budesonide on airway responsiveness and clinical asthma severity in inhaled steroid-dependent asthmatics. Eur Respir J 3:1122, 1990

Naclerio RM, Norman PS, Fish JE: In vivo methods for the study of allergy. Mucosal tests, techniques, and interpretations: Bronchial challenge testing. *In* Middleton E, Reed C, Ellis E, et al (eds): Allergy: Principles and Practice, 4th ed., St. Louis, Mosby, 1993, p 612

Ruppel G: Manual of Pulmonary Function Testing, 7th ed., St Louis, Mosby, 1998

Sterk PJ, Fabbri LM, Quanjer PH, et al: Airway responsiveness. Standardized challenge testing with pharmacological, physiological and sensitizing stimuli in man. Eur Respir J 6(Suppl 16):53, 1993

Chapter 4

Airborne Allergens

David L. Gossage

Airborne allergens are ubiquitous in most outdoor and indoor environments. Seasonal plant pollen and mold spores account for the majority of outdoor allergens. Dust mite fecal pellets, animal danders, cockroach feces, saliva and body parts and fungal spores comprise most indoor allergens. Most allergens range in size from 56 to 70 μm in diameter (Fig. 4–1). Some airborne allergens such as pollen grains can be identified microscopically as distinctive units. Others like cat dander are amorphous and are more readily quantified biochemically. Most airborne allergens are composed of a mixture of sensitizing proteins or glycoproteins that are associated with various carrier particles. Together they form aerosol units known as aeroallergens. Clinically important aeroallergens display three major characteristics. First, they contain specific antigenic determinants capable of triggering an IgE-mediated allergic response in susceptible individuals. Second, ambient exposure levels of the aeroallergens are sufficient to evoke an allergic response in sensitized subjects. Third, the sizes of the aeroallergens are of a diameter small enough to reach the respiratory mucosa.

Each aeroallergen may harbor one or more allergenic proteins that can initiate an allergic response. Proteins that bind to a majority of IgE-enriched sera from sensitized patients are called major allergens. Those proteins that bind infrequently are termed minor allergens. Allergic individuals may possess IgE antibodies to either one or both of these groups. In addition, these proteins may contain peptide epitopes that interact with specific T-cell populations.

Specific major and minor allergenic proteins from biogenic sources have been designated according to an international consensus: the first three letters of the genus name and the first letter of the species name followed by a group designation uniquely identifies an allergen. For example, a major allergen from short ragweed, *Ambrosia artemisiifolia*, is designated as Amb a 1. Many major and minor allergenic proteins have been identified and classified according to this system. Developing an understanding of a few of these proteins and the classes of outdoor and indoor aeroallergens they represent will provide the clinician with useful tools to care for allergic patients.

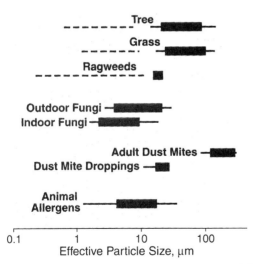

Figure 4–1. Common airborne allergen unit sizes. The broader bars denote more typical ranges in aeroallergen sizes, while dashed lines indicate pollen allergens recoverable in aerosols smaller than single intact grains. In general, depth of respiratory tract penetration rises with decreasing particle size. (From Naclerio R, Solomon W: Rhinitis and inhalant allergens. JAMA 278:1843, 1997; with permission. © 1997, American Medical Association.)

OUTDOOR AEROALLERGENS

Most outdoor aeroallergens are produced from biogenic sources that release pollen or fungal spores into the atmosphere according to specific seasonal patterns. Only a small fraction of the total aeroallergen produced achieves appreciable dispersal. Temperature, humidity, and wind speed influence airborne aeroallergen concentrations. Pollination and sporulation are optimized by warmer temperatures and usually peak during midday. These processes are suppressed in temperatures less than 10°C (40°F). Most pollen and some fungal spores are released in low humidity conditions, whereas many fungi and some pollens such as ragweed require humidity levels greater than 65% to achieve maximum dispersal. Overnight rainfall or fog may hinder or accelerate pollination or sporulation depending on the particular plant or fungus. Aeroallergen concentrations increase as wind speed increases up to 13 to 17 mph. Air speeds above this create significant air turbulence that causes mixing of upper and lower air layers and producing a drop in surface level concentrations.

Airborne allergen concentrations also are dependent on the aerodynamic properties of each particle. Smaller particles are buoyant and remain airborne longer, increasing exposure levels; in contrast, larger particles settle more quickly, except in high winds. Most pollen and fungal spores are between 20 to 60 μm in diameter. This physical restriction limits their deposition to the eyes and nasal mucosa where they elicit allergic eye and nasal symptoms, respectively. However, some patients complain of worsening asthma symptoms during pollen seasons, suggesting aeroallergen access into the lower airways. In these cases, wheezing may be induced by one or more possible mechanisms: (1) Aeroallergens deposited in the nasopharynx may stimulate receptors that trigger a nasopulmonary reflex, (2) an allergenic protein may reach the lower respiratory tract by way of the bloodstream after elution from an aeroallergen deposited in the upper airway, or (3) pollen or fungal spore fragments (<10 μm) may be inspired and penetrate deep into the lower respiratory tract.

Pollen

Pollen grains house the male gametes (sperm) and serve as vectors for fertilization of the female gamete (egg) located in the stigma of flowering plants. The pollen wall is comprised of two main layers: the outer exine (which is subdivided into external sexine and internal nexine layers) and an inner intine. The exine layer exhibits circular pores, elongate furrows, or both. When a pollen grain impacts on the mucosa of an allergic individual, allergenic proteins stored in the sexine and intine layers percolate through the pores and furrows of the exine layer, triggering an allergic response.

Only 10% of seed-producing pollinating plants rely exclusively on wind for pollen dispersal (anemophiles), yet this class of pollinators accounts for the majority of pollen-related clinical allergy. Anemophiles tend to have odorless, inconspicuous flowers. They produce copious amounts of small, nonadhesive, buoyant pollen grains that achieve very high airborne concentrations. In contrast, the majority of flowering plants use insect or animal vectors to transport pollen (entomophiles). This group produces conspicuous, fragrant flowers, but scant amounts of pollen. The pollen that is produced is often large with an adhesive coating. The entomophilous plants do not play a major role in allergy because their pollens are usually not airborne.

Simplistically, trees pollinate in the early spring, grasses in the late spring to midsummer, and weeds from late summer to autumn. For most pollinating plants, this sequence of pollination is accurate; however, some trees pollinate in the autumn and certain weeds pollinate in the early spring. Weather patterns and geographic location also influence timing of pollination. Figure 4–2 illustrates the timing of pollination for prominent allergenic trees, grasses, and weeds by region in North America.

Pollen counts may be useful in determining seasonal prevalence of common aeroallergens in a given locale. Pollen is usually quantitated visually by gravitational methods using glass slides covered with glycerin jelly or by volumetric means employing a rotor rod that houses a microscopic slide within the collecting unit. Direct correlation of pollen counts with allergy symptoms on a given day may be misleading for several reasons. First, extreme day-to-day variation of pollen counts sometimes occurs, making daily symptom prediction difficult. Second, an individual may experience allergic symptoms because of high local concentrations of pollen when the total pollen count may be low. Third, each allergic individ-

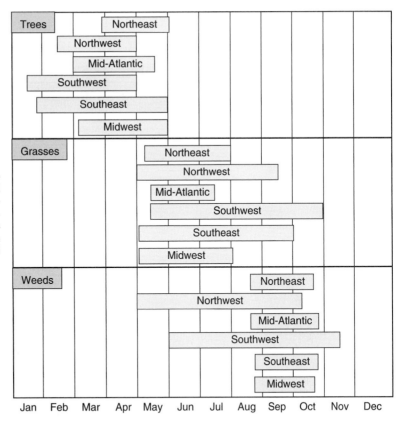

Figure 4–2. Pollen seasons by region in the continental United States. (From Sicherer SH, Eggleston PA: Environmental allergens. *In* Lieberman P, Anderson JA (eds): Allergic Diseases. Totowa, NJ, Humana Press, 1997, p 40; with permission.)

ual has a certain threshold above which allergic symptoms become manifest. Should the pollen count rise significantly, an individual may not demonstrate any allergic symptoms if the individual's allergy threshold is not exceeded. Fourth, pollen counts determined microscopically may not always correlate with allergen concentrations determined biochemically.

Despite these limitations, knowing the timing of a patient's symptoms, the prevalence and characteristics of the local fauna, and the seasonal timing of pollination, a physician can make reasonable inferences about a patient's seasonal allergic triggers. Current local pollen and fungal spore counts may be obtained free of charge by contacting the National Allergy Bureau at 1-800-9-POLLEN or via the internet at http://www.aaaai.org/nab.

Tree Pollen

There are two major classes of pollen-producing trees: the angiosperms (which include the broad-leafed trees) and the gymnosperms (which include conifers). A majority of the angiosperms produces pollen that causes significant allergy. In contrast, a large fraction of conifers including pines, firs, spruces, and hemlock are not considered clinically important because their pollen is very large in size, 50 to 90 μm, and weakly allergenic. Exceptions to this rule include the scrub-juniper, the mountain cedar, and the red cedar. These evergreens are responsible for causing significant allergic symptoms in regions where they are indigenous.

In North America, tree pollination begins in late February and extends into April. In some areas, the season may begin as early as December and in other areas it may last through the month of June. Most flowering trees may be categorized as either early, midseason, or late pollinators. Elm and red cedar are examples of early pollinators. Poplar, birch, ash, and willow pollinate in midseason; sycamore, oak, and mulberry represent late-season pollination. Table 4–1 illustrates five prominent allergenic trees in each region of North America. They are listed according to their sequence of pollination.

Table 4–1. **Selected Trees and Weeds of Allergenic Significance**

Region	Trees	Grasses	Weeds
Northeast (ME, NH, VT, NY, PA, NJ, MA, RI, CT)	Elm Maple Poplar Oak	Timothy June Sweet vernal Bluegrass	Plantain Russian thistle Giant ragweed Short ragweed
Mid-Atlantic (DE, MC, DC, VA, NC, SC)	Birch Elm Maple Hickory Oak	Orchard Timothy Bluegrass June Bermuda	Plantain Dock Sage Short ragweed Giant ragweed
North Central (OH, KY, WI, MI, IA, northern MO, IL, IN, TN)	Ash Elm Maple Willow Box elder	Orchard Timothy Bluegrass June	Plantain Dock Russian thistle Short ragweed Giant ragweed
Pacific Northwest (WA, NV, OR, northern CA)	Alder Birch Maple Oak Walnut	Timothy Bluegrass Fescue Rye Redtop	Dock Plantain Russian thistle Nettle Sagebrush
Plains (NE, MN, eastern MT, Dakotas)	Elm Oak Box elder Willow Maple	Timothy Orchard Bluegrass Bermuda Redtop	Marsh-elder Russian thistle Western hemp Short ragweed Giant ragweed
Rocky Mountains (ID, WY, CO, UT, western MT)	Cedar Elm Ash Birch Oak	Timothy Orchard Fescue Redtop June	Sagebrush Russian thistle Short ragweed Giant ragweed
Southern (FL, GA, AL, TX, AR, southern MO)	Cedar Elm Mulberry Poplar Oak	Bermuda Orchard Timothy Saltgrass	Dock Pigweed Russian thistle Giant ragweed Short ragweed
Southwest (western TX, NM, AZ)	Cedar Ash Mulberry Oak Olive	Bermuda Johnson	Sagebrush Russian thistle Saltbush Kochia Short ragweed
Southern California	Ash Walnut Elm Oak Olive	Bermuda Saltgrass Brome	Nettle Bur ragweed Russian thistle Sage Western ragweed

From Sicherer SH, Eggleston PA: Environmental allergens. *In* Lieberman P, Anderson JA (eds): Allergic Diseases. Totowa, NJ, Humana Press, 1997, p 41; with permission.

Grass Pollen

In North America, the grass pollen season begins in May, overlapping the close of the tree pollen season, and continues until the end of July. There are two main groups of grasses: the Northern grasses that grow in temperate climates and the Southern grasses that are found in the South and subtropic regions. Prominent Northern grasses include orchard, timothy, ryegrass, and bluegrass. Each grass pollen contains specific antigenic determinants, but unlike tree or weed pollen, there is a high degree of cross-allergenicity among Northern grasses. Thus, individual grass species exposure is less important than total grass pollen exposure. In contrast, the three main major Southern grasses are Bahia, Bermuda, and Johnson grass. The allergenic proteins of these grasses are antigenically distinct and demonstrate minimal cross-reactivity with the Northern grasses. In some parts of the country, Bermuda may pollinate almost year round. Table 4–1 shows the major allergenic grasses by region in North America.

Weed Pollen

Weed pollinosis generally begins in late summer and extends to October or the first killing frost. Though there is a tremendous diversity of weeds that cause allergic symptoms, ragweed species are by far the most abundant and clinically significant. There are several varieties of ragweed, each of which produces the major allergen Amb a 1. Sensitized individuals may experience out of season allergic symptoms when travelling to areas such as southern Florida, where coastal ragweed pollinates perennially. Other important weeds responsible for significant allergy symptoms include pigweed, marsh elder, dock, sorrel, plantain, and Russian thistle. Allergenically important weeds are listed in Table 4–1 by region and order of pollination.

Reducing Pollen Exposure

Because most of the allergenic pollens are well mixed throughout the lower atmosphere, strict

Table 4–2. **Pollen Avoidance Measures**

- Wear a respirator when mowing the lawn, gardening, or any prolonged outdoor activity
- When pollen counts are high, remain indoors with windows closed. Use air conditioning
- Perform essential outdoor activities in the early morning before midday when pollen counts usually peak

avoidance during pollen seasons is virtually impossible. The goal is to minimize excessive pollen exposure. Common sense dictates avoidance measures (Table 4–2). Pollen counts are usually highest around midday on warm, slightly windy days. Pollen levels are usually lower after long continued rains or in foggy conditions, but are not generally affected by brief downpours associated with thunderstorms. When outdoor exposure is unavoidable, wearing a respirator while mowing the lawn, working in the garden, or performing farm work may be an acceptable alternative. Indoor exposure to pollen can be significantly reduced by closing windows and using central air conditioning.

Patients with regional pollen allergy may contemplate moving to another region to escape symptoms. If a move is being considered, a patient should consider a temporary move of at least four weeks in the new area, preferably in more than one pollen season, to determine if symptoms will actually improve. Unfortunately, a move to a new region does not always completely resolve allergy symptoms. Over time, many of these individuals will become sensitized to the aeroallergens found in their new environment.

Outdoor Fungi

The terms fungi and mold are frequently used synonymously, although the two terms are not equivalent. Concisely, molds are a type of fungus that lack macroscopic reproductive structures but may generate visible colonies or other growth. Fungi are found in two structural forms: yeast and hyphae. They may reproduce asexually, sexually, or cycle between the two, depending on growth conditions. In general, fungi grow best in moist cool conditions. Some fungal spores can survive prolonged

Table 4–3. **Outdoor Fungi Avoidance**

- Avoid raking leaves, mowing grass, farming activities such as cutting and bailing hay, hiking in a forest
- Wear a respirator when outdoors during high fungal spore counts
- Stay indoors with windows closed when fungal spore counts are high. Use air conditioning
- Avoid exposure to cool damp areas such as composts or grain silos

cold exposures to temperatures as low as $-56°C$. At the other extreme, thermophilic varieties can thrive at temperatures as high as 71°C. When the relative humidity drops below 65%, most fungi cannot proliferate.

Common outdoor molds include *Cladosporium, Alternaria, Aspergillus, Penicillium,* and *Botrytis. Cladosporium* spore levels are the most prevalent, while *Alternaria* produces the highest degree of sensitivity among fungi-exposed subjects. Fungal spores can be detected year round except in polar regions. High levels are found in areas of crop production and in locations where bulk, decaying, biogenic debris may be found. Fungal spore levels peak in late summer and autumn and also in the spring with wet weather. Certain outdoor activities may predispose individuals to come into contact with high local concentrations of fungal spores and may elicit allergic symptoms. Outdoor activities that tend to increase outdoor fungal spore exposure include leaf ranking, lawn mowing, hiking, or farming activities. Any activity performed in the outdoors during damp weather conditions may increase fungal spore exposure. Table 4–3 lists some fungi avoidance measures.

INDOOR AEROALLERGENS

Over the past century, the indoor environment has become a potent source of airborne allergens. One factor that has contributed to this trend has been the modernization of homes and offices. Changes in home construction have decreased indoor ventilation. Addition of home furnishings such as carpets, sofas, and other upholstered furniture have increased allergen reservoirs. Together these home improvements have fostered the growth and accumulation of multiple indoor allergens. A second factor that has contributed to this

trend has been an increase in personal exposure to these indoor allergens. In contrast to earlier in this century, most individuals in modern society spend the majority of their days and nights indoors.

Indoor allergens cause perennial allergic symptoms because of chronic exposure. Symptoms may be worse in the winter because days are shorter and colder and more time is spent indoors. Occasionally, a patient's chronic symptoms may wax and wane. This fluctuation in symptoms may be related to an intermittent exposure to an indoor allergen such as cat or dog dander.

Because many of the indoor allergens are amorphous, specific allergenic proteins are measured by sensitive immunoassays. Airborne indoor allergen levels vary and are not as predictable as seasonal outdoor aeroallergen levels. Indoor allergens can be measured in reservoir dust samples or by obtaining volumetric air samples. The former has been shown to be a valid index of significant clinical exposure for larger aeroallergens such as dust mite and cockroach, while the latter may be more reliable for smaller aeroallergens such as animal danders, which remain airborne for longer periods of time. Maintaining low levels of indoor allergens in the home is important because it may help prevent development of sensitization in atopic individuals. For those already sensitized, low levels of indoor allergens may reduce allergic exacerbations.

Dust Mites

House dust mites are the major allergen found in house dust. The two predominant species are *Dermatophagoides pteronyssinus* and *Dermatophygoides farinae.* Approximately 80% to 95% of human–mite-specific IgE cross-reacts between these two species. Dust mites are microscopic (approximately 0.3 mm in length), eight-legged, eyeless acarids that share the same family as scabies. They feed on human scales and other debris. Under ideal conditions egg-to-adult metamorphoses take 3 to 4 weeks and includes a five-stage life cycle. Adult mites survive for approximately 6 weeks. Dust mites require ambient moisture to survive. They thrive at relative humidities between 75% and 80% and temperatures of 20°C to 30°C (68°F to

84°F). Viable *D. pteronyssinus* are usually not found in relative humidities below 65%, and dust mites will perish in humidities below 45%. *D. farinae* is hardier and can survive at a relative humidity of 45% at 15°C. Dust mites are rarely found in mountainous areas above 3600 feet above sea level because the relative humidity is very low. Smooth floor surfaces also retain less humidity and thus harbor few dust mites. However, in areas where humidity can be retained, such as in carpets, mattresses, blankets, pillows, and stuffed animals, dust mite concentrations may be high. Dust mites are unable to regulate their body temperature. Thus, their growth is determined by both ambient temperature and humidity.

The major allergens from each of two predominant species of dust mites have been identified and characterized as Der p 1 and Der f 1 respectively. Both are gut-associated cysteine proteases, are likely to be digestive enzymes, and are concentrated in mite fecal pellets. These fecal pellets are covered by a permeable membrane that allows rapid elution of allergenic proteins when in contact with moist mucosal surfaces. Most pellets are between 10 and 35 μm in diameter (similar to the size of some pollen grains). The pellets can become airborne but settle within minutes after a disturbance.

Several avoidance measures have been shown to significantly reduce dust mite allergens in the home. They include (1) covering mattress and pillow case with an airtight, impermeable cover, (2) washing bedding weekly at 130°F, (3) reducing the relative humidity to less than 45%, and (4) removing carpet, stuffed animals, and clutter from the bedroom (Table 4–4).

There are other available treatments that may decrease dust mite allergen loads, but their clinical effectiveness is uncertain. Applying benzyl benzoate (Acarosan, Center

Laboratories, Port Washington, NY) or 3% tannic acid to carpets may reduce dust mite allergens for weeks to a few months. The former product is acaricidal and very expensive. The latter product is inexpensive but does not kill dust mites; it denatures the dust mite allergenic proteins. A drawback of tannic acid is that it may stain light-colored carpets. Stuffed animals that children refuse to remove from their beds and that cannot withstand hot water washing can be placed in a freezer bag at −20°C for 24 hours. This has been shown to kill the dust mites.

There are some treatments that should be avoided because they may actually enhance dust mite proliferation. Avoid the use of humidifiers. High humidity will increase dust mite populations. Do not use water when cleaning carpets. The usual result is that the carpet and the padding underneath become damp, creating ideal growth conditions for both dust mites and fungi. Carpet should be avoided, particularly in the basement. Leakage of water from above and condensation from concrete slab floors below make it virtually impossible to keep basement carpeting completely dry. Although routine vacuuming with a unit that contains a high efficiency particulate air (HEPA) filter is encouraged, purchase of an expensive vacuum cleaner is of little added benefit.

INDOOR FUNGI

Indoor environments provide a warm, constant temperature for indoor fungal growth. If the relative humidity is high, fungal sporulation will usually occur. Leaky basements, wet bathrooms, soiled or damp upholstery, storage of damp food or clothing, and garbage containers are all excellent sites for indoor fungal growth. *Penicillium, Aspergillus, Rhizopus,* and *Cladosporium* are some examples of common fungi that thrive in a permissive indoor environment. Fungal colonies may be visible as darkly stained growths on bathroom tile, around window seals, in sinks, and on concrete walls in basements. *Penicillium* forms a greenish growth, whereas *Rhizopus* produces fluffy black colonies.

The best therapy for indoor mold avoidance is to maintain a low relative humidity. In

Table 4–4. **Dust Mite Avoidance**

- Cover mattress and pillow cases with impermeable covers
- Wash bedding weekly in 130°F water
- Remove carpets, stuffed animals, and clutter from bedrooms
- Reduce relative humidity to less than 45%
- Treat carpets with benzyl benzoate or 3% tannic acid

many areas this can be done simply by using air conditioning. Routine use of cold reservoir humidifiers should be discouraged. Frequently, mold may grow in the reservoir, allowing fungal spores to be dispersed throughout a home as the machine runs. Cleaning damp areas regularly with bleach is an effective deterrent to mold growth.

COCKROACH

Three cockroach species account for the majority of cockroaches found in the United States: *Blattella germanica* (German cockroach), *Periplaneta americana* (American cockroach), and *Blattella orientalis* (Oriental cockroach). The German cockroach is the most prevalent of the three species and inhabits most urban areas throughout the United States. It is strictly a domestic species and does not survive outdoors. The American and Oriental cockroaches are hardier and can be found in and around homes. The prevalence of cockroach allergy is inversely related to socioeconomic status. This is likely because higher levels of cockroach allergen are found in inner city housing. In this venue, cockroach allergen has been shown to be a major risk factor for emergency room visits for asthma exacerbations.

Cockroach allergens can be detected through an entire household, but the highest concentration of allergens is found in the kitchen and bathrooms. Human exposure to cockroach allergens results from inhalation of disturbed dust containing cockroach feces, saliva, and body part fragments. More than four allergenic proteins from the German cockroach have been identified, cloned, and sequenced. The two most important allergens are Bla g 1 and Bla g 2. A major allergen from the American cockroach, Per a 1, has also been identified and has been shown to cross-react with Bla g 1.

Cockroaches are difficult to eradicate from infested premises. Effective avoidance measures have not been well defined (Table 4–5). Killing roaches *per se* has not been proved to reduce cockroach allergen levels; however, a study done in a cockroach-infested dormitory revealed that extermination followed by aggressive cleaning reduced cockroach allergens by 86%. Controlled studies are

Table 4–5. **Cockroach Avoidance**

- Keep food out of the bedroom
- Store food and garbage in closed containers. Never leave food out
- Apply roach bait underneath kitchen sinks and in bathrooms, away from contact with young children and pets
- Wipe down kitchen floors and counters regularly

under way to determine if reducing cockroach allergens results in a reduction in clinical allergy and asthma symptoms.

Despite the above-mentioned uncertainties, several methods of cockroach elimination have been attempted. Spraying in the home kills few roaches, and the fumes may be irritating to patients with asthma. Traps catch only a small portion of available roaches. The use of bait is a more efficient method of killing roaches. Many different baits have been used. The two most popular baits are boric acid and hydromethanon. Boric acid is a simple bait that is nontoxic to humans and kills roaches by affecting their foregut. Hydromethanon is the most lethal of cockroach baits, but it should be used with caution in households with young children. It can be purchased for residential use as Combat Superbait (The Clorox Company, Oakland, CA). A newer agent, Fipronil, which kills by contact and ingestion, is being used professionally (Max-Force, The Clorox Company, Oakland, CA). Interestingly, the most effective control measure of cockroach allergen is a cat. Indoor cockroach allergen levels have been found to be inversely related to cat allergen levels. Homes with cats have fewer roaches, presumably because the cats ingest the roaches. Obviously, this last method of roach control could be detrimental to cat allergic patients. Regardless of the method of roach elimination used, it should coincide with frequent cleaning of kitchens and enclosing of food.

CATS

Cats are a common household pet. Survey data of an atopic population have shown that between 20% and 40% of atopic individuals are sensitized to cat allergens. More importantly, about one third of these people live with a cat.

The major cat allergenic protein is Fel d 1 *(Felis domesticus)*. Reactivities to other proteins, including cat albumin, have lesser clinical importance. More than 85% of cat-allergic individuals produce IgE antibodies to the Fel d 1 protein. All breeds of cat, both short- and long-haired varieties, produce Fel d 1. Nonneutered male cats produce more allergenic protein than female cats. Fel d 1 is produced in the sebaceous glands and dermis of the skin and is distributed by cat licking and grooming.

Unlike the vectors for dust mite and cockroach, which are relatively large, cat dander particles are generally less than 25 μm, and 10% to 30% may be smaller than 2.5 μm. These sizes approximate particles generated by therapeutic nebulizers. Because of its small size, cat dander remains airborne for longer periods of time, which increases the possibility it may penetrate deep into the lower respiratory tract.

The most effective way to control exposure to cat allergen is to remove the cat from the premises. This option is unpopular with most cat owners. Even if the cat is removed, levels of Fel d 1 may not fall below allergic thresholds for up to 4 months. The delayed clearance of Fel d 1 is due to its continued release from reservoirs such as carpets, upholstered furniture, drapes, and clothing. A second control option is to keep the cat but restrict its territory to outside the house. If the family plays with the cat and pets it regularly, there is likely to be a significant amount of Fel d 1 brought indoors by passive transfer from clothing. A third alternative is to allow the cat to remain indoors but wash it weekly. Cat washing has been used as a method to elute cat allergen for commercial extract production. Washing the cat thoroughly can reduce airborne Fel d 1 in homes by as much as 85%. To maintain these reduced levels of allergen, washing must be repeated regularly, limiting its practicality. A fourth control option is to use a HEPA filter in the bedroom. When a HEPA filter is combined with the use of pillow and mattress covers, and the cat's access to the bedroom is restricted, bedroom airborne levels of Fel d 1 can be reduced. Unfortunately, this reduction does not correspond with any improvements in clinical symptoms. Thus, it may not be possible to sufficiently reduce cat allergen exposure while a cat is

Table 4–6. **Cat Dander Avoidance**

- If possible, remove cat from the house
- Reduce reservoirs for cat dander such as carpets, sofas, etc.
- Increase indoor ventilation or obtain a HEPA air filter
- Wash cat weekly
- Female cats produce less cat allergens. Consider having male cats neutered

living in the home. At least at present, the only certain pragmatic way to reduce cat allergen exposure in cat-allergic patients is to remove the cat from the home (Table 4–6).

DOGS

Dogs may also be a potent source of allergens, although sensitivity to dogs appears to be less common than sensitivity to cats. The major allergen for dog *(Canis familiaris)* is Can f 1, which is found in dog hair and saliva. All breeds of dog produce this major allergen, but the absolute amounts may vary. Contrary to many dog owners' opinions, there is no genuine allergen-free breed. Some breed-specific allergens have been identified, but their clinical significance is unknown. Fewer studies have been performed on dog allergens. Can f 1 has been detected in homes and schools without dogs, signifying passive transfer of allergen can occur. Avoidance measures for dog allergens are likely to parallel those for cat dander.

OTHER FURRY ANIMALS

There are several mammals other than cats and dogs that are frequently chosen as pets in homes, schools, and the workplace. Gerbils, rabbits, guinea pigs, and other exotic pets such as ferrets and minks may be purchased at pet shops or from specialty breeders. Allergens from these animals have not been well characterized but are usually found in the fur, saliva, or urine. Farm animals such as pigs, horses, and cattle may also cause allergic disease. Farmers and veterinarians who care for these larger animals could be at increased risk to become sensitized to these allergens. The prevalence of allergic disease related to these allergens is unknown.

Laboratory animal dander is another potent source of indoor allergens. Between 10% to 30% of laboratory animal workers have occupational allergy to laboratory animal dander. One third of these individuals will also have symptomatic asthma. Most workers become sensitized within 3 years of employment. Workers who have the most direct contact with the animals, such as cleaning animal cages and feeding the animals, are at the highest risk for sensitization.

Mice and rats are responsible for the majority of laboratory animal allergy. The major allergen for mouse *(Mus musculis)* is Mus m 1. It is a prealbumin found in mouse urine and dander. Serum and urine levels are four times higher in males because gene expression is upregulated by testosterone. Two major allergens have been found in the rat *(Rattus norvegicus)*, Rat n 1A and Rat n1B. Both allergens are variants of the same protein, alpha$_{2u}$-globulin. This protein is also androgen-dependent and is found in rat dander, urine, and saliva.

Workers can reduce exposure to these allergens by wearing respiratory protective gear. Employing laminar flow caging and using frequent wet washing of vivaria can further reduce allergen levels. The ventilation systems for the vivaria should be carefully monitored to ensure they remain totally functional.

BIRDS

Exposure to avian proteins in occupations such as egg processing and bird breeding frequently results in respiratory disease. IgE-mediated sensitivity to feathers has been reported in canary breeders and other bird breeders although a major protein allergen has not been identified. The results of allergy skin testing to feather extract may be misleading because the feather extract may be contaminated with dust mite or mold, leading to false-positive results. Egg allergy usually is not associated with feather allergy although dual sensitization has been reported.

In contrast, individuals may develop a hypersensitivity pneumonitis after prolonged exposure to pigeons, canaries, or budgerigars (parrots). This disease process is mediated by an IgG antibody response toward avian gamma globulin; however, IgE responses have been observed in some individuals.

LATEX

Natural latex is a highly processed plant product that is used in a wide variety of household and industrial items. It is derived from the cytosol or latex of the commercial rubber tree, *Hevea brasiliensis*. The major allergen of this plant product has been identified as rubber elongation factor (Hev b 1). Most allergic symptoms triggered by latex involve tactile interaction of latex by sensitive individuals, resulting in a contact dermatitis or urticaria; however, rhinitis, asthma, and in rare cases anaphylaxis may occur.

In addition to its role as a contact allergen, latex is also a potent aeroallergen. High levels of airborne latex have been demonstrated in operating rooms and surgical clinics during working hours, but allergen levels rapidly decline and become undetectable when work activities cease. The major source of aerosolized latex comes from latex-containing rubber gloves. By simply switching to latex-free gloves in these work areas the airborne latex levels can be reduced from 100 to 200 ng/m^3 to less than 3 ng/m^3.

Latex may function as a significant outdoor aeroallergen as well. In congested urban areas numerous respirable tire fragments have been detected in the air. These tire fragments have been shown to contain latex. It is likely that as the number of automobiles in the inner cities continues to increase, the levels of latex allergen in inner city air will increase. Higher levels of latex in the air will increase latex exposure and possibly latex sensitization.

In the United States, there are currently no standardized commercially available extracts for latex skin testing diagnostics. Serum immunoassays are available but may have variable sensitivities of from 50% to 90%. For latex-sensitive individuals who are undergoing medical procedures, a latex-free clinic and hospital environment has been recommended by the Task Force on Allergic Reactions to Latex by the American Academy of Allergy, Asthma and Immunology. In high-risk latex exposure areas such as operating rooms, outpatient surgical suites, dental offices, or at the patient's bedside, personnel should wear latex-free gloves, and no latex accessories should come in direct contact with the patient. Avoidance of selected cross-reactive foods may also be necessary (see Chapter 5, Food Allergens).

MISCELLANEOUS INDOOR ALLERGENS

There are a number of other potential biogenic materials present in the indoor environment that may serve as allergens. Although less is known about these miscellaneous allergens, in certain allergic individuals, they may cause significant allergic symptoms. Several plants or plant products may produce allergic symptoms. The weeping fig tree *(Ficus benjamina)* produces a sap that when aerosolized can produce respiratory symptoms. Other plant materials such as orris root, pyrethrum, castor bean, flaxseed, psyllium, vegetable gums and ovalbumin, along with dust from cotton, kapok, coffee, and flour have shown to produce allergic symptoms.

Bacteria and protozoa may be found in the indoor environment, but there is no definitive proof that these organisms cause IgE-mediated allergy. On the other hand, it is well known that these infectious agents may exacerbate or complicate existing allergic disease.

Chapter 5

Food Allergens

Wesley Burks, Ricki Helm, Steve Stanley, and Gary A. Bannon

A number of advances in the scientific knowledge concerning adverse food reactions have been made in the last several years. Understanding about the nature of the food allergen itself, the molecular characterization of the epitopes on these allergens, the pathophysiology of the clinical reaction, and diagnostic methods for detecting allergen response have all been significantly enhanced. Part of the difficulty in understanding adverse food reactions has been the nomenclature used in this literature. Standardized definitions are beginning to ensure the scientific literature is more uniform (Table 5–1). An adverse food reaction is a generic term referring to any untoward reaction after the ingestion of a food. Adverse food reactions may be secondary to food allergy (hypersensitivity) or food intolerance. A food-allergic reaction is presumed to be the result of an abnormal immunologic response after the ingestion of a food, whereas food intolerance is the result of nonimmunologic mechanisms.

The true prevalence of adverse food reactions is unknown. In American households about one-third of families believe some family member to be affected. The best studies to date indicate that approximately 6% to 8% of young children and 1% to 2% of adults have some type of food allergy.

FOOD ALLERGENS

Foods are typically derived from animal and vegetable sources. Both animals and vegetables are classified botanically. Examples of animal groups include birds (i.e., chicken, duck), crustaceans (i.e., crab, lobster), and red meats (i.e., beef, veal). Examples of plant groups include the apple family (i.e., apple, pear), grass family (i.e., corn, wheat), legume family (i.e., lentil, peanut), and walnut family (i.e., black walnut, pecan). Allergy to one member of some food groups may result in a variable degree of clinical reactivity (a clinical reaction) to other members of the same group because of cross-reacting allergens. Much more is understood now about the differences between clinical sensitivity (evidence of immunologic sensitivity) and clinical reactivity within a group of similar foods.

Foods are composed of proteins, carbohydrates, and lipids. The major food allergens have been identified as water-soluble glycoproteins having molecular weights ranging from 10,000 to 60,000 daltons. There are no known, unique biochemical or immunochemical characteristics of food allergens. Comparisons of primary amino acid sequences of allergenic proteins have not revealed conserved patterns. However, food allergens tend to be resistant to usual food processing and preparation conditions. Thus, these proteins are comparatively resistant to heat and acid treatment, proteolysis, and digestion. The treatment of food allergens with acid concentrations simulating stom-

Table 5–1. Definitions of Adverse Food Reactions

Adverse food reaction—generic term referring to any untoward reaction after the ingestion of a food

Food allergy (hypersensitivity)—the result of an abnormal immunologic response after the ingestion of a food

Food intolerance—the result of nonimmunologic mechanisms after the ingestion of a food

ach conditions typically has little effect on the specific IgE binding of the allergen. There are, however, important exceptions, such as the major allergens in fresh fruits and some vegetables.

The food allergens, in general, are soluble in water or saline solutions, or both, and thus belong to the classes known as albumins (water soluble) or globulins (saline soluble). Although the level of exposure to a specific protein necessary to sensitize an individual is unknown, extremely low levels of the offending food can initiate a reaction in individuals with pre-existing IgE-mediated food allergies. Microgram to milligram quantities of peanut have elicited an adverse reaction in food challenges in selected individuals. The immunochemical or physicochemical properties that account for such unique allergenicity of food allergens are poorly understood.

MAJOR FOOD ALLERGENS

The most common foods to cause documented IgE-mediated reactions in childhood are cow's milk, eggs, peanuts, soybeans, wheat, fish, and tree nuts (Table 5–2). Approximately 80% of these reactions are secondary to either milk, eggs, or peanuts. In adulthood, the most common food allergens are peanuts, tree nuts, fish, and shellfish. Worldwide there are some differences in which foods cause problems in both children and adults in different countries, primarily because of the diet of the population.

Cow's Milk

The prevalence of cow's milk allergy in infants and children, worldwide, is estimated at be-

Table 5–2. **Major Food Allergens in Children and Adults**

Children	Adults
Milk	Peanuts
Egg	Tree nuts
Peanuts	Fish
Soybeans	Shellfish
Wheat	
Fish	
Tree nuts	

tween 2.0% and 2.5%. Allergic symptoms related to cow's milk often begin in early childhood, but children typically lose their sensitivity in the first 3 to 5 years of life. Cow's milk is composed of a number of different proteins, traditionally divided into caseins, which make up 80% of the total protein, and whey proteins, which comprise the remainder. Most patients who are allergic to cow's milk have specific-IgE antibodies to more than one of the milk proteins. Caseins were originally defined as phosphoproteins that precipitate from raw skim milk upon acidification to pH 4.6 at 20°C; whey proteins are those proteins remaining in the milk after precipitation of caseins. The nomenclature of specific milk proteins uses a Greek letter with or without a subscript preceding the class name to identify the family of proteins. The genetic variant of the milk protein is indicated by an upper case Arabic letter with or without a numerical superscript following the class name. Post-translational modifications are added in sequence (Table 5–3).

A number of milk proteins have been identified as allergens in humans. By either skin prick testing or oral challenge many patients have reactivity to multiple cow's milk proteins. Caseins and beta-lactoglobulin appear to be the major allergens in cow's milk. The caseins are a family of proteins (alpha, beta, and kappa) that are chemically related. The major alpha- and beta-caseins have a molecular weight of approximately 23 kD. There are several genetic variants of each of these caseins. Beta-lactoglobulin (17 kD), the most abundant whey protein, also has several genetic variants. Alpha-lactalbumin (14 kD) and bovine serum albumin (67 kD), both whey proteins, appear to be minor cow's milk allergens. Bovine serum albumin (BSA) has also been identified as a distinct milk allergen. This protein is heterogeneous in nature and has a molecular weight of 67 kD, comprising approximately 1% of the total milk protein.

Eggs

Egg is one of the most commonly implicated causes of food allergic reactions both in the United States and Europe. Eggs from chickens *(Gallus domesticus)* are widely used for human

Table 5–3. **Purified Antigens in Foods**

Protein Fraction	Molecular Weight (kD)
Cow's Milk	
Caseins	19,000–24,000
α-casein	27,000
α$_S$-casein	23,000
β-casein	24,000
κ-casein	19,000
γ-casein	21,000
Whey	
β-lactoglobulin	36,000
α-lactoglobulin	14,400
Bovine serum albumin	69,000
Chicken Egg White	
Ovalbumin	45,000
Ovomucoid	28,000
Ovotransferrin	77,700
Lysozyme	14,300
Peanut	
Ara h 1	63,500
Ara h 2	17,500
Ara h 3	56,000
Soybean	
Gly m 1	34,000
Soybean trypsin inhibitor	20,500
Fish	
Allergen M [Gad c 1]	12,328
Shrimp	
Antigen I	42,000
Antigen II	38,000
Pen a 1	36,000

consumption. Although there is extensive cross-reactivity among the various birds, hen eggs tend to be slightly more allergenic than duck eggs. Eggs are composed of egg white and egg yolk. The egg white (albumin) appears to be more allergenic than the yolk. The major protein in the egg white is ovalbumin, with other proteins including ovotransferrin, ovomucoid, ovomucin, and lysozyme. Egg yolk can be separated into two fractions using ultracentrifugation. This results in a granular fraction that contains primarily protein and a supernatant fraction that contains primarily lipid. The granular fraction contains lipovitellin, phosvitin, and low-density lipoprotein.

Ovomucoid (Gal d 1), a glycoprotein with a molecular weight of 28 kD and an acidic isoelectric point, has been implicated as the major allergen in egg. In a recent study, purified ovomucoid was found to be a more potent allergen than purified ovalbumin by skin prick testing and with radioallergosorbent testing

(RAST) in a group of children with egg allergy. Although previous studies had shown that ovalbumin was the major egg allergen, this recent work demonstrated ovomucoid contamination in the previously isolated ovalbumin.

Ovalbumin (Gal d 2) is a monomeric phosphoglycoprotein with a molecular weight of 43 to 45 kD and an acidic isoelectric point. Purified ovalbumin has three primary variants, A$_1$, A$_2$, and A$_3$. Because of the previous ovomucoid contamination of ovalbumin, it is difficult to determine the exact role of this allergen. Ovotransferrin (Gal d 3) (conalbumin) has a molecular weight of 77 kD and an acidic isoelectric point. It has antimicrobial activity and iron-binding properties. Lysozyme (Gal d 4) is a lower molecular weight allergen (14.3 kD) that has appeared to be a major allergen in some studies, but in other studies it has been thought to be a minor allergen. Other minor allergens in eggs include apovitellin, ovomucin, and phosvitin. Additional studies have shown that the carbohydrate portion of the glycoproteins in eggs, particularly in ovomucoid, does not have a primary role in specific IgE binding. B- and T-cell epitopes have been mapped in a limited way for both ovalbumin and ovomucoid.

Peanuts

The peanut is an annual plant in the family Leguminosae. In the United States several varieties, including the Virginia, Spanish, and runner, are grown. Most of the peanut crop in the United States is used for production of peanut butter. Runner types are used most frequently for oil production and peanut butter. Children are increasingly being exposed to peanut products at an early age. Allergic reactions to peanuts are often very acute and severe, accounting for many of the cases of food-induced anaphylaxis documented each year.

Peanut proteins are customarily classified as albumins (water soluble) and globulins (saline soluble). The globulin proteins are made up of two major fractions, arachin and conarachin (also known as legumine and vicilin, respectively). In its native state, arachin exists as a molecule of at least 600 kD and readily dissociates into a 340- to 360-kD dimer and a monomer of approximately 170 to 180 kD. Conarachin can be divided by ultracentrifugation into two fractions, one 2S and one 8.4S.

There have been a number of peanut allergens identified and characterized. Peanut-1 and concanavalin A-reactive glycoprotein (CARG) were two of the first peanut allergens partially characterized. Ara h 1 is a 63.5-kD glycoprotein identified as a major peanut allergen using immunoblotting and enzyme-linked immunosorbent assay (ELISA) methods. This allergen has an acidic isoelectric point and is relatively resistant to enzyme degradation. Molecular studies have identified multiple IgE binding sites in the amino acid sequence of Ara h 1. This peanut allergen has at least 23 specific-IgE binding epitopes along its amino acid sequence. Ara h 1 has been identified as a member of the vicilin family of seed storage proteins. Ara h 2 is a 17-kD allergen with a acidic isoelectric point. This allergen has at least 10 specific-IgE binding epitopes along its amino acid sequence. Ara h 2 appears to be a member of the conglutin family of seed storage proteins. Ara h 3 is another peanut allergen of 56 kD and is a member of the glycinin family of seed storage proteins.

Soybeans

Soybeans, although not implicated as often as milk, eggs, and peanuts, are one of five major allergens in the United States that cause food-allergic reactions in children. Soybean globulins are the major proteins of the soybean. The soybean globulins can be separated into ultracentrifugation components identified as 2S, 7S, 11S, and 15S fractions. Alpha-conglycinin is a primary protein of the 2S fraction, beta-conglycinin is the primary fraction of the 7S component, and glycinin is the primary component of the 11S ultracentrifugation fraction.

Soybeans, like peanuts, are legumes that have multiple allergens. While examining specific-IgE to the ultracentrifugation components, authors have primarily identified either the 2S or the 7S fraction as containing the primary allergens. Gly m 1 is a 30-kD allergen that is a component of the 7S fraction. In one study the majority of patients had soybean-specific IgE to Gly m 1. Gly m 1 has an acidic

isoelectric point. It has sequence homology to a soybean seed 34 kD oil–body-associated protein (called soybean vacuolar protein P34). There appear to be at least 16 distinct soybean-specific IgE binding epitopes along the amino acid sequence of this allergen. The Kunitz soybean trypsin inhibitor has also been shown in several studies to bind soybean-specific IgE in soybean-allergic patients although only in a minority of patients (making it likely a minor allergen).

Wheat

Although not the most common sources of food allergy, wheat and other cereal grains are often implicated as food allergens, particularly in children. The proteins of wheat include the water-soluble albumins, the saline-soluble globulins, the ethanol-soluble prolamins, and the glutelins. It is not uncommon for children to have multiple positive prick skin test reactions to various cereal grains while having clinical reactivity to only one of the foods. This extensive cross-reactivity is most likely caused by nonspecific IgE binding to the lectin fractions in cereal grains. Patients with wheat allergy apparently have specific IgE binding to wheat fractions of 47 kD and 20 kD (proteins not recognized by the serum from patients with grass allergy). Additional studies have shown the wheat alpha amylase inhibitor (15 kD) to be a major wheat allergen. This protein does not bind IgE from wheat-tolerant control patients, including those with grass allergy.

Fish

The consumption or inhalation of fish allergen is a common cause of IgE-mediated food reactions. The incidence of fish allergy is believed to be much higher in countries where fish consumption is greatest. For example, codfish allergy is extremely common in the Scandinavian countries. One of the most comprehensive descriptions of a food allergen has been the work by Aas and Elsayed on the codfish allergen, Gad c 1 (originally designated Allergen M). Gad c 1 belongs to a group of muscle proteins known as parvalbumins.

The parvalbumins control the flow of calcium in and out of cells and are found only in the muscles of amphibians and fish. This allergen has an acidic isoelectric point and a molecular weight of 12 kD. The tertiary structure of Gad c 1 exhibits three domains. There are at least five IgE-binding sites on the allergen, and the carbohydrate moiety does not appear to be important in its allergenicity.

Tree Nuts

Tree nuts are common causes of food allergic reactions in both children and adults. Like allergic reactions to fish and peanuts, reactions to tree nuts tend to persist throughout the lifetime of an individual. Two major allergens have been identified in almonds. The allergens are a 70-kD heat-labile protein and a 45- to 50-kD heat-stable protein. In Brazil nuts, the major allergen is Ber e 1, a high-methionine, 12-kD protein. Work with the walnut allergens has identified a major allergen as a 65-kD glycoprotein similar to other plant vicilins.

Shrimp

Shrimp is the most studied of the crustacea. The original two allergen fractions characterized in shrimp were antigen I (45 kD) and antigen II (38 kD). SA-II was the next major allergen characterized in shrimp and studies revealed that SA-II was similar to antigen I, which had been previously described. Pen a 1 was identified as a major allergen from boiled brown shrimp (isolated in the boiled water), and thus was thought to be similar to SA-II. This allergen has a molecular weight of 36 kD and constitutes 20% of the soluble protein in crude cooked shrimp. Pen a 1 binds shrimp-specific IgE in over 85% of patients with shrimp allergy studied to date. Another shrimp allergen, Met e 1, has been isolated from another species of shrimp and has a molecular weight of 34 kD. Studies of the Pen a 1 and Met a 1 allergens have shown them to be highly homologous with tropomyosin from a variety of species.

FOOD ALLERGEN CROSS-REACTIVITY (Table 5–4)

Cow's Milk

Immunoblotting and crossed-radioimmuno-electrophoresis studies have shown extensive milk-specific IgE cross-reactivity among milk proteins in cows, goats, and sheep. Earlier studies showed that at least 50% of cow's milk allergic individuals were also allergic to goat's milk. Clinical practice indicates that patients who are allergic to one type of milk protein will not tolerate milk proteins of other species.

Legumes

Extensive *in vitro* allergenic cross-reactivity in the legume family has been documented. A clinical study of 57 patients with legume sensitivity to peanuts, soybeans, peas, and lima beans revealed extensive *in vitro* IgE cross-reactivity but minimal *in vivo* clinical cross-reactivity. Specifically 59% of skin test–positive patients reacted to oral challenge with one of the legumes but only 5% of the patients reacted to oral challenge with more than one legume. Although patients with peanut-specific IgE may have clinical reactions to other legumes, these reactions will be quite uncommon and should be evaluated on an individual basis.

Wheat

Serum from patients with cereal grain allergies exhibits extensive cross-reactivity *in vitro* among the different cereal grains. One-hun-

Table 5–4. **Food Allergen Cross-Reactivity**

Allergen	Specific IgE to Multiple Members of the Family	Clinical Cross-Reactivity
Milk	Common	Common
Legumes	Common	Uncommon
Wheat	Common	Uncommon
Fish	Common	Uncommon
Crustacea–mollusks	Common	?
Tree nuts	Common	Uncommon
Egg–chicken	Occasional	Rare
Milk–beef	Occasional	Uncommon

dred forty-five children with food sensitivity were found to have at least one positive prick skin test response to one of the cereal grains (i.e., wheat, oat, rye, barley, corn, and rice). Thirty-one children (21%) experienced clinical symptoms during food challenges (wheat, 26; rye, 4; barley, 4; oat, 5; rice, 1; and corn, 5). Of the children reacting to cereal grains, only 20% reacted to more than one. Approximately 70% of these patients also showed positive prick skin test responses to grass pollens (i.e., timothy, orchard, and Bermuda). Overall, about 20% of patients with positive prick skin test responses to cereal grains will react when ingesting the grain, and about 4% will react to more than one grain.

Fish

Several studies have assessed the reactivity of fish-allergic subjects to different species of fish. Of 11 children allergic to fish on blinded oral challenge, one reacted to 2 fish, two reacted to 3 fish, and one patient did not react to any fish. In general, fish-allergic adults have more *in vivo* cross-reactivity than do children. Not only do adults have fish-specific IgE to multiple species of fish, they are also more likely to have adverse reactions to more than one species on oral challenges.

Crustacea and Mollusks

Patients who have positive prick skin tests or RAST to the crustacea tend to react positively to multiple members of this family. In particular, individuals with shrimp allergy exhibit positive responses to skin tests and RAST to other crustaceans. Studies have shown extracts from shrimp, blue crab, and crawfish all inhibit Pen a 1 RAST to a similar extent. There is little oral challenge data to reveal the extent of clinical reactivity among the different crustacea.

Although mollusks are much less commonly allergenic than crustacea, there are studies to show some *in vitro* cross-reactivity among oysters (mollusks) and the crustacea. Shrimp, blue crab, spiny lobster, and crawfish were all highly cross-reactive with oyster. Again, the extent of clinical cross-reactivity has not

been studied sufficiently. Therefore, clinical advice to patients must be individualized.

Tree Nuts

A variety of nuts have caused anaphylactic reactions in children and adults. In one study, 14 children underwent 19 blinded challenges to nuts; one patient reacted to 5 nuts, one to 2 nuts, and the remaining 12 children to 1 nut each. Overall, there were 7 reactions to walnuts, 6 to cashews, 3 to pecans, 2 to pistachios, and 1 to filbert. Adults allergic to nuts generally do not need to avoid peanuts (a legume), and vice versa, although children with peanut allergy appear to be more likely to develop allergy to tree nuts than the general population.

Egg and Chicken

Egg-allergic patients older than 3 years of age may react (i.e., <5%) following the ingestion of chicken, and similarly chicken-allergic patients may react to eggs. An association also has been reported between allergic reactions to egg and respiratory symptoms in bird keepers exposed to their birds.

Milk and Beef

Of 335 children with atopic dermatitis evaluated by blinded challenges for possible food hypersensitivity, 11 reacted to beef; 8 of these children were also sensitive to milk on previous double-blind, placebo-controlled food challenge (DBPCFC). Three of the patients could tolerate well-cooked beef and experienced symptoms only when they ingested partially cooked beef. IgE immunoblots in these patients revealed the presence of both heat-labile and heat-stable protein fractions.

Tree Nuts and Pollen Allergy

Patients allergic to tree pollen may also have an allergic reaction on the ingestion of nuts from the same tree. For example, some patients with birch pollen-specific IgE also react to hazelnut. Through a series of elegant studies it has been determined that a profilin with a molecular weight of 14 kD is responsible for the cross-reactivity between a variety of fruits and vegetables. Profilins are highly conserved, ubiquitous proteins that are found in almost all eukaryotic organisms. Profilins have been isolated from a variety of pollens including timothy grass, rye grass, and mugwort. Pollen profilins also appear to share cross-reactivity with a number of foods. As an example, cross-reactivity has been demonstrated among mugwort pollen, celery, and carrots. Birch profilin has been associated with the fruits of rosaceae including apple, pear, cherry, and peach. For most of these studies it is felt that exposure to tree pollens can lead to the development of IgE antibodies that recognize epitopes on a variety of food proteins that contain similar amino acid sequences. The primary sensitization appears to be to the pollen and not to the food. There are patients though that do have clinical reactivity to fruits with IgE to fruit-specific allergens. These allergens are different than the cross-reacting pollen–fruit allergens.

Food and Nonpollen Allergens

A number of surveys have reported an association between latex allergy and allergic reactions to bananas, avocado, kiwi, chestnut, and papaya. In a series of 25 patients diagnosed with latex allergy (by history and prick skin testing), approximately one-half of these patients were diagnosed with food allergies (based on positive prick skin test results and history of at least two reactions within the previous 5 years). Overall, 42 reactions (systemic anaphylaxis in 23) were diagnosed in 13 patients: avocado, 9; chestnut, 9; banana, 7; kiwi, 5; and papaya, 3.

DIAGNOSIS AND DIETARY CONTROL

As with all medical disorders, the diagnostic approach to the patient with a suspected adverse food reaction begins with the medical

history and physical examination. Based on the information derived from these initial steps, various laboratory studies may be helpful.

The true value of the medical history is largely dependent on the patient's recollection of symptoms and the examiner's ability to differentiate disorders provoked by food hypersensitivity and other etiologies. The history may be directly useful in diagnosing food allergy in acute events (e.g., systemic anaphylaxis following the ingestion of fish). In many series though, fewer than 50% of reported food-allergic reactions could be substantiated by DBPCFC. Several pieces of information are important to establish that a food-allergic reaction occurred (Table 5–5): (1) the food suspected to have provoked the reaction, (2) the quantity of the food ingested, (3) the length of time between ingestion and development of symptoms, (4) a description of the symptoms provoked, (5) the knowledge of whether similar symptoms developed on other occasions when the food was eaten, (6) other factors (e.g., exercise) necessary to cause the reaction, and (7) the length of time since the last reaction. Any food may cause an allergic reaction, although only a few foods account for 90% of the reactions. In children, these foods are egg, milk, peanuts, soy, and wheat (fish in Scandinavian countries). In chronic disorders like atopic dermatitis the history is often an unreliable indicator of the offending allergen.

A diet diary has been frequently used as an adjunct to the medical history. Patients are asked to keep a chronologic record of all foods ingested over a specified period of time and to record any symptoms they experience during this time. The diary can then be reviewed during a patient visit to determine if there is

Table 5–5. **Important Information from Medical History**

The food suspected to have provoked the reaction
The quantity of the food ingested
The length of time between ingestion and development of symptoms
A description of the symptoms provoked
Whether similar symptoms developed on other occasions when the food was eaten
Whether other factors (e.g., exercise) are necessary for the reaction to occur
The length of time since the last reaction

any relationship between the foods ingested and the symptoms experienced. It is uncommon for this method to detect an unrecognized association between a food and a patient's symptoms.

An elimination diet is frequently used in both diagnosis and management of adverse food reactions. If a certain food or foods are suspected of provoking the reaction, they are completely eliminated from the diet. The success of an elimination diet depends on several factors, including the correct identification of the allergen(s) involved, the ability of the patient to maintain a diet completely free of all forms of the possible offending allergen, and the assumption that other factors will not provoke similar symptoms during the study period. The likelihood of all of these conditions being met is often slim. For example, in a young infant who is reacting to cow's milk formula, resolution of symptoms following substitution of cow's milk formula with a soy formula or casein hydrolysate formula (Alimentum Ross Laboratories, Nutramigen Mead Johnson) is highly suggestive of cow's milk allergy, but the reaction also could be caused by lactose intolerance. Avoidance of suspected food allergens prior to blinded challenge is recommended so the reactions occuring during the challenge may be heightened and more obvious. Elimination diets though are rarely diagnostic of food allergy, particularly in chronic disorders such as atopic dermatitis or asthma.

Allergy prick skin tests are highly reproducible and are often used to screen patients with suspected IgE-mediated food allergies. The criteria established by May and Bock have proved useful to many investigators and clinicians. The glycerinated food extracts (1:10 or 1:20 w/v) and appropriate positive (histamine) and negative (saline) controls are applied by either the prick or puncture technique. A food allergen eliciting a wheal at least 3 mm greater than the negative control is considered a positive response; anything else is considered negative. A positive skin test result to a food indicates only the possibility that the patient has symptomatic reactivity to that specific food (overall the positive predictive accuracy is less than 50%). A negative skin test result confirms the absence of an IgE-mediated reaction (overall negative predictive accuracy is greater than 95%). Both of these statements are justified if appropriate and good quality food extracts are used.

The prick skin test should be considered an excellent means of excluding IgE-mediated food allergies, but only suggestive of the presence of a clinical food allergy. There are some minor exceptions to the general statement: (1) IgE-mediated sensitivity to several fruits and vegetables (apples, oranges, bananas, pears, melons, potatoes, carrots, celery, etc.) is frequently not detected with commercial reagents, presumably secondary to the lability of the responsible allergen in the food; (2) children younger than 1 year of age may have IgE-mediated food allergy without a positive skin test response, and children younger than 2 years of age may have smaller wheals, possibly because of the lack of skin reactivity and conversely, (3) a positive skin test response to a food ingested in isolation that provokes a serious systemic anaphylactic reaction may be considered diagnostic.

An intradermal skin test is a more sensitive tool than the prick skin test but is much less specific when compared to a blinded food challenge. In one study, no patient who had a negative prick skin test result but a positive intradermal skin test result to a specific food had a positive DBPCFC to that food. In addition, intradermal skin testing has a greater risk of inducing a systemic reaction than does prick skin testing.

Radioallergosorbent tests and similar *in vitro* assays (including ELISA) are used for the identification of food-specific IgE antibodies. These tests are often used to screen for IgE-mediated food allergies. Although these assays are slightly less sensitive than skin tests, one study comparing RAST with DBPCFCs found prick skin tests and RASTs to have similar sensitivity and specificity when a RAST score of three or greater was considered a positive result. In this study, if a two was considered a positive result, there was a slight improvement in sensitivity while the specificity decreased significantly. In general, *in vitro* measurement of serum food-specific IgE performed in high quality laboratories provides information similar to that available from prick skin tests. Recent studies have used the CAP-RAST to give better positive and negative predictive values for the major food allergens. The study indicated that if the patient had a CAP-RAST value above a certain point then there was an either 90% or 95% likelihood that the patient would have a positive food challenge response. The cut-off value was different for each of the food allergens.

Basophil histamine release assays (BHR) have generally been reserved for research and academic settings. Newer, semiautomated methods that use small amounts of whole blood have been developed and are being promoted for screening multiple food allergens. The use of whole blood in the assays should circumvent the problem of high spontaneous basophil histamine release, which occurs in food-allergic individuals who continue to ingest the responsible allergen. One such method was employed in a study that compared BHR to prick skin tests, RASTs, food antigen-induced intestinal mast cell histamine release, and food challenges in suspected food-allergic children. As found in earlier studies, the food allergen-induced BHR correlated most closely with RAST results. The BHR did not appear to be any more predictive of clinical sensitivity than the prick skin test or RAST.

The double-blind placebo-controlled food challenge (DBPCFC) has been labeled the gold standard for the diagnosis of food allergies. This test has been used successfully by many investigators for the last several years to examine a wide variety of food-related complaints in both children and adults. The foods to be tested in the oral challenge are based on history and prick skin test (or RAST) results. Foods thought to be unlikely to provoke a food-allergic reaction may be screened by open or single blind challenges. It is necessary though, except in very young infants, to confirm multiple positive reactions by DBPCFC. Prior to undertaking a DBPCFC, several conditions should be established: (1) suspect foods should be eliminated for 7 to 14 days prior to challenge; (2) antihistamines should be discontinued long enough to establish a normal histamine skin test; (3) other medication use should be reduced to minimal levels sufficient to prevent breakthrough of acute symptoms, and (4) in some patients with asthma, short bursts of corticosteroids may be necessary to obtain adequate pulmonary reserve for testing (FEV_1 >70% predicted).

The food challenge should be administered with the patient in a fasting state. The challenge is started with a dose of food that is unlikely to provoke symptoms (generally 125 mg to 500 mg of lyophilized food) (Table 5–6). This dose is then doubled every 15 to 60 minutes, depending on the type of reaction that was suspected to occur. A similar scheme is followed with the placebo portion of the study. Clinical reactivity is generally ruled out when the patient who is blinded to the ingested food has tolerated 10 gms of lyophilized food in capsules or liquid. If the blinded portion of the challenge is negative, however, *it must be confirmed by an open feeding under observation* to rule out the rare false-negative challenge result.

A DBPCFC is the best means of controlling for the variability of chronic disorders (e.g., chronic urticaria, atopic dermatitis, and so forth), any potential temporal effects, and acute exacerbations secondary to reducing or discontinuing medications. Particularly, psychogenic factors and observer bias are eliminated. There are rare false-negative challenges in a DBPCFC. A false-negative result may occur when a patient receives insufficient challenge material during the challenge to provoke the reaction or the lyophilization of the food antigen has altered the relevant allergenic epitopes (e.g., fish). Overall, the DBPCFC has proved to be the most accurate means of diagnosing food allergy at the present time.

DBPCFCs should be conducted in a clinic or hospital setting, especially if an IgE-mediated reaction is suspected. Trained personnel and equipment for treating systemic anaphylaxis should be present. If life-threatening anaphylaxis is suspected and the causative agent cannot be identified conclusively by history, a challenge should be conducted in the inten-

Table 5–6. **Sample Schedule for Double-Blind, Placebo-Controlled Food Challenge**

Food		Placebo	
Time	Dose	Time	Dose
0:00	500 mg	3:00	500 mg
0:15	1 gm	3:15	1 gm
0:30	2 gm	3:30	2 gm
0:45	3 gm	3:45	3 gm
1:00	3.5 gm	4:00	3.5 gm

sive care unit of a center that frequently deals with food-allergy reactions. The evaluation of suspected delayed reactions can be conducted safely on an outpatient basis, provided the symptoms have not been severe and there is no concern about the patient breaking the blinding by opening capsules. There are some possible adverse food reactions in which the proposed symptoms are largely subjective. Three cross-over trials with reactions developing only during the allergen challenge are necessary to conclude that a cause-and-effect relationship exists.

PRACTICAL APPROACH TO DIAGNOSING FOOD ALLERGY

The diagnosis of food allergy remains a clinical exercise that uses a careful history, selective prick skin tests or RAST (if an IgE-mediated disorder is suspected), an appropriate exclusion diet, and food challenges (Table 5–7). Other diagnostic tests, which do not appear to be of significant value, include measurement of food-specific IgG or IgG4 antibody levels, food–antigen–antibody complexes, evidence of lymphocyte activation (^{3}H-thymidine uptake, interleukin 2 production, leukocyte inhibitory factor, and so forth), and sublingual or intracutaneous provocation. Blinded challenges may not be necessary in suspected gastrointestinal disorders; pre- and postchallenge laboratory values and biopsy specimens are often useful in these cases.

An exclusion diet eliminating all foods suspected by history or prick skin testing (or RAST) should be conducted for at least 1 to 2 weeks prior to challenge. To detect some gastrointestinal disorders the exclusion diet

Table 5–7. **Practical Approach to Diagnosing and Managing Food Allergy**

1. Medical history
2. Appropriate laboratory evaluation—selective prick skin tests or RAST
3. Exclusion diet based on laboratory and test results
4. Food challenge(s)
5. Appropriate diet based on information generated
6. Adequate follow-up history and future challenges

may have to be extended for up to 12 weeks following appropriate biopsy studies. If no improvement is noted while the patient is following the diet, it is unlikely that food allergy is involved. In the case of some chronic diseases, such as atopic dermatitis or chronic asthma, other precipitating factors may make it difficult to discriminate between the effects of the food allergen and other provocative factors.

Single-blind challenges (in which the food being challenged is known only to the individuals administering the challenge) in a clinic setting may be helpful to screen suspected food allergens. Positive challenge responses should be confirmed by a DBPCFC unless a single major allergen (egg, milk, soy, wheat) provoked classic allergic symptoms. A patient with multiple food allergies is rare and, if multiple allergies are suspected, the diagnoses should be confirmed by DBPCFC. Many dry foods can be obtained through grocery stores, health food stores, and camping outlets. The presumptive diagnosis of food allergy based on a patient's history and prick skin tests or RAST results is not acceptable. There are exceptions to this, such as the patients with severe anaphylaxis following the isolated ingestion of a specific food, particularly peanuts, tree nuts, fish, and shellfish. It is important that the physician make an unequivocal diagnosis of food allergy so that the patient and family are aware of which foods they should specifically avoid.

After the diagnosis of food hypersensitivity is established, the only proved therapy is strict elimination of the offending allergen. It is important to remember that prescribing an elimination diet is like prescribing a medication; both can have positive effects and unwarranted side-effects. Elimination diets may lead to malnutrition, or eating disorders, especially if they include a large number of foods or are used for extended periods. Patients and parents should be taught and given educational material to help them detect potential sources of hidden food allergens by appropriately reading food labels. Education of the patient and family is vital to the success of the elimination diet. Families should be given instructional material to help them remember what foods contain the allergen they are to avoid. It is often difficult to determine what foods will contain an allergen without careful reading of the label. Studies in both children and adults indicate that symptomatic reactivity to food allergens is often lost over time, except possibly for peanuts, tree nuts, and seafood.

Symptomatic reactivity to food allergens is generally very specific. Patients rarely react to more than one member of a botanical family or animal species. Importantly, initiation of an elimination diet totally excluding only foods identified to provoke food allergic reactions will result in symptomatic improvement. This treatment generally will lead to resolution of the food allergy within a few years and is unlikely to induce malnutrition or other eating disorders.

Suggested Reading

Bernhisel-Broadbent J, Dintzis HM, Dintzis RZ, et al: Allergenicity and antigenicity of chicken egg ovomucoid (Gal d III) compared to ovalbumin (Gald d I) in children with egg allergy and in mice. J Allergy Clin Immunol 93:1047, 1994.

Bernhisel-Broadbent J, Sampson HA: Cross-allergenicity in the legume botanical family in children with food hypersensitivity. J Allergy Clin Immunol 83:435, 1989.

Bock SA: Prospective appraisal of complaints of adverse reaction to foods in children during the first 3 years of life. Pediatrics 79:683, 1987.

Burks AW, Cockrell G, Stanley JS, et al: Recombinant peanut allergen *Ara h* I expression and IgE binding in patients with peanut hypersensitivity. J Clin Invest 96:1715, 1995.

Elsayed S, Apol J: Immunochemical analysis of cod fish Allergen M: Locations of the immunoglobulin binding sites as demonstrated by the native and synthetic peptides. Allergy 38:449, 1983.

Host A, Halken S: A prospective study of cow milk allergy in Danish infants during the first 3 years of life. Allergy 45:587, 1990.

Jones SM, Magnolfi CF, Cooke SK, et al: Immunologic cross-reactivity among cereal grains and grasses in children with food hypersensitivity. J Allergy Clin Immunol 96:341, 1995.

Sampson HA: Food allergy. J Allergy Clin Immunol 84:1062, 1989.

Valenta R, Duchene M, Vrtala S, et al: Profilin, a novel pan-allergen. Int Arch Allergy Immunol 99:271, 1992.

Yunginger JW, Sweeney KG, Sturner WQ, et al: Fatal food-induced anaphylaxis. J Am Med Assoc 260:1450, 1988.

Chapter 6

Controversial Techniques in Allergy

Abba I. Terr

Over the past century, an enormous body of laboratory and clinical research has established a strong scientific basis for understanding the mechanisms of allergic diseases. Accurate diagnostic procedures and effective treatment modalities for managing patients with allergy based on this firm scientific foundation are readily available for the sizable portion of the population suffering from all forms of allergy.

Ironically, unscientific theories and procedures continue to flourish and attract a certain number of patients, especially those who espouse nontraditional approaches to health care. Some of these methods have been investigated and found to be useless. Others have not been tested. Certain methods discussed here are offered exclusively for allergy diagnosis and treatment, but there are unscientific schools of practice or healing promoted for allergy as well as for a variety of other diseases.

Table 6–1 lists some unproven and controversial diagnoses and procedures. The list is not exhaustive, but it does provide those unconventional diagnostic and therapeutic techniques most prevalent today. It includes procedures that are inherently useless for diagnosis or therapy for any disease, as well as some that may be indicated for certain medical conditions (e.g., the pulse test, lymphocyte analyses) but are not appropriate for diagnosis or treatment of allergic disorders.

CONTROVERSIAL THEORIES AND DIAGNOSES

In general, the controversial and unproved methods for allergy diagnosis and treatment that exist today are grounded in theories that are not supported by scientific studies. Some of the most prevalent of these combine concepts of hypersensitivity (allergy) and toxicity, two very different mechanisms with different clinical effects (Table 6–2).

Allergic toxemia, also called the *allergic tension-fatigue syndrome,* is based on the idea that fatigue, lethargy, and difficulty in concentration in the absence of any localized form of inflammation are primary allergic manifestations. As with many other unproved and disproved concepts in this field, allergic toxemia is usually attributed to foods. Allergic toxemia is often diagnosed in children with symptomatic complaints and behavior problems. Food elimination diets are used as a diagnostic tool, but symptoms occurring hours, days, or even weeks after food ingestion are accepted as diagnostic. This is contrary to double-blind studies, which have failed to confirm the existence of delayed food allergy. Fatigue and the many other symptoms ascribed to delayed food allergy are common in some children without a specific illness and are more likely caused by psychological or social factors.

Many controversial theories and methods focus on foods and food additives as allergens. As mentioned earlier, *delayed food allergy* is a commonly mistaken explanation for nonspecific symptoms, but it has also been considered to cause or exacerbate other conditions, including arthritis, colds, and even pneumonia. Multiple foods are often implicated, because elimination diets rarely have a sustained therapeutic benefit, leading to the progressive elimination of additional foods. *Food-additive sensi-*

Table 6–1. **Controversial Procedures in Allergy**

Diagnoses

Allergic toxemia
Allergic tension-fatigue syndrome
Delayed food allergy
Food additive–induced attention deficit
  hyperactivity disorder
Multiple chemical sensitivities (environmental
  illness)
Chronic fatigue immune dysfunction syndrome
Candida hypersensitivity syndrome

Tests

Skin end-point titration
Provocation–neutralization (injected or sublingual)
Pulse test
Applied kinesiology
Electrodermal testing
Cytotoxic (leukocytotoxic) test
IgG antibody or immune complex analysis for food
  allergy
Quantitative measurements of xenobiotic chemicals,
  nutrients, lymphocyte subsets, lymphocyte
  mitogenic response, cytokines, or their receptors

Treatments

Neutralization (symptom-relieving) injections or
  sublingual application of allergens
Enzyme-potentiated desensitization
Excessive dietary restrictions
Excessive environmental restrictions
Nutritional supplements or vitamins
Autogenous urine injections

Practice Systems

Acupuncture
Homeopathy
Herbal therapy
Chiropractic manipulations

tivity has been alleged to cause attention deficit hyperactivity disorder, chronic urticaria, and many other diseases, in spite of substantial evidence to the contrary.

The concept of multiple food allergies causing nonspecific symptoms evolved into a currently popular term *multiple chemical sensitivities (MCS),* originally called *environmental ill-*

ness. Numerous other names have been applied as theories to explain this concept change (Table 6–3). The condition is said to be an acquired disease caused by the large scale release into the environment of synthetic industrial chemicals in recent years. Originally the illness was conceived in general terms as a failure of adaptation to these chemicals, with the symptoms representing a new form of allergy. Later theories proposed that in this condition environmental chemicals were immunotoxins rather than allergens, and the symptoms were then explained as manifestations of immunodeficiency or autoimmunity. Research has failed to confirm any role for the immune system in environmental illness, so more recently the focus has been on the central nervous system, because of the commonly reported difficulties in cognition and memory reported by affected patients.

The condition of multiple chemical sensitivities is characterized by subjective symptomatology without objective findings on physical examination or diagnostic testing. Symptoms are wide-ranging, suggesting illness in multiple organ systems, even though objective examinations fail to reveal any structural or functional abnormalities. The patient reports that symptoms are triggered by exposure to numerous environmental "chemicals," which are, in fact, common everyday items that typically are detected by a distinctive odor. The most commonly reported trigger items are perfumes, scented body and household products, organic solvents, pesticides, vehicular fuels, exhaust fumes, new carpets, and building materials. Some patients attribute illness to physical phenomena such as electromagnetic fields. Most patients with this condition report

Table 6–2. **Clinical Distinctions of Hypersensitivity and Toxicity**

Characteristic	Hypersensitivity	Toxicity
Mechanism	Immunologically mediated inflammation	Direct tissue damage
Genetic predisposition	Usually required	Usually not required
Sensitization	Necessary	Unnecessary
Tissue reaction	Independent of allergen properties	Dependent on toxin properties

Table 6–3. **Synonyms for Multiple Chemical Sensitivities**

20th century disease
Cerebral allergy
Chemical AIDS
Chemical hypersensitivity syndrome
Chemically induced immune dysregulation
Ecologic illness
Environmental hypersensitivity
Environmental maladaptation syndrome
Idiopathic environmental intolerances
Total allergy syndrome
Toxic chemical encephalopathy
Universal allergy

that their symptoms are provoked by many foods and by almost all drugs, so it is more accurately termed *multiple food, chemical and drug sensitivities.*

There exist today a group of closely related, controversial conditions referred to as syndromes. The patients diagnosed as having multiple chemical sensitivities are clinically similar if not indistinguishable from those with the diagnosis of chronic fatigue syndrome, except that in the former condition the symptomatology is attributed to environmental chemical exposures. Some prefer to label the latter condition as chronic fatigue immune dysfunction syndrome (CFIDS), in spite of the lack of evidence for an immune abnormality. A certain number of patients with the equally controversial Gulf War syndrome are also believed to have sensitivities to multiple chemicals.

Recently, a committee convened by the World Health Organization recommended that the name be changed once again to *Idiopathic Environmental Intolerances,* because there has been no evidence to date that chemicals are involved in the symptomatology and because there is no proof of a hypersensitivity mechanism.

A related theory offered to explain the same clinical phenomenon of multiple symptomatology in the absence of objective illness is the *Candida hypersensitivity syndrome.* In this case the illness is attributed to the presence of *Candida albicans* which is frequently found as a commensal organism in portions of the gastrointestinal tract and in the vagina. Although this commensal colonization is recognized as a normal occurrence in healthy persons, a *Candida*-producing immunotoxin has been proposed to explain the same symptomatology attributed to chemicals in multiple chemical sensitivity. Like multiple chemical sensitivity, *Candida* hypersensitivity is said by its proponents to cause or potentiate a number of diseases with as yet undetermined causes, such as multiple sclerosis, rheumatoid arthritis, psoriasis, schizophrenia, depression, and many others.

The small group of physicians who diagnose these conditions form a practice entity known for many years as clinical ecology, whose thesis is that any chemical synthesized by industrial processes is toxic, whereas a chemical produced by natural processes is not, even if the two should be identical molecular species. The toxicity of synthetic chemicals is believed to occur at any concentration, in marked contrast to well-established principles of clinical toxicology based on the axiom that the dose makes the toxin. Suspect chemicals include all those commonly used for many years with no apparent ill effects. Explanations for chemical toxicity include toxic induction of hypersensitivity, immunologic dysfunction, central nervous system dysfunction, and general cell toxicity. Regardless of the proposed pathophysiologic mechanism, the result is a subjective intolerance to numerous chemicals, a condition referred to also as universal allergy. The prevailing opinion of those who have investigated these theories and evaluated the clinical conditions of the patients is that the symptomatology believed to be triggered by chemical exposure cannot be reproduced in controlled trials and is best explained by psychiatric mechanisms.

Those clinicians who base their practice on this theory now prefer to be called specialists in environmental medicine, rather than clinical ecologists.

A recently emerging concept implicates atmospheric *mold sensitivity* as the cause of a variety of subjective complaints in individuals who display no consistent pattern of illness. The diagnosis is usually made in persons living in homes or working in buildings subject to recent flooding or excessive humidity that promotes indoor mold growth. The diagnosis in these cases rests on the presence of low levels of antifungal antibodies in serum. These antibodies, however, have not yet been shown to be different from those in persons who are well. As in the case of multiple chemical sensitivities, a combination of toxicity and hypersensitivity is intertwined in explanations of this proposed new disease whose existence has yet to be proved or even defined.

In contrast, thoroughly documented and widely accepted allergic diseases caused by fungal allergy include respiratory illness, especially asthma, caused by certain mold allergens, some cases of hypersensitivity pneumonitis, allergic bronchopulmonary aspergillosis, and allergic fungal sinusitis. These can be identified by localized symptomatology and objective physical findings, functional and imaging studies that confirm pathology, and the presence of the relevant immune response by the patient.

CONTROVERSIAL DIAGNOSTIC TESTS

Controversial and unproved allergy tests are best understood by comparison with those diagnostic procedures with proved validity for recognized, well-established allergic diseases.

Allergy testing is often equated with immediate wheal-and-flare skin tests. In fact, the diagnosis of allergic disease is an algorithmic process that starts with the patient's history and physical examination to determine whether the patient's clinical condition is consistent with the known effects of allergy. If necessary, the examination may require appropriate imaging and functional studies to supplement the objective physical findings. If these data suggest that the patient has an allergic disease, identification of the relevant allergens responsible for that disease is accomplished by detecting evidence that the patient has mounted an immune response of the type known to cause that disease (Table 6–4). This information must correlate with the history and other clinical information to be diagnostic of allergic disease. The presence of immune responses to an allergen in the absence of allergic disease manifestations on exposure to the allergen does not constitute disease.

The success of this protocol for allergy diagnosis has spawned a number of controversial procedures that are typically used without regard for clinical correlation. One variation of skin testing for atopy is known as *skin end-*

point titration, in which serial five-fold increasing concentrations of allergen are injected intradermally to establish for each allergen the threshold of a positive test, known as the endpoint. Although the procedure itself is theoretically sound, the value of the end-point has been misinterpreted as indicating both a safe dose for initiating immunotherapy and the optimal dose for maintaining the treatment. The method is conservative enough to be safe, but it underestimates the maintenance dose, resulting in treatment that is no more effective than placebo injections. In addition, the method used for reading test results is the presence of a cutaneous wheal at 10 minutes after allergen injection without regard for a concomitant erythematous flare. The absence of erythema may lead to a false-positive result, and the short time interval for reading the test may lead to a false-negative diagnosis.

The serial end-point titration skin test has been modified to a procedure called *provocation–neutralization.* In this case, testing of a variety of substances such as environmental chemicals, hormones, and microbial products, as well as inhalant allergens and food extracts, is performed by intradermal or subcutaneous injection followed by the patient's self-report of symptoms and sensations during the 10 minutes following the injection. In practice, any reported symptom, whether consistent with an allergic disease or not, is judged to be a positive response. Once such a positive result occurs, further injections of the same substance are administered, using either a lower or higher dose than that causing symptoms, until the patient reports the absence of symptoms, at which time the symptoms are said to be neutralized. There is no theoretical or empiric justification for the procedure of symptom-provocation or neutralization. Since no proper controls are used in practice, results can occur by chance or by suggestion. In fact, a carefully performed double-blind placebo-controlled study showed that results are no different whether the patients are given an active extract or a placebo.

Sublingual provocation–neutralization is a variation in which the test substance is administered as a drop under the tongue. Regardless of the method used, these procedures have been employed mostly by clinicians who espouse the idea of multiple food and chemical

Table 6–4. **Appropriate Testing for Allergic Diseases**

Test	Disease
Immediate wheal-and-flare skin test, or	Atopy (allergic rhinitis, asthma, atopic dermatitis)
Radioallergosorbent test (RAST) for IgE antibodies	Systemic anaphylaxis Urticaria
Precipitin test for IgG antibodies	Serum sickness Hypersensitivity pneumonitis
48-hour patch test	Allergic contact dermatitis

hypersensitivity, so that the patients who are tested are usually those with far-ranging subjective complaints not consistent with allergic disease. The use of the sublingual route to test for allergy in the patient with severe atopic or anaphylactic sensitivity is potentially dangerous in the event that the correct allergen is used.

The *pulse test* is based on the idea that an allergic reaction alters the heart rate, although this bizarre concept has never been explained in detail. The test is performed by measuring the peripheral pulse rate before and after eating a food. A change in pulse of 10 or more beats per minute, in either direction, is considered a positive test for allergy to that particular food. No formal study of this procedure has been reported. Since it can be done by the patient, there is no information on the extent to which it is actually practiced.

An unsubstantiated theory that allergy and many other disease processes can affect the normal functioning of muscles is the basis of the practice know as *applied kinesiology*. This technique is usually employed to diagnose food allergy. There are many variations on the technique, but usually the food to be tested is in a container that is placed somewhere on the patient's body while a technician subjectively tests the strength of a limb, comparing it with a similar maneuver performed before contact with the container. It is thus not necessary for the food itself to have any direct connection with the patient. Although the procedure is bizarre and clearly without merit, many patients accept the results as valid.

A similar procedure is known as *electrodermal testing* or electrodiagnosis. In this case a change in the electric potential of the skin is said to occur from allergy. Electrodermal testing is usually employed to test for food allergy. A container of food is connected to an apparatus that purportedly measures the electrical resistance of the skin. This procedure is often aligned with acupuncture, so that different forms of allergy are diagnosed if they correspond to resistance changes at various acupuncture points on the skin.

A procedure known as the *cytotoxic* (or *leukocytoxic*) *test* was introduced in 1956 and is still performed, largely through direct advertising to patients. It is based on a theory that allergic disease causes lysis of leukocytes, re-sulting in leukopenia. It is primarily used to detect food allergy, but it is performed also as a test for allergy to inhalants and drugs.

This test is performed by mixing the patient's peripheral blood leukocytes with an extract of the allergen on the surface of a microscope slide at room temperature. Changes in the observed microscopic appearance of the white cells are used to diagnose allergy. The results are judged subjectively and without rigorous control of test conditions that can affect leukocytes in vitro, such as the incubation time, pH, osmolarity, temperature, and humidity. Studies have failed to correlate the results with allergen-induced clinical disease.

Quantitative analysis of a variety of *body chemicals* is used by proponents of environmental illness or multiple chemical sensitivities. In some cases, blood or other body fluids or tissues are analyzed for the presence of such chemicals as pesticides and organic solvents in the belief that any amount, no matter how little, can be both toxic and allergenic. In fact, many environmental chemicals can be detected in all persons at quantities not known to be toxic, and there is no proof that individuals purportedly suffering from this condition are any different in this respect. In many of these cases, abnormal levels of normal body constituents such as amino acids, vitamins, minerals, and other nutrients are said to be diagnostic, but the evidence put forth is anecdotal only. No definitive studies have shown that abnormal levels of any specific body chemical correlates with such a disease.

Several technically valid methods have been employed to detect and quantitate circulating immune complexes containing food allergens. The presence of the specific allergen and the antibody isotype can be detected with the relevant labeled antibody reagents in a solid-phase immune assay. The complex can be separated from free allergen and antibody by ultracentrifugation or precipitation. These techniques, known as *food immune complex assay* (*F.I.C.A.*), are offered as clinical tests of food allergy. Both IgG-containing and IgE-containing complexes are assayed by certain commercial clinical laboratories. Although the method is technically acceptable, there is no credible evidence that the existence of such complexes indicates allergy to the food. In fact, food antigen–containing immune complexes are found in normal individuals, and these increase transiently in the circulation following a meal containing the food.

The theory that food allergy is mediated by immune complexes does not fit with the known pathophysiology of immediate atopic or anaphylactic food allergy. The existence of reactions to foods by other mechanisms similar to a serum sickness reaction has been proposed but not yet proved. Neither has the presence or quantity of such circulating complexes been shown to serve as a clinical marker of any form of adverse food reaction.

The presence of *antibodies to IgG food allergens* in serum has also been demonstrated in normal patients without a history of food allergy. The measurement of such antibodies, in contrast to food-specific IgE antibodies, has no diagnostic role in allergy.

Extensive research on basic lymphocyte physiology in recent years has identified a large number of developmentally and functionally different subsets that can be readily identified because of the presence of different surface protein markers known as clusters of differentiation (CD markers). Such markers also are useful in identifying other leukocytes, including macrophages, eosinophils, and neutrophils. Analysis of a representative sample of the leukocyte population of blood, bone marrow, bronchial alveolar and other body fluids, lymph nodes, and solid tumors has been an important advance in the diagnosis and pathophysiology of a variety of diseases.

Functional assessment of viable lymphocytes involves stimulation of these cells with the mitogens phytohemagglutinin (PHA), pokeweed mitogen (PWM), and concanavalin A (ConA) to produce uptake of tritiated thymidine and expansion of the cell population. The procedure is independent of antigen specificity and used primarily to verify a condition of cellular immune deficiency, in which low values are typical.

To date there is no place in the diagnosis or management of hypersensitivity diseases for either *lymphocyte function assay* or *leukocyte subset analysis* by quantitation of CD markers in the blood. These tests have been commonly used by environmental medicine proponents to supposedly assist in the diagnosis of environmental illness in which minor but clinically insignificant variations in cell counts are used as

evidence of an immunologic abnormality, even though the clinical status of the patient does not suggest disease.

Likewise, measurement of *cytokines* and their cellular *receptors* in serum are being offered as diagnostic tests for environmental sensitivities. There is no theoretical foundation for such tests, and there have so far been no published data supporting their use in allergy diagnosis, even on an empiric basis. Normal serum levels and abnormal findings in disease states remain to be determined, but it is unlikely that systemic levels as measured in peripheral blood samples would accurately reflect normal or abnormal functioning of these locally secreted and acting endogenous chemical activators or their receptors or inhibitors.

TREATMENTS

Logical and effective treatment of any disease must rest on an accurate diagnosis. In the case of allergic diseases, reliable diagnostic procedures are necessary to establish both the disease entity and the specific causative allergen or allergens. The foundation of allergy treatment consists of a reasonable avoidance of allergens, medications to reduce or eliminate allergic inflammation, and allergen immunotherapy. Many attempts have been made to alter the allergen or the method of administering the allergen used in immunotherapy in order to improve efficacy and lessen the chance of adverse reactions. Allergen modification by denaturing the molecule with phenol, polymerizing with gluteraldehyde, or using peptide fragments of the allergen have been promising approaches, but for various reasons these have not been successfully incorporated into practice. The use of adjuvants such as pyridine or aqueous–lipid allergen suspensions also have been tried, but they have not improved on the standard subcutaneous injections of aqueous extracts. Administration of the treatment allergen by the oral, subcutaneous, or nasal or bronchial inhalation routes has likewise been unsuccessful.

On the other hand, a number of unsubstantiated treatments that evolved from unproved testing procedures are being used for patients with controversial diagnoses as well as for allergic disease.

Sublingual drop therapy is frequently recommended for treatment of multiple chemical sensitivities and sometimes for allergy, in which case the drops contain not only extracts of allergenic inhalants and foods, but also solutions of environmental chemicals, hormones, mediators such as histamine and serotonin, and other substances with no proof of effectiveness.

Enzyme-potentiated desensitization is currently being offered by a small number of physicians for allergy treatment. It consists of the addition of a very small quantity of β-glucuronidase to a low dose of therapeutic allergen solution as a means of desensitizing the patient to the specific allergen. It is claimed that this technique requires far fewer injections, possibly only a single one each season, to achieve superior clinical results. Although recommended for allergic rhinitis and asthma, its use has been extended to other conditions not known to be treatable by standard immunotherapy, such as nasal polyposis, eczema, inflammatory and irritable bowel diseases, rheumatoid arthritis, and others. The theoretical basis for an enhancing effect of the enzyme on the induction of allergen-specific clinical tolerance is not clear, and no experimental proof of efficacy in animal models of these human diseases has been done. The results of a few reported clinical trials in patients with aeroallergen sensitivity are not convincing.

Symptom-neutralization is a form of treatment in which extracts of allergen or other substance are either injected or taken sublingually with the intent of promptly relieving ongoing symptoms. Typically this process follows the provocation–neutralization testing procedure during which a neutralizing or relieving dose is determined. There is no rationale for symptom-neutralization. It cannot be explained immunologically, and typically the patient who responds favorably has nonspecific symptoms rather than those of a recognized allergic disease. A double-blind placebo-controlled clinical trial showed that prompt symptom provocation and neutralization cannot be distinguished from placebo responses, and therefore they occur only because of an expectation of a particular response.

This form of therapy must not be confused with conventional allergen immunotherapy for atopy or anaphylaxis, in which the therapeutic response is determined by an overall improvement in the disease rather than by immediate symptom relief and for which there is extensive validation.

Conventional allergy management emphasizes avoidance of allergens where possible. This recommendation places a premium on accurate identification of each patient's specific allergic sensitivities in order to prevent unnecessary lifestyle restrictions. The diagnosis of so-called environmental illness or multiple chemical sensitivities, however, is accompanied by excessive and at times extreme *environmental restrictions*. Patients are typically advised to avoid exposure to any and all synthetic chemicals to the extent of living an isolated life in specially constructed and furnished quarters. This is coupled with extreme dietary restrictions and inappropriate avoidance of medications. Such a major lifestyle disruption is predicated on unproved concepts and diagnostic methods.

Unnecessary *diet restrictions* are a consequence of any unproved method for determining allergy to foods. Some of these procedures, such as provocation–neutralization, the cytotoxic test and the use of IgG food antibodies, are capable of suggesting food intolerance where it does not exist and which is then difficult to erase from the patient's mind. This often leads to a pattern of even more food restrictions, because the underlying condition, whether physical or psychological, is not solved by a change in diet. In cases in which the diet is so restricted that nutritional adequacy is threatened, a *rotary diet* is recommended. This is designed to limit but not totally restrict foods by allowing the patient to eat each food on a 5-day cycle of food rotations. The rotary diet also is recommended by some practitioners who believe that many foods are toxic or that excessive exposure to a substance, such as a food, makes it allergenic, a concept with no scientific basis.

Many unproved allergy practices include recommendations that the patient take daily *nutritional supplements* such as multiple vitamins, minerals, and antioxidants either to treat the presumed allergic disease or to prevent the development of allergies. There is no theoretical basis for the use of any of these supplements to treat or prevent allergy, and there have been no controlled studies to establish that they are necessary.

Allergen immunotherapy has a long track record of benefit for patients with respiratory atopic allergy or *Hymenoptera* venom anaphylaxis, supported by an impressive number of controlled clinical trials validating its use in properly selected patients. This success may be responsible partly for a proliferation of controversial treatments with superficial resemblances to, but critical differences from, immunotherapy.

Allergists have not yet been successful in immunizing patients with life-threatening anaphylaxis to specific foods, even though this treatment is highly successful in venom-induced anaphylaxis. A demonstrated IgE hypersensitivity to foods, whether the result is systemic anaphylaxis, nonfatal urticaria, allergic gastroenteropathy, or exacerbation of atopic dermatitis or asthma is satisfactorily managed by avoidance of the specific food allergen. Fortunately, the vast majority of patients with this problem suffer from a single or at most a small number of food sensitivities, so that the necessary diet rarely has significant nutritional consequences. Some practitioners who diagnose multiple food allergies based on inappropriate methods recommend *food injection therapy,* which has never been examined for efficacy by controlled trials. In almost all such cases the patient's reported symptoms are not consistent with those of allergy and the symptoms' relationship to foods is speculative and not proved.

Another variation of allergen immunotherapy is *autogenous urine injections,* a bizarre procedure that is fortunately of only historic interest today. It consisted of intradermal or subcutaneous injections of the patient's urine after it was chemically treated to extract a substance called proteose, alleged to be the metabolized form of the patient's inhaled or ingested allergens. This substance was considered to be more efficacious for immunization than the allergen extract itself. The treatment was not only of unproved value but potentially dangerous.

CONTROVERSIAL PRACTICE SYSTEMS

A number of practice systems that claim to diagnose and treat diseases as well as to promote health and a sense of well-being are being increasingly pursued by many people as alternatives to scientific evidence-based medical practice. Scientific medicine has been enormously successful in understanding normal body structure, function, and disease pathology, as well as in developing effective diagnostic tools and therapy. The alternative practice systems on the other hand are purely empiric, and they are not consistent with established principles of anatomy, physiology, and disease pathology. None of them have survived controlled trials of efficacy. Some persons today question or even reject the established scientific approach to medical care in favor of unproved practices. The reasons for this are many and complex. The clinician must recognize this trend without acquiescing to it. Knowledge of these practices is helpful for providing informed advice as part of managing allergic disease in those patients who choose to supplement effective treatment with one or more of these modalities.

Practitioners of these alternative systems frequently combine features of more than one of them in their treatments. When used for allergy, these frequently include diets that are said to have a beneficial effect on the functioning of the immune system. There are literally thousands of untested practice modalities, but only a few of the more common ones will be mentioned here.

Acupuncture is probably one of the most popular of the ineffective procedures used to deal with allergic problems. It involves insertion of needles into the skin at certain defined points on the body with some presumed relationship to a particular organ or disease. Many patients report trying acupuncture for allergy, usually reporting no results or temporary subjective improvement that is not sustained. There is no scientific rationale for acupuncture, and there are no controlled clinical trials in allergy. It is a component of *Chinese medicine,* which typically includes *herbal therapy.* The herbs used may or may not have pharmacologically active components. Such active chemicals in herbs could be isolated, purified, analyzed chemically, tested both in vitro and in vivo for possible inhibition of allergic reactions, and finally subjected to controlled clinical trials for safety and efficacy. If such activity were found, it would then be necessary to compare it with similar activity of existing drugs. This has not been done. Nonetheless, many patients believe that ingesting an herb is a more natural treatment and therefore must be safer and more effective than an approved drug, even if it contains no demonstrated anti-allergic pharmacologic activity.

Homeopathy is a practice system based on the unproved principle of like treats like, that is, the administration of an agent that allegedly produces the disease is therapeutic for that disease if given in infinitesimally small amounts. It presumes that the disease cause is known and identifiable as a substance that can be safely tolerated by the patient. Its use as treatment for allergy is rationalized in part on a superficial resemblance to allergen immunotherapy or infectious disease immunization, except that the latter are based on techniques that generate a protective immune response, which has never been demonstrated for homeopathic remedies. These remedies are given in vanishingly small amounts, predicated on the theory that the molecule of remedy impresses a mirror image of itself upon water molecules in solution. The means by which these putative altered molecules treat the disease are purely speculative.

RISKS

No treatment or mode of practice is without risk. In medical practice the risk/benefit ratio must be constantly monitored for each patient by the physician who undertakes the management of a chronic disease, including allergy. For example, the benefit of extreme measures to avoid eating even trace amounts of peanut protein in a patient with peanut-induced anaphylaxis is worth the substantial risk of death. Reasonable house dust mite avoidance measures are warranted for the benefit of lessening the extent of nonfatal atopic eczema in a mite-sensitive child. Similar risk/benefit analyses are inherent in the decisions made

routinely in an allergist's practice, and the principle applies equally to the primary care physician.

In a practice that uses unproved testing and treatment and resulting in incorrect diagnoses, the risk/benefit ratio is always infinitely high and therefore indefensible. Even if the treatment provides nothing more than a placebo response that the patient perceives as beneficial, there remains a real danger of missing the opportunity to uncover a treatable disease. Furthermore, dependence solely on a placebo effect for relief of symptoms is an illusion, because it is typically transient. The reappearance of the patient's symptoms creates a need for more treatment, without ever achieving a permanent resolution of the problem.

The patient may develop a psychological dependence on an unproved mode of treatment. The extreme lifestyle changes recommended for the so-called multiple chemical sensitivities may impact adversely on the patient's family as well.

Specific and predictable side-effects and toxicities are well recognized in the cases of sublingual exposure to an allergen and high-dose vitamin therapy. Adverse responses should be considered for all other forms of unconventional practices as well.

Suggested Reading

American Academy of Allergy and Clinical Immunology Executive Committee: Position statement: Controversial techniques. J Allergy Clin Immunol 67:333, 1981

Grieco MH: Controversial techniques in allergy. JAMA 253:842, 1985

Jewett DL, Fein G, Greenberg MH: A double-blind study of symptom provocation to determine food sensitivity. N Engl J Med 323:429, 1990

Sparks PJ, Daniell W, Black DW, et al: Multiple chemical sensitivity syndrome: A clinical perspective. I. Case definition, theories of pathogenesis, and research need. J Occup Med 36:718, 1994

Terr AI: Unconventional theories and unproved methods in allergy. In Middleton E Jr, Reed CE, Ellis EF, et al (eds): Allergy, Principles and Practice, 5th ed. St. Louis, Mosby, 1998, pp 1235–1249

Chapter 7

Conjunctivitis

Mitchell H. Friedlaender

The eye is a frequent target of inflammation in both local and systemic allergic reactions. The vast majority of ocular allergy affects the conjunctiva, the mucous membrane of the eye. Therefore, we usually speak of ocular allergy and allergic conjunctivitis almost interchangeably. There are several types of allergic conjunctivitis. The largest group is associated with environmental allergens, and is the ocular component of allergic rhinoconjunctivitis. A smaller group is associated with atopic dermatitis and is usually referred to as atopic keratoconjunctivitis. An unusual syndrome that occurs mainly in children and has impressive allergic features is vernal keratoconjunctivitis. The popularity of contact lenses has spawned another category of ocular allergy known as giant papillary conjunctivitis (GPC). The exact cause of this condition is of considerable interest to ophthalmologists, their patients, and contact lens manufacturers. Ophthalmologists tend to be treaters of disease, and when patients complain eye drops are generally prescribed. This tendency has led to a variety of contact allergy reactions caused by a wide array of medications and their preservatives.

The importance of ocular allergy is more because of its frequency than its severity. From the ophthalmologist's perspective ocular allergy is rarely a blinding disease, although some cases of atopic and vernal keratoconjunctivitis have produced severe corneal scarring and loss of vision. From the practicing allergist's point of view the question often arises whether to treat or not treat the red, itchy eye and whether to refer the patient to an ophthalmologist. From the patient's point of view the symptoms of ocular allergy are usually mild but moderately annoying. When

the condition is seasonal, patients usually learn to live with their symptoms. Others may experience symptoms year round, and, occasionally, the ocular features are the most prominent part of the allergic patient's disease, particularly in patients with vernal keratoconjunctivitis and atopic keratoconjunctivitis.

As in other medical specialties, over-medication is a significant problem in ophthalmology. The indiscriminate use of antibiotics, antivirals, and anti-inflammatory agents has led to a high incidence of contact allergic reactions in routine ophthalmic practice. It is often difficult to pinpoint the allergen in patients who are using a variety of medications or solutions, and also to separate the toxic from the allergic components. The use of thimerosal and other preservatives in eye drops and contact lens solutions has been partially responsible for the high incidence of contact allergy in patients with and without previous ocular inflammation.

ALLERGIC RHINOCONJUNCTIVITIS

The conjunctiva, like the nasal mucosa, can be affected by allergies to airborne pollens, animal dander, and other environmental antigens. The most important allergens vary from one location to another, but the symptoms and signs appear to be similar throughout the world. Often symptoms are not severe enough to precipitate a visit to the allergist or the ophthalmologist. Of patients who seek help, some may not require treatment and others may simply need to avoid certain allergens.

Ocular Features

Symptoms usually consist of low-grade ocular and periocular itching, tearing, burning, stinging, photophobia, and watery discharge. Redness and itching seem to be the most consistent symptoms. Although symptoms persist throughout the allergy season, they are subject to exacerbations and remissions depending on the weather and the patient's activities. Pollen-induced symptoms are generally worse when the weather is warm and dry. Cooler temperatures and rain tend to alleviate symptoms. Although itching is generally mild, occasionally it can be severe, and rarely patients may be incapacitated by their symptoms.

The conjunctiva usually shows mild or moderate edema and injection (Fig. 7–1). The combination of these two features gives the conjunctiva a pinkish to milky appearance. Because the conjunctival blood vessels are partially obscured, they are best evaluated with a slit lamp microscope. Occasionally, chemosis is so marked that it is obvious without magnification. If edema is severe, patients also will show periorbital edema. This edema is more prominent around the lower lids because of gravity. Ecchymoses, or the allergic shiner, also has been described in allergic patients and is thought to be the result of impaired venous return from the skin and subcutaneous tissues, although proof of this is lacking.

A proper diagnosis can generally be made by taking a careful history. Often patients are not aware that they are allergic until symptoms develop during a severe allergy season. Scratch or prick tests are helpful in establishing a definite diagnosis. Instillation of an offending pollen into the conjunctival sac will also produce the typical symptoms of hay fever conjunctivitis; however, this type of conjunctival testing is rarely necessary.

Scraping the conjunctival surface to look for eosinophils is a helpful diagnostic test. The procedure is done by placing a drop of topical anesthetic, such as tetracaine hydrochloride 0.5%, in the lower conjunctival sac. The anesthetic takes effect within 10 seconds. The inner surface of the lower lid is gently scraped several times with a platinum spatula. The material is then spread on a microscope slide. The slide is stained with Hansel stain or Giemsa. Slides are examined for the presence of eosinophils or eosinophil granules. Eosinophils are not ordinarily found in conjunctival scrapings from nonallergic individuals. The presence of even one eosinophil or eosinophil granule is considerable evidence in favor of a diagnosis of allergic conjunctivitis. The absence of eosinophils should not rule out a diagnosis of allergy. Eosinophils are often present in the deeper layers of the conjunctiva and may be absent or undetectable in the upper layers. The frequency of eosinophils in the conjunctival scrapings from patients with allergic conjunctivitis may be as high as 80%.

Treatment

Antihistamines may be given systemically to relieve allergic symptoms. They may only partially relieve ocular symptoms, and patients often complain of side effects such as drowsiness

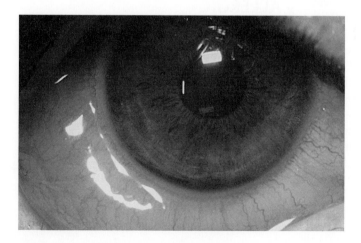

Figure 7–1. Allergic conjunctivitis caused by animal dander.

and dryness of the eyes, nose, and mouth. Antihistamines such as antazoline and pheniramine are available as eye drops and are usually combined with a topical vasoconstrictor such as naphazoline hydrochloride. These antihistamine–vasoconstrictor eye drops are useful in treating mild allergic conjunctivitis. Most are used four times a day, and the side-effects are minimal. They whiten the eyes by constricting the conjunctival blood vessels. They also relieve itching in the majority of patients.

Four percent cromolyn (Bausch & Lomb, Crolom) can be a useful addition to the other drugs available for treating allergic conjunctivitis. Several studies have confirmed the therapeutic value of cromolyn in allergic conjunctivitis. Usually 10 to 14 days of treatment are necessary before optimal relief is obtained. Occasionally, patients notice improvement within 24 to 48 hours. Cromolyn is most useful for relief of mild and moderate symptoms of allergic conjunctivitis. More severe cases may require the addition of topical corticosteroids. Unlike corticosteroids, cromolyn has minimal ocular side-effects. An acute chemotic reaction to cromolyn has been reported in two patients, but as in the treatment of asthma, cromolyn-related side-effects are rare. An extra benefit of cromolyn eye drops is the relief of nasal symptoms caused by the drainage of the tear fluid into the nasal passages. Other mast cell stabilizers, such as lodoxamide (Alcon Laboratories, Alomide) and olopatadine (Alcon Laboratories, Patanol) (which also has an antihistamine effect), also are available for ophthalmic use.

Corticosteroids may be extremely effective in relieving symptoms of allergic rhinitis and conjunctivitis, but since the disease is a chronic, recurrent, benign condition, these drugs should be used only in extreme situations. Topical steroids are associated with glaucoma, cataract formation, and infections of the cornea and conjunctiva. They should, therefore, be used with the greatest caution, and preferably the patient should be monitored by an ophthalmologist. Under no circumstances should patients be allowed to use corticosteroid eye drops without medical supervision; nor should they be given prescriptions for unlimited refills.

ATOPIC KERATOCONJUNCTIVITIS

The skin of the eyelids can be affected in atopic dermatitis just as the skin elsewhere can. There are some unique ocular features of atopic dermatitis that make this condition interesting and challenging from the ophthalmologist's point of view.

Ocular Features

Erythematous and exudative lesions may be found on the eyelid skin. In later stages crusting and scaling can occur. Secondary staphylococcal blepharitis may also develop and require treatment (Fig. 7–2). In fact, *Staphylococcus aureus* can be cultured from the eyelids of a high percentage of atopic patients. The

Figure 7–2. Staphylococcal blepharitis in an atopic patient.

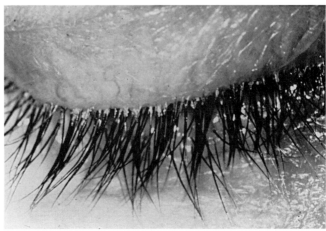

conjunctiva may show hyperemia, chemosis, and filamentous discharge. Less commonly, giant papillary hypertrophy may be observed on the palpebral conjunctiva. Trantas dots (small white dots rich in eosinophils) can sometimes be seen at the limbus, especially superiorly. Atopic keratoconjunctivitis may persist for many years, and, occasionally, the ocular component of this disease may be the predominant feature. Patients with these severe cases show tremendous photophobia, redness, and tearing. Many patients have difficulty opening their eyes outdoors and are constantly bothered by ocular irritation, itching, and discharge. In long-standing disease there may be significant conjunctival scarring. This can be manifested as stellate scars, most visible on the upper palpebral conjunctiva. Rarely shrinkage of the fornices can occur.

Punctuate staining of the cornea can be demonstrated by putting a drop of fluorescein in the eye, and if the disease is severe, scarring and vascularization of the cornea may be evident. Some corneal changes may be related to atopic scarring of the ocular surface; others may be due to effects of staphylococci (and their toxins), which populate the lids of atopic individuals. Keratoconus (Fig. 7–3) is an unusual cone-shaped ectasia of the cornea that is sometimes associated with atopic dermatitis. In one series, 16% of keratoconus patients had atopic dermatitis and an additional 16% had other forms of cutaneous inflammation. It has been suggested, although not proved, that excessive eye rubbing coupled with a congenitally thinned and weakened cornea may lead to the development of keratoconus.

Atopic cataracts are another complication seen in 8% to 10% of atopic dermatitis patients. Cataracts are seen mainly in the severe, chronic forms of the disease, especially in children and young adults. Atopic cataracts usually appear at least 10 years after the onset of skin involvement. Once a cataract is detected, however, it may evolve rapidly into complete opacification within 6 months. These cataracts are frequently bilateral and may be symmetric. Occasionally, a unilateral cataract is seen. Classically atopic cataracts have a shield-like opacification affecting the anterior cortex (Fig. 7–4). Frequently the cataract begins as a posterior subcapsular opacity. Since this form of cataract is identical to the type induced by corticosteroids, it may be impossible to determine whether the cataract was caused by the treatment or the disease.

Spontaneous retinal detachment is said to be more common in patients with atopic dermatitis than in the general population. This is a rare complication of ocular allergic disease.

Atopic keratoconjunctivitis patients have elevated levels of serum IgE; however, the pattern of total and specific IgE antibodies does not help distinguish atopic keratoconjunctivitis patients from other groups of patients with allergic conjunctivitis.

Treatment

Topical corticosteroids may be used for short periods; however, their long-term use should be avoided. Some success has been obtained with 4% cromolyn eye drops and other mast

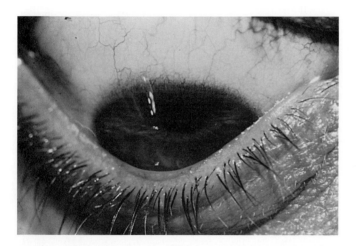

Figure 7–3. Keratoconus in an atopic patient.

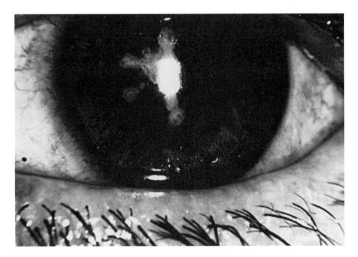

Figure 7–4. Atopic cataract.

cell stabilizers. Often supplemental topical steroids must be used, especially during periods of heightened disease activity. If an inciting antigen can be identified, it should be eliminated. The eyelid lesions should be treated as atopic skin lesions elsewhere on the body.

Surgery for atopic cataracts should not be undertaken lightly since complications, including hemorrhage, retinal detachment, iridocyclitis, and corneal edema can occur. Keratoconus can be treated successfully with contact lenses or in advanced cases by corneal transplantation.

VERNAL KERATOCONJUNCTIVITIS

Vernal keratoconjunctivitis is a bilateral and often severe disease, occurring mainly in children and associated with climatic factors. It is characterized by a stringy mucinous discharge and giant papillae of the upper palpebral conjunctiva (Fig. 7–5). Many features of vernal keratoconjunctivitis suggest an allergic cause.

Patients with vernal keratoconjunctivitis frequently have a history of atopic disease such as hay fever, atopic eczema, or asthma. Sometimes a history of atopy can be elicited only in a member of the patient's family. Increased levels of IgE can be detected in the tears of patients with vernal keratoconjunctivitis, and even when the mean level of IgE in tears is not significantly greater than in control subjects, the serum levels are significantly elevated. In patients with vernal keratoconjunctivitis it has been shown that IgA, IgD, and IgE are synthesized locally by conjunctival plasma cells in a ratio of approximately 4:1:2, respectively. Allergen-specific IgE antibodies have

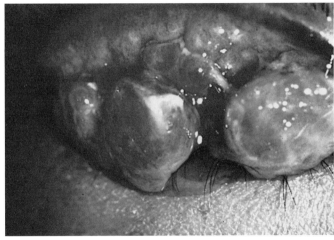

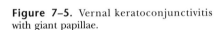

Figure 7–5. Vernal keratoconjunctivitis with giant papillae.

been demonstrated in the tears and serum of vernal conjunctivitis patients. Positive reactions to pollens, house dust mites, and cat epithelium have been demonstrated in some patients. Presently, it is unclear whether vernal keratoconjunctivitis is associated with one allergen or is the end result of ocular sensitization to a wide variety of allergens.

Histologically the conjunctiva contains many eosinophils, plasma cells, and tissue mast cells. Eosinophils and mast cells also can be demonstrated in scrapings from the conjunctiva obtained with a platinum spatula. Additional histologic features have recently been described, including the presence of basophils, microvascular alterations of endothelial cells, and deposition of fibrin. Other histologic features of vernal keratoconjunctivitis include infiltration by lymphocytes and neutrophils and epithelial invasion by mast cells and eosinophils.

Ocular Features

Vernal keratoconjunctivitis begins in the prepubertal years, at which time it is more common in males than in females. After puberty, the incidence in the two sexes is about equal. The peak incidence is between the ages of 11 and 13, and the disease is rare after the age of 20. Vernal keratoconjunctivitis is more common in warm climates than in temperate zones and is rarely seen in cold climates. Because of its geographic pattern, heat and other physical factors have been felt to contribute to the pathogenesis of the disease.

Patients complain of extreme itching, photophobia, and a ropy, mucous discharge. The hallmark of vernal keratoconjunctivitis is the presence of giant papillae on the palpebral conjunctiva. These papillae are polygonal and flat-topped and contain tufts of capillaries. The conjunctiva has a milky appearance, and many fine papillae may be present on the lower palpebral conjunctiva.

Corneal findings include superficial corneal ulcers and plaque-like deposits in the anterior cornea (Fig. 7–6). These deposits contain mucus and many compacted layers of epithelial cells. Trantas dots may be found at the limbus, especially during periods of heightened disease activity. Other corneal complications include diffuse epithelial keratitis and an arcus-like deposit that may be adjacent to limbal papillae.

The limbal form of vernal keratoconjunctivitis (Fig. 7–7) is characterized by several gelatinous swellings at the limbus. These swellings may be associated with a variable amount of giant papillae on the upper tarsal conjunctiva. This form of vernal keratoconjunctivitis is more common in dark-skinned people.

Treatment

Vernal keratoconjunctivitis is a self-limited disease that runs a 5- to 10-year course. Treatment should be conservative and aimed at relieving symptoms without producing serious iatrogenic side-effects. Topical and systemic corticosteroids are frequently employed in treating this condition. Although they de-

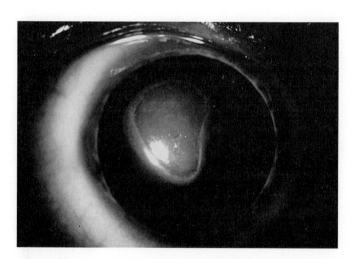

Figure 7–6. Corneal plaque in vernal keratoconjunctivitis.

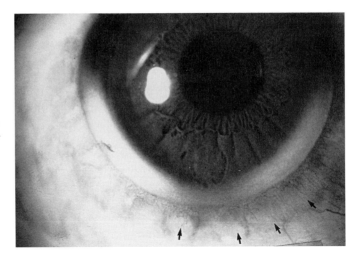

Figure 7–7. Limbal vernal keratoconjunctivitis with an arcus-like deposit. Note swellings at the limbus.

crease symptoms, corticosteroids do not significantly affect the corneal complications or shorten the duration of the disease. They may also be associated with serious side-effects. A short course of topical steroids is useful in breaking the inflammatory cycle. Steroid use should be supplemented with vasoconstrictors, cold compresses, ice packs, and climatotherapy. In many cases, patients may experience marked relief of symptoms if they move to a cool moist climate or sleep in a cool or air-conditioned room. Cromolyn eye drops in a 1% to 4% solution have recently been used topically with good results. Lodoxamide hydrochloride drops also appear to show promise. These drugs reduce itching, hyperemia, and mucous discharge. The giant papillae may remain large for months or years despite therapy, yet symptoms are markedly improved. Often supplemental topical corticosteroids are required for satisfactory relief of symptoms.

Hyposensitization therapy with grass pollens and other antigens may be helpful in some instances but in general has not been rewarding. Systemic antihistamines also may be helpful.

The corneal plaques are usually resistant to medical therapy, and in most cases they must be surgically removed. These plaques may be associated with some scarring and may lead to a permanent reduction in the patient's vision.

GIANT PAPILLARY CONJUNCTIVITIS

A condition similar in appearance to vernal keratoconjunctivitis is seen in contact lens wearers and has become known as giant papillary conjunctivitis (GPC). This condition (Fig. 7–8) is seen mostly in individuals who wear

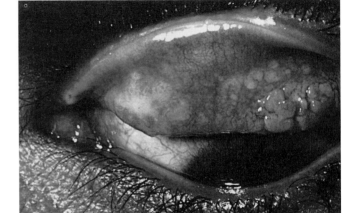

Figure 7–8. Giant papillary conjunctivitis (GPC) associated with contact lens wear.

soft contact lenses, but it has been observed in hard contact lens wearers and in people who wear ocular prostheses after an eye has been enucleated. In mild cases the papillae are not really giant, and the upper tarsal conjunctiva has a red, fine papillary response. Trantas dots have been reported, but these are rare in GPC.

The cause of GPC is unclear. There may be some predisposition among allergic patients, but this is difficult to prove. The offending antigen could be the contact lens polymer, deposits on the surface of the lens, or chemicals in the contact lens solutions. It is likely that nonallergic irritative factors play a major role in the formation of giant papillae. Inert stimuli, such as nylon sutures, cyanoacrylate tissue adhesive, ocular prostheses, and even limbal dermoid tumors can cause GPC.

It is easy to treat GPC by discontinuing contact lens wear. Many patients will not accept this alternative and are tenaciously attached to their contact lenses. It may be possible to continue contact lens wear if the patient's wearing time is reduced, but usually symptoms persist. Prescribing a new contact lens is often helpful but only temporarily. Some success has been obtained by switching to a different contact lens material, such as silicone. Improvement has also been reported with cromolyn eye drops. Many contact lens cleaning and wetting solutions contain thimerosal, and this substance has been implicated in contact lens intolerance. It may be helpful to use a nonthimerosal cleaner, and unpreserved saline can be used if the patient is cautious about his or her hygiene.

Symptoms of GPC include redness, burning, itching, pain, and discharge. Affected patients find it difficult to wear their contact lenses more than a few hours at a time. This produces considerable visual and emotional problems for many people, and a great deal of time and effort can be expended in trying to eliminate the signs and symptoms of this condition. Mechanically removing contact lens deposits with a polishing wheel may be helpful, and disposable contact lenses worn on a daily wear basis have relieved most signs and symptoms in a large percentage of GPC sufferers.

CONTACT ALLERGY

The eye is a frequent site of involvement in contact dermatitis. Ocular preparations containing neomycin sulfate, atropine and its derivatives, and thimerosal are effective sensitizers. A typical victim of conjunctivitis medicamentosa is the patient who is treated for a red eye. Eye drops are prescribed and the patient's symptoms begin to improve. The medication is continued for one reason or another, and the eye starts to become redder. More eye drops (or sometimes a different eye drop) are used, and a vicious cycle of inflammation is begun. It becomes difficult to tell whether the conjunctivitis is related to the original disease or the medication. Usually the best treatment is to stop all eye drops, see the patient in a few days, and perform cultures and conjunctival scrapings.

The skin of the eyelids may be red, edema-

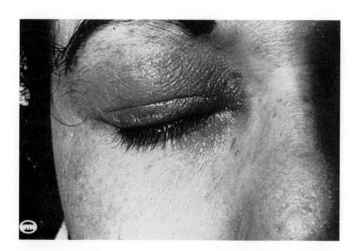

Figure 7–9. Contact allergy (conjunctivitis medicamentosa) related to pilocarpine eye drops.

tous, and ulcerated (Fig. 7–9). Conjunctivitis characterized by a papillary response, pronounced vasodilation, chemosis, and watery discharge may be present. In severe cases, a keratitis can develop and is typified by small to large epithelial defects and corneal opacities. Some of the most severe responses are associated with topical anesthetics. Some long-standing cases have also occurred with glaucoma medications.

Rubbing the eyes after handling soaps, detergents, or chemicals may provoke a contact dermatitis reaction. Allergic reactions to cosmetics affect primarily the eyebrows and upper lids because of the method of application. Mascara, eyebrow pencil, and face creams all may act as allergens. Nail polish can cause sensitization around the eye if the patient accidentally touches the area. Lip gloss and eye gloss cosmetics contain lanolin fractions that may also act as sensitizers.

A diagnosis of allergic contact sensitivity can be made by patch testing. More often a different eye drop, ointment, or contact lens solution is prescribed. For acute skin lesions, cold compresses can be applied to the eyelids. Corticosteroids are rarely necessary; however, systemic corticosteroids are sometimes used in severe poison ivy dermatitis involving the eyes. For the conjunctivitis or keratitis associated with drugs, the best treatment is withdrawal of the drug and substitution of an appropriate, nonsensitizing medication.

CONCLUSION

Allergic conjunctivitis, unlike many ocular conditions, is rarely associated with permanent visual impairment. It is, however, a common and extremely uncomfortable problem for those who are affected. Since patients with allergic conjunctivitis may be seen by a variety of physicians, it is important that physicians recognize the hallmarks of allergic conjunctivitis and understand the different therapeutic alternatives for the management of this condition.

RESOURCES

American Academy of Ophthalmology
655 Beach Street
San Francisco, CA 94109-1336

Sjögren's Syndrome Foundation
333 North Broadway
Jericho, NY 11753

Francis I. Proctor Foundation
95 Kirkham Street
San Francisco, CA 94122

Suggested Reading

Friedlaender MH: Corticosteroid therapy of ocular inflammation. Int Ophthalmol Clin 23:175, 1983
Friedlaender MH: Some unusual nonallergic causes of giant papillary conjunctivitis. Trans Am Ophthalmol Soc 88:343, 1991
Friedlaender MH: Allergy and Immunology of the Eye. New York, Raven, 1993
Friedlaender MH, Ohashi Y, Kelley J: Diagnosis of allergic conjunctivitis. Arch Ophthalmol 102:1198, 1984
Sampolinsky D, Samra Z, Zavaro A, et al: Allergen-specific immunoglobulin E antibodies in tears and serum of vernal conjunctivitis patients. Int Arch Allergy Appl Immunol 75:317, 1984
Tuft SJ, Kemeny DM, Dart JKG, et al: Clinical features of atopic keratoconjunctivitis. Ophthalmology 98:150, 1991
Wiens JJ, Jackson WB: New directions in therapy for ocular allergy. Int Ophthalmol Clin 28:332, 1988

KEY POINTS

▶ The main manifestation of ocular allergy in the eye is conjunctivitis.
▶ Most ocular allergy is mild and seasonal, but rare conditions such as vernal and atopic conjunctivitis may be severe.
▶ A wide variety of ophthalmic antiallergic drugs are available, including antihistamines, mast cell stabilizers, and nonsteroidal anti-inflammatory drugs.
▶ Corticosteroids are the most potent topical antiallergic drugs. They may be associated with serious side-effects, although safer preparations are being developed.

Chapter 8

Allergic and Nonallergic Rhinitides

Mary V. Lasley

Rhinitis is a term used to describe diseases that involve inflammation of the nasal epithelium and can be accompanied by symptoms of sneezing, rhinorrhea, and nasal congestion. It is difficult to know the precise number of patients that are affected with rhinitis symptoms. Many patients may not seek medical care, whereas others suffer severely. Rhinitis can be divided into two general categories: allergic and nonallergic as shown in Table 8–1. This chapter will review the rhinitides, describing the pathophysiology, presentation, and treatment of each disease state. Allergic rhinitis, the most common of the rhinitides, affects 15% to 25% of the population. Also, there are many patients with chronic rhinitis symptoms who undergo allergy evaluation and no identifiable allergen is found. These patients are classified as having nonallergic rhinitis and the prevalence varies from one-quarter to one-half of all rhinitis patients.

ALLERGIC RHINITIS

Presentation and Progression

Pathophysiology

Genetic predisposition and environmental exposure are important factors in the development of allergic rhinitis. When an atopic person inhales airborne allergens, these proteins penetrate the nasal mucosal epithelium and interact with allergen-specific IgE bound to high-affinity receptors on mast cells and basophils and to low-affinity receptors on other cells, such as eosinophils, monocytes, and platelets. The early allergic phase occurs when mast cells and basophils degranulate and release pre-formed chemical mediators such as histamine and tryptase, and newly generated mediators such as leukotrienes, prostaglandins, cytokines, kinins, and platelet activating factor. These chemical mediators alter nasal mucosal permeability and cause rhinorrhea and nasal congestion. Histamine stimulates sensory fibers of the vidian nerve, leading to sneezing and itching. Pharyngitis, hoarseness, and chronic cough may develop from posterior pharyngeal mucus drainage. Following the early phase, there is a quiescent period of a few hours followed by a late phase reaction which occurs approximately 4 to 8 hours later. Inflammatory cells, such as eosinophils, basophils, CD4+ T cells, monocytes, and neutrophils, infiltrate the nasal mucosa. Activation of these inflammatory cells leads to release of chemical mediators and a perpetuation of chronic inflammation and nasal hyper-reactivity, resulting in symptoms of nasal congestion and rhinorrhea.

If one parent has allergies, the risk is 25% to 40% that their child will also develop allergic disease. If both parents have allergies, the risk increases to 50% to 70%. Also, the same allergic diseases tend to occur in families.

Clinical Presentation

Allergic rhinitis may be seasonal, perennial, episodic, or occupational depending on the

Table 8–1. **Differential Diagnosis of Rhinitis**

| | Non-Allergic | |
Allergic	Nonanatomic	Anatomic
Seasonal	Atrophic rhinitis	Adenoidal hypertrophy
Perennial	Drug-induced rhinitis	Cerebrospinal fluid rhinorrhea
Episodic	Hormonal rhinitis	Choanal atresia
Occupational	Idiopathic (vasomotor) rhinitis	Foreign bodies
	Infectious rhinosinusitis	Granulomas
	NARES (Nonallergic rhinitis with eosinophilia syndrome)	Nasal polyps
	Physical rhinitis	Septal deviation
	Rhinitis medicamentosa	Tumors
		Turbinate hypertrophy

patient's exposure. Some patients will experience perennial symptoms with seasonal exacerbations.

Seasonal Allergic Rhinitis. Seasonal allergic rhinitis is caused by airborne allergens that have a seasonal pattern. For example, trees usually pollinate in the spring, grasses in late spring to summer, and weeds in summer and fall. It is important to consider climate variation when evaluating patients with rhinitis. In warmer climates, such as California and the deep South, trees may pollinate during the winter months. The regional flora determines pollen exposure. Most flora that cause significant allergic reactions are wind-pollinated, and their pollen can travel many miles. Because of this factor and the tendency of some pollens to cross-react with related species, a move to a different climate usually does not help the patient with allergic rhinitis.

Perennial Allergic Rhinitis. The most important perennial allergens include house dust mites, animal proteins, molds, and cockroach. Dust mites, or *Dermatophagoides pteronyssinus* and *Dermatophagoides farinae* species, are microscopic arachnids that live on human skin scales. The highest concentration of dust mites is found in indoor areas where people spend the most amount of time. They accumulate in high concentrations in bedding, mattresses, upholstered furniture, and carpet. The mite's fecal pellet is the major source of the allergen found in house dust. These microscopic particles are easily inhaled into the nose and lung, where they can trigger an allergic response. Studies have shown a direct quantitative correlation between mite allergen exposure and the development of allergic sensitization.

The major cat allergen, found primarily in the sebaceous glands and dermis of the cat, has been well characterized. It is primarily distributed by cat saliva and dander and is found in all breeds of cats. The primary antigen is a charged molecule and can remain airborne for long periods of time. Even after the cat has been removed from the home, cat allergen can be measured several months later. The major antigen found in dog dander has also been identified. Animals shed dander at different rates, and hair length is only a minor factor in the amount of dander made and shed. Nonallergenic breeds of cats or dogs do not exist. Even hairless cats and nonshedding dogs have significant amounts of dander and are potentially allergenic.

Mold is a cause of both perennial and seasonal allergic rhinitis. *Aspergillus* and *Penicillium* mold species are found most commonly in basements, crawl spaces, and bedding. *Alternaria, Cladosporium, Helminthosporum,* and *Fusarium* mold species are prevalent during the summer and fall months and usually disappear with the first frost. These outdoor molds can gain access to homes through open windows and doors.

Episodic Rhinitis. Episodic rhinitis usually occurs with intermittent exposure to antigens that do not follow seasonal or work-related trends. Episodic disease is mostly related to intermittent exposure to animals or dusty environments. Visiting the home of a cat owner can trigger acute allergic rhinitis symptoms even when the cat is absent.

Occupational Rhinitis. The incidence of occupational rhinitis is not known. The patient's history often helps diagnose this type of rhinitis, usually revealing a temporal relationship between nasal symptoms and on-the-job exposure. Occupations associated with on-the-job allergen exposures include bakers and agricultural workers (grains), veterinarians and laboratory workers (animals), woodworkers (wood dust), and health care workers (latex). Other common causes of occupational rhinitis include exposures to irritants (paint fumes, tobacco smoke, exhaust) or corrosives (ammonia, chlorine). Occupational rhinitis often precedes the development of occupational asthma. This topic is more thoroughly reviewed in Chapter 13, Occupational Asthma.

The typical patient with allergic rhinitis will complain of clear rhinorrhea, nasal congestion, paroxysms of sneezing, itching of the nose, eyes, ears, or palate, and postnasal drip. Mucus draining into the posterior pharynx may result in frequent attempts to clear the throat, nocturnal cough, or hoarseness. Other concerns the patient may have include ear popping, ear plugging, loss of smell, mouth breathing, snoring, fatigue, or headache.

It is also important to identify the onset, duration, and severity of symptoms with emphasis on exposure to allergens or nonspecific irritants such as tobacco smoke as well as changes in the home or work environment. Inquiring about a family history of atopy can also yield helpful information.

Although classic physical findings are often described, physical findings may be subtle. There are no pathognomonic features for allergic rhinitis. The classic nasal examination reveals pale-pink or bluish-gray, swollen, boggy nasal turbinates with clear, watery secretions. Frequent nasal itching and rubbing can lead to a transverse nasal crease found across the lower bridge of the nose. Oropharyngeal examination may reveal lymphoid hyperplasia of the soft palate and posterior pharynx or visible mucus. Ocular findings include allergic shiners, which are dark, swollen areas under the eyes caused by venous congestion. The eyelids may be swollen and erythematous with conjunctival injection. Retracted tympanic membranes from eustachian tube dysfunction or serous otitis media also may be noted. Sinus palpation may reveal tenderness when sinusitis is present. Evidence of other atopic diseases such as asthma or eczema will help lead the clinician to the correct diagnosis.

Diagnosis

For patients who suffer from seasonal allergic rhinitis, the history and physical examination provide excellent clues. Further evaluation may be warranted, however, particularly for patients with multiseasonal and perennial allergic rhinitis, or for patients who suffer from adverse effects or complications of rhinitis.

An allergist offers the special skill of administering and interpreting skin tests to determine immediate hypersensitivity to aeroallergens in the diagnosis of allergic rhinitis. Percutaneous tests (prick or puncture) provide immediate and accurate results. They are quick, safe, and cost-effective. Positive skin test results correlate strongly with nasal and bronchial allergen provocative challenges. Patients should be tested for sensitivity to allergens found in their environment.

Intradermal testing may be necessary for patients with a strong clinical and atopic history but who have negative results of percutaneous tests. The predictive value of intradermal testing is less than that of percutaneous tests because there is an associated higher false-positive rate.

Radioallergosorbent tests (RAST) or the enzyme-linked immunosorbent assay (ELISA) are *in vitro* tests that measure specific IgE antibody directed against an allergen. These tests are useful for patients with extensive skin disease or dermatographism, with anaphylaxis tendency, or who are taking medications (e.g., antihistamines) that interfere with skin testing. Disadvantages of RAST or ELISA include increased cost, lack of laboratory standardization, inability to obtain immediate results, and reduced sensitivity as compared to skin tests. Widespread screening with *in vitro* testing without regard for a patient's symptoms is not recommended.

Measurement of total serum IgE or blood eosinophils is generally not helpful in the differential diagnosis of rhinitis.

Nasal smears may add useful information to the history and physical examination findings. Nasal secretions are obtained and then stained with Wright's or Hansel's stains. The presence of eosinophils on the nasal smear suggests a diagnosis of allergy, but eosinophils can also be found in patients with nonallergic rhinitis with eosinophilia syndrome (NARES) which will be discussed later in this chapter. Nasal smear eosinophilia is often predictive of a good clinical response to nasal steroid sprays.

Fiberoptic rhinoscopy allows direct visualization of the upper airway, which may be helpful for patients who do not respond to medical therapy or if there is suspicion of an anatomic or pathologic abnormality. Referral to a physician well trained in recognizing abnormalities of the airway is advocated. Observations also can be recorded on videotape to provide a permanent record.

Natural History

Allergic rhinitis is the most common atopic disease. The incidence of allergic rhinitis has increased over the past 20 years, most notably in industrialized countries. Although allergic rhinitis usually begins during childhood or young adulthood, 30% of patients may develop initial symptoms after the age of 30 years. In the United States, allergic rhinitis outranks heart disease as the sixth most prevalent chronic illness. Patients with allergic rhinitis may experience sleep disturbances, activity limitations, irritability, mood changes, and cognitive disorders that adversely impact their performance at work and school and their sense of well-being. A reliable and accurate quality of life questionnaire for children, adolescents, and adults with seasonal allergic rhinitis has been developed to assess this impact. Other airway disorders, such as asthma, otitis media, chronic sinusitis, and nasal polyposis are found frequently to coexist with allergic rhinitis. Conjunctivitis symptoms related to allergic disease can be particularly severe and difficult to control.

Treatment

The management of allergic rhinitis is based on three therapeutic interventions: allergen avoidance, pharmacologic therapy, and immunotherapy.

Allergen Avoidance

Steps to minimize exposure to known allergens should be taken whenever possible. Avoidance measures are easier to accomplish for indoor than for outdoor allergens; however, a long-term commitment is required. Complete avoidance of the allergen can be curative for some patients.

For dust mite–sensitive patients, the bedding should be washed weekly in hot water (>130°F). Dust mite–impermeable zippered mattress and pillow encasements should be used, and feather pillows and down comforters, and other dust collectors such as stuffed animals, books, and magazines should be removed. These are vital steps that can reduce the dust mite load. Mold-allergic patients should avoid damp, musty basements, barns, hay, or piles of leaves. Installing fans in the bathroom and kitchen and using a dehumidifier to reduce the home's relative humidity to < 50% are helpful in controlling both dust mite and mold growth.

For pet-allergic patients, avoidance must be emphasized. It is often difficult, however, to convince patients to remove their pet from the home. Immediate benefit may not be observed after the pet is removed because dander levels decrease slowly over several months. If removal of the pet is unacceptable, then minimally, the pet should not be allowed into the bedroom and use of a high-efficiency particulate air (HEPA) filter may reduce the amount of airborne dander. A frank discussion should be held with the patient and the family about reduced expectations for successful therapy if the pet is not eliminated from the environment. Varying opinions exist as to whether weekly pet washing can reduce the amount of dander that an animal sheds.

Patients who suffer from pollen allergies may benefit from keeping bedroom and car windows closed and using air conditioning while indoors, especially when pollen counts are high during midday and afternoon. However, such restrictions may have a negative impact on the overall quality of life, making these unreasonable recommendations for many patients and their families.

Medications

Antihistamines are the most frequently used medications for treatment of allergic rhinitis and have been available for over 50 years. They work by competitive inhibition of the H1 receptor site. They are very useful in treating the symptoms of rhinorrhea, sneezing, and nasal and ocular itching, less so with nasal congestion. The antihistamines are usually divided into two classes: first and second generation as shown in Table 8–2. The first-generation antihistamines are lipophilic compounds and easily cross the blood–brain barrier. Drowsiness is reported in one-fourth of adults who use first-generation antihistamines. Subtle impairment of performance has been documented with their use, which may go unrecognized by the patient, similar to a driver not recognizing impairment due to alcohol ingestion. Other side-effects include anticholinergic actions such as blurred vision, urinary retention, dry mouth, tachycardia, and constipation as well as paradoxical stimulatory effects of the central nervous system resulting in irritability and restlessness. These effects may be more frequently observed in very young or elderly patients.

The second-generation antihistamines are more lipophobic, less able to cross the blood–brain barrier, and considerably less sedating. Astemizole (Hismanal, Janssen Pharmaceutica, Titusville, NJ) and terfenadine (Seldane, Hoechst Marion Roussel, Inc., Kansas City, MO) can be cardiotoxic when taken in excess or co-administered with other medications such as erythromycin, clarithromycin, troleandomycin, ketoconazole, itraconazole, micona-

zole, nefazodone, fluvoxamine, and ritonavir. Terfenadine and astemizole have been voluntarily withdrawn from the U.S. market. Typically, the antihistamines are available in tablet or pill form. Cetirizine (Zyrtec, Pfizer, Inc., UCB Pharma, Inc.) and loratadine (Claritin, Schering Corporation, Kenilworth, NJ) are also available in syrup formulation. Cetirizine is approved for children older than 2 years of age, and loratadine is approved for children older than 6 years of age. Azelastine (Astelin, Wallace Laboratories, Cranbury, NJ), a topical nasal antihistamine spray, is also available and effective for seasonal allergic rhinitis for children over the age of 12 years.

Decongestants are used to relieve nasal congestion and can be taken orally or intranasally. Oral medications, such as pseudoephedrine, phenylpropanolamine, and phenylephrine, are available either alone or in combination with antihistamines. Side-effects of oral decongestants include insomnia, nervousness, irritability, tachycardia, tremors, and palpitations. For patients participating in organized sports, the use of oral decongestants may be restricted because of their performance-enhancing effect. Contraindications for the use of oral decongestants include hypertension, coronary heart disease, hyperthyroidism, glaucoma, diabetes mellitus, and prostatic hypertrophy. Monoamine oxidase inhibitors combined with oral decongestants can cause a hypertensive crisis. Topical nasal decongestant

Table 8–2. **Comparison of Selected Antihistamines**

Generic Name	Trade Name	Onset	Sedation	Possible Cardiac Side-Effects	Pregnancy Category	Age	Dosing Schedule
First Generation Antihistamines							
Brompheniramine	Dimetapp	1 hr	Yes	No	C	<6*	TID-QID
Chlorpheniramine	Chlor-Trimeton	1 hr	Yes	No	B	>2	TID-QID
Clemastine	Tavist	1 hr	Yes	No	B	>6	BID
Cyproheptadine	Periactin	1 hr	Yes	No	B	>2	BID-TID
Diphenhydramine	Benadryl	1 hr	Yes	No	B	>2	TID-QID
Hydroxyzine	Atarax	1 hr	Yes	No	C	<6*	TID-QID
Triprolidine	Actidil	1 hr	Yes	No	C	<6*	TID-QID
Second Generation Antihistamines							
Acrivastine	Semprex-D†	1–2 hrs	Yes	No	B	>12	QID
Azelastine‡	Astelin	1 hr	Yes	No	C	>12	BID
Cetirizine	Zyrtec	1–2 hrs	Yes	No	B	>2	QD
Fexofenadine	Allegra	1–2 hrs	No	No	C	>12	BID
Loratadine	Claritin	1–2 hrs	No	No	B	>6	QD

*Consult a physician.
†SemprexD = Acrivastine + Pseudoephedrine.
‡Intranasal application.

sprays are very effective for immediate relief of nasal obstruction, but should be used for fewer than 5 to 7 days to prevent occurrence of rebound nasal congestion (rhinitis medicamentosa).

The most potent pharmacologic agents for treating allergic rhinitis are the intranasal corticosteroids. Table 8–3 lists the topical nasal corticosteroid sprays available in the United States. They work topically to decrease inflammation, edema, and mucus production and are effective during both the early and late phases of an allergic reaction. They are less effective for ocular symptoms, but are very effective in controlling symptoms of nasal congestion, postnasal drip, rhinorrhea, itching, and sneezing. Nasal steroid sprays have been safely used in long term therapy. Deleterious effects on adrenal function or nasal membranes have not been reported if used appropriately. The most common side-effects include local irritation, burning, and sneezing in 10% of the population. Nasal bleeding from improperly spraying the nasal septum also can occur. Rare cases of nasal septal perforation have been reported.

Generally, topical nasal steroid sprays provide relief within a few days to a week and are most effective when used regularly. Most nasal sprays are recommended for use in children older than 6 years with fluticasone (Flonase, Glaxo-Wellcome, Inc.) recently approved for use in children older than 4 years and mometasone (Nasonex) for children older than 3 years. They are available as aqueous or aerosol sprays, and each formulation has its advantages and disadvantages. The aqueous sprays produce less intranasal drying and do not contain chlorofluorocarbon propellants. Conversely, the aerosols produce less dripping into the pharynx after spraying, which often make them better tolerated by youngsters, and therefore improve compliance. When patients have severe nasal congestion, a short course of oral corticosteroids may be helpful. Typically, prednisone is prescribed at 30 to 40 mg for a 5- to 7-day course. Prolonged oral corticosteroid therapy is not recommended because of serious side-effects associated with long-term use such as cataracts, glaucoma, osteoporosis, aseptic necrosis of the femoral head, hypertension, hypothalamic-pituitary-axis suppression, and glucose intolerance.

Similar caution is indicated regarding depot injections of corticosteroids. Although quite effective for nasal congestion, the side-effects of these injections can be serious. Depot injections cannot be reversed, and patients who have steroid psychosis will need to wait until the drug washes out. They also can suppress adrenal cortex function for long periods of time. And lastly, the incidence of severe complications is correlated with a lifetime cumulative dose of corticosteroids. Therefore, minimizing the amount of exposure will help reduce or avoid steroid complications.

Cromolyn sodium (Nasalcrom, Pharmacia and Upjohn), a topical anti-inflammatory nasal spray that is less potent than inhaled corticosteroids, is now available over the counter. It is helpful in reducing symptoms of sneezing, rhinorrhea, and pruritus with minimal side-effects. An important limitation of this medication is its short duration of action so that frequent dosing of 4 to 6 times per day is required. It has been approved for use in chil-

Table 8–3. **Topical Nasal Steroid Sprays Available in the United States**

Generic Name	Trade Name	Formulation	Age	HPA Axis Suppression
Beclomethasone	Beconase AQ	Aqueous	≥6	No
	Beconase	Aerosol		
	Vancenase AQ	Aqueous		
	Vancenase Pockethaler	Aerosol		
	Vancenase AQ DS	Aqueous		
Budesonide	Rhinocort	Aerosol	≥6	No
Dexamethasone	Dexacort	Aerosol	≥6	Yes
Flunisolide	Nasarel/Nasalide	Aqueous	≥6	No
Fluticasone	Flonase	Aqueous	≥4	No
Mometasone	Nasonex	Aqueous	≥3	No
Triamcinolone	Nasacort AQ	Aqueous	≥6	No
	Nasacort	Aerosol		

dren older than 6 years of age and may be safely used in even younger children. Pregnant women and elderly patients may also benefit from this medication.

Ipratropium bromide is a topical anticholinergic nasal spray. It is very effective in the treatment of anterior rhinorrhea. It has been recommended for use in children older than 12 years.

Immunotherapy

If environmental control measures and medication intervention are only partially effective or produce unacceptable side-effects, immunotherapy may be recommended. The mechanism of action for allergen immunotherapy is complex. It includes an increased production of an IgG blocking antibody, decreased production of allergen-specific IgE, and a shifting of cytokine production from T helper 2 (Th2) to T helper 1 (Th1) cells. This alteration in cytokine expression results in diminished interleukin 4 and interleukin 5 levels, a reduction in recruitment and activation of eosinophils, and mast cell proliferation. Double-blind controlled studies have shown immunotherapy to be quite effective for desensitization to pollens, dust mites, cat and dog protein, and some mold spores. Most patients who respond to immunotherapy will receive maintenance injections for a period of 3 to 5 years.

In 1994, the American Academy of Allergy, Asthma, and Immunology published a position statement that gave guidelines to minimize the risk of systemic reactions from injections of allergenic extracts. It was recommended that all patients be observed for a minimum of 20 minutes after the allergen injection and for higher risk patients (patients with asthma or patients with prior systemic reactions), this period should be extended to 30 minutes or more. Epinephrine, oxygen, and resuscitative equipment must be available, and injections should be given only in settings with trained personnel under the direct supervision of a physician.

When to Refer

Many treatment options are available to the clinician for treating patients who suffer from allergies. Each patient's treatment must be individualized based on the frequency, duration, and severity of symptoms as well as the degree of allergic sensitization. Those who may benefit from a referral to an allergy–immunology specialist include:

- Patients with other comorbid airway diseases (asthma, sinusitis, otitis media, nasal polyps)
- Patients with intolerable side-effects from medications
- Patients who do not respond to typical medical management
- Patients with occupational rhinitis
- Patients whose diagnosis is in question

NONALLERGIC RHINITIS

Nonallergic rhinitis is a term for a group of nasal diseases in which there are rhinitis symptoms without evidence of allergic cause. Some researchers have suggested that nonallergic rhinitis can account for one-quarter to one-half of the patients presenting to the physician with chronic nasal symptoms. Nonallergic rhinitis can be further divided into nonanatomic and anatomic causes.

Nonanatomic—Presentation and Progression

Clinical Presentation

Atrophic rhinitis. Atrophic rhinitis is an infrequent cause of rhinitis symptoms. Extensive loss or resection of nasal tissue can create a paradoxical nasal obstruction because of crusting and drainage. This condition results in the clinical presentation termed ozena (foulsmelling discharge). There is progressive atrophy of the nasal mucosa and in severe cases, loss of underlying bone. Primary atrophic rhinitis appears to result from *Klebsiella* colonization, and is most frequently encountered in underdeveloped countries. Secondary atrophic rhinitis may develop after overaggressive nasal surgery. The surgeon operating on the nasal turbinate tissue must take care to preserve sufficient mucosa.

Drug-induced Rhinitis. Medications prescribed for non-nasal indications can cause nasal symptoms. The most notorious offenders are antihypertensive medications (Table 8–4). These medications are available alone or in combination with diuretics. Aspirin and other nonsteroidal anti-inflammatory agents, oral contraceptives, and conjugated estrogens can also cause rhinitis.

Rhinitis Medicamentosa. Rhinitis medicamentosa describes abuse of decongestants, usually topically applied, such as oxymetazoline, phenylephrine, or cocaine. Upon initial use, intense vasoconstriction results in a dramatically clear nasal passage. Withdrawal of the medication results in rebound nasal congestion, encouraging repeated medication use. Rhinitis medicamentosa usually occurs if topical decongestant nasal sprays are used for longer than 5 to 7 days. The nasal mucosa becomes hyperemic and congested, and punctate bleeding may be seen. The pathophysiology of rhinitis medicamentosa is not known. Treatment requires that the patient discontinue the offending decongestant spray and the underlying nasal disease be evaluated and treated. The addition of topical steroid nasal sprays, and frequently a short course of oral steroids will help the patient break this vicious circle.

Hormonal Rhinitis. Significant nasal symptoms can affect approximately one-third of all pregnant women. The cause of nasal symptoms has been attributed to elevated hormone levels affecting the nasal mucosa as well as an increase in nasal vascular pooling because of increased circulating blood volume. However, the exact mechanism is not known. Rhinitis

Table 8–4. **Antihypertensive Medications Associated with Nasal Symptoms**

Class of Antihypertensive Medication	Examples
Antiadrenergic blockers	
Centrally acting	Clonidine, guanabenz, methyldopa
Peripherally acting	Guanethidine, prazosin, reserpine, terazosin
Alpha or beta adrenergic blockers	Labetalol
Vasodilators	Hydralazine, isosorbide mononitrate
Other	Indapamide

usually occurs at the end of the first trimester and resolves shortly after delivery. Oral contraceptives and conjugated estrogens can also contribute to nasal symptoms.

Patients with hypothyroidism may present with nasal congestion, rhinorrhea, or both. Thyroid function tests should be obtained especially in elderly patients with negative skin test results who have persistent nasal symptoms.

Idiopathic (Vasomotor) Rhinitis. A better term for vasomotor rhinitis is noninfectious, nonallergic, idiopathic rhinitis. Patients with idiopathic rhinitis have year-round symptoms of nasal congestion, rhinorrhea, and postnasal drainage with minimal sneezing, pruritus, or conjunctival symptoms. The pathophysiology is not proved, but the nasal mucosa reacts dramatically to relatively mild, nonimmunologic stimuli such as strong smells (perfumes, solvents, bleach), irritants (cigarette smoke, dusts, exhaust fumes), alcohol ingestion, and changes in temperature or humidity. The nasal smear does not show eosinophilia, and allergy skin testing results are negative. Often, treatment is not satisfactory but should be tailored to the patient's symptoms. Oral decongestants, topical ipratropium, topical nasal steroid sprays, and saline irrigation can help alleviate symptoms, with varying success.

Infectious Rhinitis. The most common condition causing rhinitis is the common cold. More than 200 viruses can cause colds. Symptoms typically resolve within 7 to 10 days. An average child has three to six common colds per year, with younger children and those attending day care the most affected. Persistence of nasal symptoms beyond 10 days can lead to sinusitis. The term rhinosinusitis is more exact than sinusitis, as rhinitis frequently precedes and complicates sinusitis. Sinusitis can easily be mistaken for perennial allergic rhinitis. Although history is important, imaging studies and allergy testing may be needed to differentiate between these conditions. Further information regarding sinusitis is available in Chapter 9, Sinusitis, Otitis Media, and Nasal Polyps.

Nonallergic Rhinitis with Eosinophilia Syndrome. Nonallergic rhinitis with eosinophilia syndrome (NARES) was first described in 1981 and is characterized by abundant eosinophils on nasal smear without evidence of allergic disease. Patients have year-round symptoms of rhinorrhea, nasal congestion, mild pruritus, sneezing, and occasionally anosmia. Nasal polyps and sinusitis are a common complication. Some researchers have suggested that nasal eosinophilia may represent an early stage of nasal polyps and aspirin sensitivity. The mechanism of NARES is unknown. Topical nasal steroid sprays are the most effective therapy.

Physical Rhinitis. Physical triggers of rhinitis symptoms include cold air (skier's nose), hot or spicy food ingestion (gustatory rhinitis), and exposure to bright light (reflex rhinitis). Gustatory rhinitis is a glandular response induced by a cholinergic reflex. It is unknown why some patients suffer from this more than others. Treatment with topical anticholinergic agents (ipratropium) and decongestants are the treatment of choice.

Anatomic—Presentation and Progression

Clinical Presentation

Approximately 5% to 10% of chronic nasal problems are due to anatomic causes. The varying etiologies of anatomic problems depend upon the age of the person affected.

Adenoidal Hypertrophy. The most common anatomic problem seen in young children is obstruction caused by adenoidal hypertrophy. Adenoidal hypertrophy can be suspected from symptoms such as mouth breathing, snoring, hyponasal speech, and persistent rhinitis with or without chronic otitis media. Infection of the nasopharynx may be related to infected hypertrophied adenoid tissue. A recent study reported that simple clinical assessment of a child's nasopharyngeal airway by observation of mouth breathing and hyponasal speech provides satisfactory assessment of the presence and degree of adenoidal obstruction. Further diagnostic tests to visualize the adenoids include a lateral soft-tissue neck film, indirect mirror evaluation of the nasopharynx, or direct rhinoscopy.

Cerebrospinal Fluid Rhinorrhea. Cerebrospinal fluid (CSF) rhinorrhea is usually post-traumatic or post-surgical, although spontaneous cases have been reported. CSF leaks caused by trauma usually present within the first 48 hours after injury, but can be delayed for up to 3 months. There is clear, watery rhinorrhea, often unilateral. Since CSF contains glucose, an easy test is to check a glucose dipstick; however, more definitive diagnostic tests should be performed. Analysis for beta-2 transferrin, a CSF protein, is a highly specific assay. Another definitive test includes the use of a radioactive tracer. The tracer is injected intrathecally by spinal tap, and nasal pledgets are placed, then removed and scanned for the presence of radioactivity.

Choanal Atresia. Choanal atresia, the most common congenital anomaly of the nose, consists of a bony or membranous septum between the nose and pharynx, either unilateral or bilateral. Bilateral choanal atresia classically presents in neonates as cyclic cyanosis because neonates are preferential nose breathers. Airway obstruction and cyanosis are relieved when the mouth is opened to cry and recurs when the calming infant tries to breathe through the nose. Some newborns only demonstrate respiratory difficulty while feeding. Unilateral choanal atresia may go undiagnosed until later in life and presents with symptoms of unilateral nasal obstruction and discharge.

Foreign Bodies. Foreign bodies also more commonly occur in young children who hide food, small toys, stones, or erasers in their noses. Psychiatric patients and senile adults are also at risk. The index of suspicion should be raised by a history of unilateral, purulent nasal discharge. The foreign body can often be seen on examination with a nasal speculum.

Granulomas. Patients with Wegener's granulomatosis, sarcoidosis, relapsing polychondritis, and midline granuloma may have chronic rhinitis symptoms. For some patients, the systemic disease may not be evident at the time the patient presents with nasal complaints. Granulomatous nasal lesions also may be caused by infections, such as tuberculosis, syphilis, leprosy, sporotrichosis, blastomycosis, histoplasmosis, and coccidioidomycosis.

Nasal Polyps. Nasal polyps typically appear as bilateral, gray-glistening sacs originating from the ethmoid sinuses. The pathogenesis of polyp formation is unknown. For adults, they represent one of the most common causes of nasal obstruction and are frequently associated with aspirin sensitivity and asthma (Samter's triad). Nasal polyps are rare in children younger than 10 years old, and if polyps are seen in children, an evaluation for an underlying disease process such as cystic fibrosis is warranted. The incidence of nasal polyposis has been reported to range from 6% to 48% of patients with cystic fibrosis. Nasal polyposis also can occur in patients with primary ciliary dyskinesia. Chronic sinusitis may result from sinonasal outlet obstruction. Systemic corticosteroids are often tried before surgical polypectomy because nasal polyps frequently recur. Topical nasal steroid sprays are advised to shrink small polyps and to prevent recurrence after surgery.

Septal Deviation and Turbinate Hypertrophy. Septal deviation and turbinate hypertrophy are common anatomic causes of nasal obstruction. In infants, nasal septal deviation can be congenital or caused by birth trauma. In older children and adults, facial trauma from sports, or automobile or bicycle accidents can result in septal deformity. Nasal septal deformity also can occur with normal nasal growth and does not always imply trauma. Hypertrophy of the turbinates also can cause nasal obstruction and can be aggravated by concomitant rhinitis. Severe anatomic abnormalities of the septum or turbinates may benefit from surgical intervention.

Tumors. Tumors, such as chordoma, chemodectoma, neurofibroma, inverting papilloma, squamous cell carcinoma, sarcoma, lymphoma, and olfactory neuroblastoma, are extremely rare causes of anatomic obstruction. Other unusual congenital lesions include dermoid cysts, teratomas, gliomas, encephaloceles, and meningoceles that present as insidious nasal obstruction in children. In adolescent boys, nasal obstruction and severe, recurring nosebleeds may be a sign of angiofibroma, a benign tumor. Imaging and referral are recommended prior to biopsy of nasal tumors, as serious morbidity can accompany office biopsy of angiofibroma, meningoceles, or encephaloceles.

When to Refer

Any patient with a suspected anatomic reason for rhinitis should be referred to the otolaryngology specialist for a complete examination of the upper respiratory tract. Certainly, patients with life-threatening causes for rhinitis such as choanal atresia, CSF leaks, and tumors require prompt referral. The patient who has a nonallergic, nonanatomic cause of rhinitis may benefit from evaluation by either the allergy-immunology specialist or otolaryngology specialist. For optimal care, these specialists should work closely in conjunction with the primary care doctor in taking care of the many patients who suffer from rhinitis.

RESOURCES

American Academy of Allergy, Asthma & Immunology
611 East Wells Street
Milwaukee, WI 53202
(414)-272-6071

American College of Allergy, Asthma & Immunology
85 West Algonquin Road, Suite 550
Arlington Heights, IL 60005
(708)-427-1200

Suggested Reading

AAAI Board of Directors: Position statement. Guidelines to minimize the risk from systemic reactions caused by immunotherapy with allergenic extracts. J Allergy Clin Immunol 93:811, 1994

Baraniuk JN: Pathogenesis of allergic rhinitis. J Allergy Clin Immunol 99:S763, 1997

Druce HM: Allergic and nonallergic rhinitis. In Middleton E Jr, Reed CE, Ellis EF, et al (eds): Allergy: Principles and Practice. 5th ed. St. Louis, Mosby-Year Book, 1998, pp 1005–1016

Executive Summary: The impact of allergic rhinitis on quality of life and other airway diseases. Summary of a European conference. Allergy 53(Suppl 41):1, 1998

Grossman J: One airway, one disease. Chest 111:11S, 1997

Juniper EF: Impact of upper respiratory allergic diseases on quality of life. J Allergy Clin Immunol 101:S396, 1998

Meltzer EO: Treatment options for the child with allergic rhinitis. Clin Pediatr 37:1, 1998

Milgrom H, Bender B: Adverse effects of medications for rhinitis. Ann Allergy Asthma Immunol 78:439, 1997

Naclerio R: Allergic rhinitis. N Engl J Med 325:860, 1991

Nelson HS: Immunotherapy for inhalant allergens. In Middleton E Jr, Reed CE, Ellis EF, et al (eds.): Allergy: Principles and Practice. 5th ed. St. Louis, Mosby-Year Book 1998, pp 1050–1062

Settipane RA, Settipane GA: Nonallergic rhinitis. Immunol Allergy Clin North Am 16:49, 1996

Simons FER, Simon KJ: The pharmacology and use of H1-receptor-antagonist drugs. N Engl J Med 330:1663, 1994

Slavin RG: Occupational rhinitis. Immunol Allergy Clin North Am 12:769, 1992

Solomon WR, Platts-Mills TAE: Aerobiology and inhalant allergen. *In* Middleton E Jr, Reed CE, Ellis EF, et al (eds): Allergy: Principles and Practice. 5th ed. St. Louis, Mosby-Year Book, 1998, pp 367–403

Spector SL: Overview of comorbid associations of allergic rhinitis. J Allergy Clin Immunol 99:S773, 1997

KEY POINTS

▶ Allergic rhinitis, the most common atopic disease, affects 15% to 25% of the U.S. population.

▶ The diagnosis of allergic rhinitis is based on history, physical examination, and allergy testing (either *in vivo* or *in vitro*).

▶ Nonallergic rhinitis, a diagnosis of exclusion, is assigned to patients with chronic nasal complaints who undergo allergy evaluation and no identifiable allergen is found. Anatomic and other identifiable causes should be considered and referred appropriately.

▶ Differentiating between allergic and nonallergic rhinitis will guide the clinician in choosing appropriate therapy for the patient.

▶ Patients who have other comorbid airway diseases, have severe side-effects from medications, are not responding to typical medical management, or have occupational rhinitis may benefit from a referral to the allergy-immunology specialist. Patients whose diagnosis is in question also should be referred.

Chapter 9

Sinusitis, Otitis Media, and Nasal Polyps

Frank S. Virant

For any clinician treating allergic patients, sinusitis, otitis media, and nasal polyps are common complications. Accordingly, when routine therapy for allergic rhinitis is not successful, it is important to be vigilant for subtle clinical signs of these new, secondary problems. The opposite is also true: when presented with recurrent sinusitis, recurrent otitis media, and nasal polyps, underlying allergic rhinitis should be considered and appropriately evaluated.

This chapter reviews sinusitis, otitis media, and nasal polyps with emphasis on clinical presentation, diagnosis, treatment, and when to refer for appropriate subspecialty care.

SINUSITIS

Clinical Presentation

Pathophysiology

Sinusitis develops when normal mucociliary clearance of secretions from the sinuses is disrupted. Obstruction of the sinus ostia is often critical in this pathway, leading to stasis within the sinus cavities. Maxillary sinus ostia are usually 2.5 to 4 mm in diameter and are located in the middle meatus between the inferior and middle turbinate bones; typically the highest point of the entrance to these ostia is near the orbital floor. With this in mind, it is easy to understand why the maxillary ostia do not benefit from gravity-dependent drainage while the patient is upright. The ethmoid sinus ostia

are generally very small, increasing their likelihood for occlusion when local mucosal edema occurs. The ostia of the frontal and sphenoid sinuses are significantly larger and thus less likely to be obstructed; exceptions are when there are accessory frontal sinuses with independent ostia and when the sphenoid ostium is several millimeters superior to the sphenoid sinus floor.

Several factors may increase the likelihood of ostial obstruction; these can be loosely divided into those that cause mucosal swelling and others that are direct mechanical factors (Table 9–1). Mucosal swelling is typically related to inflammation, e.g., secondary to a systemic disease such as cystic fibrosis or immunodeficiency, or related to tissue irritation, e.g., barotrauma or cigarette smoke. As a practical point, viral upper respiratory infections,

Table 9–1. **Sources of Sinus Ostial Obstruction***

Mucosal Swelling	Mechanical Factors
Viral upper respiratory tract infections	Choanal atresia
Allergic rhinitis	Septal deviation
Asthma	Polyps
Cystic fibrosis	Foreign bodies
Immunodeficiency	Tumor
Immotile cilia syndrome	
Down's syndrome	
Trauma, barotrauma	
Dental infections	
Cigarette smoke (?)	
Pollution (?)	

*From Rachelefsky GS, Katz RM, Siegel SC: Curr Probl Pediatr 12:1–57, 1982; used by permission.

allergic rhinitis, and nasal polyps are the most common causes of ostial obstruction. Prolonged sinus ostial obstruction promotes the development of bacterial sinusitis by inducing negative intranasal pressure and congestion. Ironically, when this occurs, patients often respond by blowing and sniffing, which may actually increase the chance of bacteria entering the sinuses. Risk for sinusitis is further enhanced when the ostia transiently open and are exposed to higher atmospheric pressures. With nasal congestion and subsequent mouth breathing, the sinus cavities become a more anaerobic environment, which favors the growth of many pathogens.

Mucociliary dysfunction also can be an important factor increasing the chances for sinusitis. The mucociliary apparatus includes cilia, thin hairlike projections from the surface of the columnar respiratory epithelia, and the overlying mucus layer. There are well-described congenital abnormalities of ciliary structure that can lead to abnormal synchrony of ciliary movement and hence related decreased mucus mobility. Clinically, it is much more common for external factors such as viral upper respiratory infections, cold or dry air, or any source of inflammation to impair mucociliary function.

Bacteriology

Ideally, antibiotic therapy for sinusitis should be based on direct culture results. The most direct access is a transnasal approach into the maxillary sinus; this procedure is painful and time consuming, and rarely done in routine practice. In select patients, in whom culture-guided therapy might obviate the need for surgical intervention, cultures are obtained by first sterilizing the nasal site to prevent contamination from beneath the inferior turbinate. Topical 4% cocaine is an ideal pretreatment agent because this solution is not irritating, provides local anesthesia, and is a good antiseptic. Culture results that best correlate with clinical infection are those with $\geq 10^4$ colony forming units/ml (cfu/ml). Another alternative to quantitative culture is a semiquantitative Gram stain of the aspirate. Generally, the appearance of an organism on such a stain equates to $\geq 10^5$ cfu/ml. Patients with

chronic or protracted disease also may need a sinus biopsy procedure to obtain specimens for careful anerobic and fungal cultures and appropriate stains.

Pathogens in Pediatric Patients. Regrettably, there have not been many good clinical studies of microbiology in pediatric sinusitis.

A major study by Wald and colleagues, in 1979, involved sinus punctures in children aged 2 to 16 years with a history of at least a 10-day (but less than 30-day) history of upper respiratory symptoms. Sinus aspirates were obtained only if the patient demonstrated radiographic opacification, air–fluid level or ≥ 4 mm mucosal thickening of either side. Significant levels of bacteria ($\geq 10^4$) were recovered in 70%. The relative prevalence of bacterial species obtained from 79 aspirates in 50 children is shown in Table 9–2. *Streptococcus pneumoniae, Moraxella catarrhalis,* and *Haemophilus influenzae* were the most prevalent. The *Moraxella* and *Haemophilus* species were frequently β-lactamase–positive. This study also confirmed that the *Haemophilus* organisms were always nontypeable, similar to the pattern observed in otitis media. Other studies in pediatric patients with acute or subacute sinusitis have confirmed that *Streptococcus, Moraxella,* and *Haemophilus* are the three most common isolates (although the rank order varies from study to study).

In contrast, results of microbiologic studies in children with chronic sinusitis have been discordant. A 1981 study by Brook evaluated 40 children with chronic sinusitis, noting that the most common organisms were anaerobic gram-positive cocci, *Bacteroides* species, and fu-

Table 9–2. **Bacterial Isolates in Acute Pediatric Sinusitis**∗

Organism	Single Isolate	Multiple Isolates	Total
Streptococcus pneumoniae	14	8	22
Moraxella catarrhalis	13	2	15
Haemophilus influenzae	10	5	15
Eikenella corrodens	1	0	1
Group A *Streptococci*	1	0	1
Group C *Streptococci*	0	0	1
α-Hemolytic *Streptococcus*	1	1	2
Peptostreptococcus	0	1	1
Moraxella species	1	0	1

∗From Wald ER, Reilly JS, Casselbrant M, et al: J Pediatr 104:297–302, 1984; used by permission.

sobacteria. Another study by Muntz and Lusk involved culture of ethmoid bullae in children with chronic sinus disease. This group also found α-hemolytic streptococci and staphylococci, but also isolated *Moraxella catarrhalis, Haemophilus influenzae,* and *Streptococcus pneumoniae,* the organisms usually seen in more acute disease. Three other studies, despite very heterogeneous patient groups, all found that the most common isolates were the same as those seen in acute or subacute disease, with streptococci and staphylococci only rarely.

Children with cystic fibrosis are a unique patient group in whom chronic sinusitis (particularly in patients over 5 years of age) is almost universally observed. Cultures in this setting suggest that the most common organisms are *Pseudomonas aeruginosa, Haemophilus influenzae,* and α-hemolytic streptococci.

Pathogens in Adult Patients. A long-term study by Gwaltney et al indicates that the most common causes of acute community-acquired sinusitis in adults are *Streptococcus pneumoniae* and *Haemophilus influenzae* (Table 9–3). Similar to the findings in children, *Staphylococcus aureus* and *Streptococcus pyogenes* were rare isolates. A study by O'Reilly et al examined acute nosocomial sinusitis, particularly in patients with nasotracheal intubation and found gram-negative enteric bacteria: *Pseudomonas aeruginosa, Klebsiella pneumoniae, Serratia marcescens, Proteus mirabilis,* and *Enterobacter* species.

Mirroring the situation in children, the microbiology of chronic sinusitis in adults is controversial, with some studies showing the typical acute organisms, and others suggesting that anaerobes and staphylococci are more im-

portant. Perhaps the best explanation for these results is that chronic sinusitis is a heterogeneous disease in which all patients have chronic inflammation. Despite a similar clinical picture, some patients may have acute infectious exacerbations, others low-grade, subtle infections, and others no infection at all; culture results simply depend on when you see the patient.

Fungal sinusitis, although rare, should be considered in patients with chronic refractory disease. Although literally dozens of fungi have been reported to cause disease, *Aspergillus* species, particularly *A. fumigatus,* are most common. In immunosuppressed patients, such organisms can be quite invasive and also can lead to formation of an intracranial mass, pneumonitis, hepatitis, or meningitis.

Unique organisms to consider in the immune-compromised host include: atypical mycobacteria, *Mycobacterium chelonae,* protozoa such as *Cryptosporidium,* parasites such as *Acanthamoeba* and *Pneumocystis carinii.*

History

The clinical history that best correlates with infectious sinusitis is that of a typical upper respiratory infection that hasn't run its course over 7 to 10 days. The most predictable, persistent symptoms in this setting are nasal congestion and cough. Rhinorrhea is variable it may not be apparent if congestion is severe, and may be either clear or purulent. In the pediatric patient, who frequently has more difficulty handling secretions, a common symptom of sinusitis is cough, particularly at night, and often to the point of vomiting.

Associated symptoms in affected patients may include halitosis, sore throat, irritability, and fatigue. Fever, sinus discomfort, and headache are relatively less common, particularly in patients with a more prolonged history.

It is important to realize that because symptoms are nonspecific, patients with sinusitis may not appreciate that they have a new problem, but rather complain that their usual therapy for known conditions such as allergic rhinitis or asthma is no longer effective. If the clinical history does not support a diagnosis of straightforward, severe allergic rhinitis or offer another obvious reason for asthma exacerba-

Table 9–3. **Bacterial Causes of Acute Maxillary Sinusitis from 383 Aspirates in Charlottesville from 1975–1990**∗

Causes	No.	Percent
Streptococcus pneumoniae	92	41
Haemophilus influenzae	79	35
Anaerobes	16	7
Streptococcal species	16	7
Moraxella catarrhalis	8	4
Staphylococcus aureus	7	3
Other	8	4

∗From Gwaltney JM Jr, Scheld WM, Sande MA, et al: J Allergy Clin Immunol 90S:457–461, 1992; used by permission.

tion, the possibility of sinusitis should be considered strongly.

Physical Examination

Examination of the patient with suspected sinusitis begins with documenting general appearance. Frequently patients will exhibit signs of upper airway congestion and edema, manifest as facial pallor and associated dark infraorbital circles and swelling. This picture is intensified if nocturnal coughing and extreme congestion have interrupted normal sleep patterns.

Sinusitis typically causes the nasal mucosa to be edematous and hyperemic. Mucopurulent drainage often can be observed in the nasal passages and on the nasopharynx floor. At the same time, it is important to remember that these clinical signs of sinusitis will obscure the underlying features of uncomplicated allergic rhinitis, pale, boggy mucosa with watery rhinorrhea. Accordingly, if underlying allergy is suspected, the clinician must rely more on nasal cytology results and clinical history in assessing the likelihood of atopy.

The middle ear should also be carefully examined, particularly in children, in whom sinusitis is associated nearly 50% of the time with serous otitis and eustachian tube dysfunction. If the sinusitis resolves but the middle ear fluid does not, underlying rhinitis should be suspected and evaluated.

Sinusitis may exacerbate asthma by increasing the need for mouth breathing and inducing bronchial hyper-responsiveness through neural pathways. This effect may be subtle because cough is a nearly universal clinical sign in sinusitis. To avoid overlooking this secondary problem, it is important to listen to the patient's chest for wheezing and to measure baseline pulmonary function.

Diagnosis

The diagnosis of sinusitis is largely clinical, based on a careful review of the history and a detailed physical examination. At the same time, many of the signs and symptoms of sinusitis are nonspecific and, ironically, are often shared with underlying disorders (see Table

9–1). Therefore it may be helpful to add various ancillary studies to clarify the clinical picture. The following section reviews several potential supportive tests with comments regarding the clinical value and limitations of each test.

Nasal Cytology

Examination of nasal secretions frequently provides useful clues about the cause of upper respiratory complaints (Table 9–4). Sinusitis is associated with a predominance of neutrophils, often with intracellular bacteria. Neutrophils also are observed with upper respiratory infections or other irritant forms of rhinitis; thus, it is crucial to view nasal cytology results in the context of the history. The appearance of ≥10% eosinophils strongly suggests the possibility of an allergic component, particularly in children. The presence of eosinophils can be an important finding in the patient with recurrent or refractory sinus disease. At the same time, absence of eosinophils in the upper airway on a single sample in the sinusitis patient does not exclude the possibility of allergic rhinitis.

Transillumination

Unfortunately, considering the simple, rapid, noninvasive nature of the technique, transillumination of the sinuses is neither specific nor sensitive. Frequently, patients will have congenital asymmetry in sinus development; transillumination can falsely suggest this to be unilateral sinusitis. Similarly, given the wide spectrum of normal maxillary contour and size, transillumination cannot easily discriminate between mild, bilateral mucosal thickening and normal, smaller sinuses.

Fiberoptic Rhinoscopy

Rhinoscopy could be considered the gold standard for the diagnosis of sinusitis in cases in which the examiner can directly document purulent secretions escaping from the sinus ostia. Drawbacks of this technique include significant preparation time, the requirement for

Table 9–4. **Differential Diagnosis of Rhinitis***

	Eosinophilic Allergic	Eosinophilic Nonallergic	Neutrophilic	Vasomotor
Clinical findings	Typically during childhood	Adulthood, early	Any age	Adulthood, rare in children
	Sneezing, nasal pruritus, clear rhinorrhea	Severe obstruction; anosmia, polyps common	Purulent secretions, sinus tenderness, nocturnal cough	Congestion, minimal rhinorrhea
	Episodic or perennial	Perennial symptoms	Appearance most common during fall and winter	Variable presentation
	Triggers are often obvious (e.g., dust mites, animals, pollens)	Aspirin sensitive often; frequent asthma and sinus disease	Infection typical; can be caused by irritation (e.g., cigarette or wood smoke)	Can be hormonal (e.g., thyroid disease, pregnancy)
Nasal cytology	Eosinophils	Eosinophils	Neutrophils often with intracellular bacteria	Unremarkable generally
	± Basophils	± Basophils		
	± Neutrophils	± Neutrophils		

*From Virant FS, Shapiro GG: Medical management of sinusitis in children. *In* Druce HM (ed): Sinusitis: Pathophysiology and Treatment. New York, Marcel Dekker, 1993, pp 87–106. By courtesy of Marcel Dekker, Inc.

patient cooperation, and moderate discomfort. Accordingly, this is not a practical study for most children, and probably should be reserved for adults with simultaneous concerns regarding upper airway anatomy, e.g., nasal polyps, septal deviation, and so forth.

Ultrasound

Sinus ultrasound is diagnostic only in the presence of complete opacification or air–fluid levels, and requires complete patient cooperation. As with transillumination, mild mucosal thickening cannot be differentiated from normal smaller anatomy. With these limitations, it is not surprising that the sensitivity and specificity of sinus ultrasound is about 50% to 60%.

Radiographic Imaging

Standard radiographs are still commonly used to assist in the evaluation of suspected new-onset sinusitis. In practice, radiographic imaging is reasonable because maxillary sinuses are nearly always involved in acute or subacute disease. For this group of patients, a Waters view is often adequate. In contrast, patients with chronic sinusitis almost uniformly have ethmoid disease; in fact after prolonged treatment they may have *only* ethmoid disease. In this setting, standard radiographic views are rarely helpful because the fine details of the

ethmoids are typically obscured by structural superimposition.

Computed tomography (CT) provides an ideal study of all of the paranasal sinuses and related anatomy. CT is the technique of choice in patients in whom maximal medical therapy has failed or in whom occult isolated ethmoid disease is suspected. The result of the coronal CT provides crucial information that allows the clinician to make appropriate decisions regarding therapy: surgical intervention versus additional aggressive medication versus consideration of unrelated nasal disorders.

The clinical value of the coronal sinus CT scan is enhanced if the patient with chronic disease has been already treated with a prolonged period of antibiotics, decongestants, corticosteroids, and so forth, so that underlying obstructing anatomy can be differentiated from local edema or fluid. In this setting, extra 1-mm cuts should be included through the osteomeatal complex (OMC), a critical drainage area for the anterior ethmoid, maxillary, and frontal sinuses. A more limited study with simple 3-mm cuts is appropriate for excluding occult ethmoid sinusitis; in many centers, the cost of this type of CT scan is comparable to that of a standard radiographic series (Caldwell, Waters, and lateral).

Axial CT scanning should be performed to exclude orbital complications when a patient presents with periorbital swelling or proptosis. Magnetic resonance imaging (MRI) should be considered to provide optimal visualization of soft tissues when the CT image or the clinical picture suggests intracranial involvement.

Associated Factors

Allergic Rhinitis

Underlying allergic rhinitis should be considered in any patient with recurrent or refractory sinusitis. The odds of upper airway allergy are significantly increased when nasal eosinophilia and a positive family history of atopy are present. Prior to exploring possible allergic rhinitis, an environmental history should be obtained with emphasis on exposure to perennial allergens such as dust mites, animals, and molds, or a suggestion of a seasonal component compatible with tree, grass, or weed pollen allergy.

Evaluation for allergic rhinitis includes prick or puncture skin tests for relevant inhalant allergens. In the younger child, testing should focus on perennial exposures that can be influenced by environmental controls such as dust mites, pets, and indoor mold. In the older child and adult, evaluation should also include pollens, and selected intradermal tests should be considered to enhance sensitivity. This comprehensive approach also provides a framework for specific immunotherapy if the patient's response to environmental control and medication is not adequate.

Testing for foods is not appropriate unless there is a strong history of a food consistently provoking upper respiratory symptoms. Without such a history, the predictive value of a positive skin test result for a food is only 40 to 50%.

Multiple clinical studies suggest that the incidence of allergic rhinitis is much higher in patients with sinusitis than in the general population. Challenge studies have demonstrated that nasal exposure to allergens can provoke a surprisingly rapid change in sinus mucosal edema (even opacification). Other *in vitro* studies strongly suggest that the eosinophil, more specifically major basic protein, may be an important pathologic link by altering mucosal surfaces and inhibiting ciliary function.

Considering that viruses may also directly and indirectly cause mucosal dysfunction, it is not difficult to envision how the combination of an upper respiratory infection and allergic rhinitis might provide the ideal environment for subsequent bacterial sinusitis.

Nasal Polyps

In a subset of patients with chronic sinusitis, nasal polyps represent a frustrating, frequently recurring associated problem. This important phenomenon is discussed in detail as a separate section later in this chapter.

Immunodeficiency

The possibility of immunodeficiency should be considered in patients with persistent or refractory sinus disease. This is particularly true for children in whom surgical intervention for sinusitis is planned; if immunodeficiency is present and undiagnosed, the operation will rarely be of long-term benefit.

Typically, the nature of immunodeficiency that occurs with recurrent or persistent sinusitis involves defects of antibody production. An appropriate screen therefore includes measurements of serum IgG, IgA, IgM, and IgE. Occasionally, more subtle forms of immune dysfunction will prompt the need for more detailed evaluation.

In patients over 2 years of age, the possibility of a lacunar immune defect should be considered, for example, poor response to polysaccharide antigens, even if the serum total immunoglobulins are normal. Rarely, such a defect will be diagnosed by a deficiency of an IgG subclass, such as IgG_2, being low or absent. Unfortunately, IgG subclass determinations are not very specific; low levels can occur in immunocompetent, normal patients and in those with clinically important immune deficits. With this in mind, a more valuable test is a qualitative challenge, for example, response to pneumococcal vaccine, measuring pre- and 4 weeks postvaccine specific antibody titers.

Some children with recurrent sinusitis will have transient developmental immunodeficiency, suboptimal but not absent polysaccharide responses. The use of prophylactic antibiotics may be a viable alternative therapy for such children. In contrast, most immunodeficient adolescents or adults will not outgrow their immune problem. Ideal treatment for these patients involves replacement therapy with monthly intravenous immunoglobulin (IVIG) at 400 mg/kg/dose. IVIG solutions should not be used empirically, but only after demonstrating *bona fide* immunodeficiency; these products are extremely expensive and have significant potential side effects.

Dysmotile Cilia

Although rare, the possibility of abnormal ciliary function should be considered in patients with persistent or recurrent sinusitis. Ciliary dysmotility should be suspected when patients' conditions have not improved despite optimal medical and surgical therapy for sinusitis, particularly in the absence of associated rhinitis or polyps.

In addition to virtually universal productive cough and recurrent or chronic sinusitis, nearly half of patients with dysmotile cilia will have *situs inversus* and bronchiectasis. This constellation of symptoms, Kartagener's syndrome, occurs in 1 of 15,000 to 30,000 births. A separate clue to possible ciliary dysfunction in men is infertility (secondary to ultrastructural defects of cilia in spermatozoa).

Abnormal ciliary function is primarily caused by ultrastructural defects. Normally the cilium axoneme extends from the cell membrane in a typical 9 + 2 arrangement of microtubules (Fig. 9–1). Centrally, a pair of two microtubules is surrounded by a helical sheath. The central section is surrounded by nine pairs of microtubules. Cilial integrity results from the action of nexin links and radial spokes. Dynein arms reach clockwise from one doublet to the adjacent doublet. Although all structures are important, the dynein arms are critical because they contain enzymes that ensure proper energy release for sliding and bending of the microtubules and subsequent ciliary motility. Electron microscopy has documented several ciliary defects including absent dynein arms, collapsed radial spokes, absence of central sheaths, and absence of one or both central microtubules.

A reasonable screening assessment for ciliary function is the saccharin test. This simple

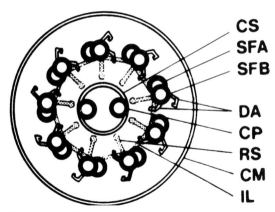

Figure 9–1. Diagram of a ciliary axoneme in cross section. *CS* = central sheath; *SFA* = subfiber A; *SFB* = subfiber B; *DA* = dynein arm; *CP* = central pair of microtubules; *RS* = radial spoke; *CM* = cell membrane; *IL* = interdoublet link (nexin). (From Rossman CM, Newhouse MT: Primary ciliary dyskinesia: Evaluation and management. Pediatric Pulmonol 5:36–50. © 1988. Reprinted by permission of Wiley-Liss, Inc., a subsidiary of John Wiley & Sons, Inc.)

procedure measures the time required for a patient to perceive sweetness after placing saccharin on the anterior surface of the inferior turbinate. Normally this takes about 19 minutes; if no taste is appreciated by 60 minutes, the test is terminated. Exogenous factors may alter any ciliary function test result, so it is important that a patient not have had an upper respiratory infection for at least 6 weeks before assessment; abstinence from smoking or caffeine for at least 3 hours before testing is also appropriate. When the saccharin test result appears abnormal, results can be confirmed by examining cilia (brush sample) for motion analysis and also ultrastructure by electron microscopy.

Effective daily saline nasal lavage and vigorous pulmonary toilet along with early antibiotic therapy for infections are the treatments of choice for ciliary dysfunction. Associated rhinorrhea can be effectively controlled with nasal ipratropium bromide up to 4 times daily.

Medical Therapy

Antibiotics

The primary treatment for acute, subacute, and chronic sinusitis is antibiotics (Table 9–5). In clinical practice, a direct sinus sample is rarely obtained for culture. Accordingly,

Table 9–5. **Antibiotics for Sinusitis***

Antibiotic	Pediatric Dosage	Adult Dosage
Amoxicillin	13 mg/kg TID	250–500 mg TID
Amoxicillin/potassium clavulanate	13 mg/kg TID†	250–500 mg TID†
	22.5 mg/kg BID†	500–875 mg BID†
Erythromycin/sulfisoxazole	12.5/37.5 mg/kg QID	–
Sulfamethoxazole/trimethoprim	20/4 mg/kg BID	800/160 BID
Cefaclor	13 mg/kg TID	250–500 mg TID
Cefadroxil	15 mg/kg BID	500–1000 mg BID
Cefuroxime	7.5 mg/kg BID	250–500 mg BID
Cefpodoxime	5 mg/kg BID	200–400 mg BID
Cefprozil	15 mg/kg BID	250–500 mg BID
Cefixime	8 mg/kg QD	400 mg QD
Ceftibuten	9 mg/kg QD	400 mg QD
Loracarbef	7.5 mg/kg BID	200–400 mg BID
Azithromycin	5 mg/kg QD‡	250 mg QD‡
Clarithromycin	7.5 mg/kg BID	500 mg BID
Ciprofloxacin	–	500–700 mg BID
Levofloxacin	–	500 mg QD
Grepafloxacin	–	400 QD
Trovafloxacin	–	200 mg QD
Sparfloxacin	–	100 mg QD§
Clindamycin	5 mg/kg TID	150–450 mg TID, QID
Metronidazole	7.5 mg/kg TID	250–500 mg TID, QID

*Modified from Virant FS, Shapiro GG. Sinusitis. *In* Tierney DF (ed): Current Pulmonology. Chicago, Mosby-Year Book, 1994.
†Based on amoxicillin component.
‡Typically, 5-day course after 10 mg/kg (pediatric) or 500 mg (adult) load equals 10 days total therapy.
§After 200-mg loading dose.

choice of antibiotic is based on a knowledge of likely causative microorganisms. As noted earlier, regardless of disease duration, the most common bacteria cultured from infected sinuses are *S. pneumoniae, M. catarrhalis,* and *H. influenzae.* Owing to altered penicillin binding proteins in *S. pneumoniae* strains (20%–30%), and the presence of β-lactamase in *Moraxella* (90%–100%) and *Haemophilus* strains (30%–40%), nearly 30% to 40% of cultured organisms are resistant to amoxicillin. Despite this, amoxicillin remains a reasonable initial choice for uncomplicated sinusitis; it is usually effective, relatively inexpensive, and well tolerated.

Alternative initial antibiotics for sinusitis include sulfamethoxazole–trimethoprim (SMX–TMP), first-generation cephalosporins such as cephalexin, or the second-generation cephalosporin cefaclor. Again, some resistance is seen, but these less expensive generically available agents deserve consideration.

Poor response to initial therapy prompts consideration of agents with a broader spectrum of activity. The addition of potassium clavulanate to amoxicillin provides one such agent with improved resistance to β-lactamase–producing organisms. Newer cephalosporins, including cefpodoxime, cefuroxime, and cef-

prozil, also have the advantages of enhanced activity, twice daily administration, and suspension availability for pediatric use. Cefixime and ceftibuten are recent third generation cephalosporins with even better activity against β-lactamase producers and are administered orally once daily. With the emergence of more resistant *S. pneumoniae* strains (unrelated to β-lactamase), however, the clinical value of these agents may be compromised because they have less gram-positive activity. Additional appropriate broader spectrum antibiotics include the newer macrolides azithromycin and clarithromycin, and loracarbef (a carbacefem). In adults, several quinolones including ciprofloxacin, levofloxacin, grepafloxacin, and trovafloxacin, have a specific indication for sinusitis. Sparfloxacin also appears to have an appropriate spectrum but has a significant risk for phototoxicity. As a group, the quinolones appear to adversely affect developing joints and are accordingly contraindicated in children under 18 years of age.

As sinusitis becomes protracted, the possibility of anaerobic pathogens should be considered. Amoxicillin combined with clavulanate covers most of these organisms adequately including *Bacteroides* species. Alternatives include clindamycin or metronidazole either alone or in combination with one of the broader spectrum agents.

Duration of antibiotic therapy is not well defined. A 14-day course of antibiotics is usually adequate for most cases of acute sinusitis. If there is little clinical improvement within 5 days of initiating therapy, an alternative antibiotic should be considered. With subacute or chronic sinusitis in which drainage is often less than optimal, more prolonged therapy may be needed. Empirically extending antibiotics for at least 1 week beyond the time when symptoms have resolved seems appropriate.

Antibiotic prophylaxis may be a consideration in some patients with recurrent sinusitis, particularly those with borderline immune or anatomic abnormalities. One approach is initiating antibiotics at the first sign of an upper respiratory infection. If this fails, the next step would include once daily antibiotics through the fall and winter when more virulent organisms are more likely to compromise OMC drainage.

Alpha-Adrenergic Decongestants

Most studies suggest that α-adrenergic decongestants are a useful adjunctive therapy because of their ability to reduce nasal mucosal edema and airway resistance. These effects are clinically most useful early in the course of sinusitis to relieve congestive symptoms. Some authors express concern about prolonged use of decongestants especially topically, because such use could decrease local delivery of antibiotics and create a more anaerobic environment.

Corticosteroids

Regrettably, there are no conclusive studies regarding the use of corticosteroids in treating sinusitis. Although some studies suggest a trend favoring more rapid clinical improvement in patients treated with nasal corticosteroids as an adjunct to antibiotics, this finding has not been statistically significant. Neither is there any difference in patient groups at longer term follow-up. Criticisms of prior studies include failure to exclude patients with refractory anatomic problems, lack of patient stratification on the basis of underlying rhinitis, and choice and duration of concomittant antibiotic use. Pending the results of well-designed studies, the use of corticosteroids intuitively makes good clinical sense: a significant percentage of patients have underlying eosinophilic rhinitis or polyps that will be responsive to treatment and encourage better ostial drainage.

Saline and Mucolytics

Nasal irrigation with a buffered saline solution theoretically should improve mucus flow and provide a less satisfactory environment for many bacteria. The efficacy of this technique is limited in smaller children, because cooperation is required for lavage with either a bulb syringe or WaterPic attachment.

There are no adequate, controlled sinusitis studies addressing the utility of mucolytic or mucokinetic agents. Considering the similarities of sinus and bronchial respiratory epithelia, it's tempting to extrapolate from chronic bronchitis studies, which do suggest value in the use of *N*-acetylcysteine and iodinated glycerol.

Surgical Therapy

When aggressive medical therapy fails to achieve a good clinical response, surgical intervention should be contemplated. Medical therapy should include appropriate long-term antibiotics, saline nasal irrigation, decongestants, topical or oral corticosteroids, and adequate treatment of allergic rhinitis. Surgery should be strongly considered when the patient also suffers from related disorders that have a significant effect on quality of life, for example, severe nasal polyposis with complete nasal obstruction and anosmia, or severe persistent asthma.

When surgery is contemplated, a full coronal sinus CT scan should be performed to provide information about the extent of disease and OMC anatomy in particular. Often this study will show unique anatomic areas of concern that can be further elucidated with rhinoscopy.

Primary surgery for refractory sinusitis in young children (under age 4) generally includes maxillary lavage and adenoidectomy. Despite ethmoid involvement in many children, enhancing maxillary drainage and removing chronically infected adenoids often provides enough aeration that gravity-dependent ethmoid drainage will occur.

In older children, adolescents, and adults, intervention typically involves functional endoscopic sinus surgery (FESS). Commonly FESS involves the following procedures designed to enhance OMC drainage: uncinate process removal, ethmoid bullae and anterior ethmoid removal, enlargement of the natural maxillary ostia, and perforation of the basal lamina (posterior ethmoid disease). When sphenoid disease is present, the natural sphenoid ostium can be removed to create a large sphenoethmoid cavity. Surgical follow-up is critical during the 4 to 6 weeks after FESS to debride adhesions and prevent scarring until normal ciliary function is established. Patients with a history of recurrent polyp formation need close observation over time so that aggressive medical and minor surgical intervention can be instituted early in the course.

Subspecialty Referral

Allergist/Immunologist

Referral to an allergist/immunologist should be considered with the following clinical patterns:

- Seasonal sinusitis
- Prior significant perennial eosinophilic rhinitis
- Sinusitis refractory to prolonged antibiotic use
- Recurrent sinusitis (≥3 episodes/year)
- Sinusitis caused by low pathogenicity organisms
- Sinusitis and associated otitis media, asthma, nasal polyps, recurrent pneumonias, immunodeficiency, fungal sinus disease, granulomatous disease
- Multiple antibiotic allergies

Otorhinolaryngologist

Referral to an otorhinolaryngologist should be considered with the following clinical patterns:

- Failure of medical therapy for sinusitis leading to a need for endoscopic surgery to relieve obstruction of the OMC or chronic adenoid infection
- Anatomic airway obstruction caused by nasal polyps, concha bullosa, septal deviation, turbinate hypertrophy, or enlarged adenoids
- Need for maxillary antral diagnostic or therapeutic lavage
- Need for nasal biopsy for suspected neoplasm, fungal disease, granulomatous disease, or abnormal ciliary structure or function
- Endoscopic evaluation of sinus disease particularly in patients with borderline anatomy based on CT or those with immune dysfunction

KEY POINTS

▸ Sinusitis occurs after prolonged ostial obstruction; common causes include viral upper respiratory infections, eosinophilic rhinitis, and nasal polyps

▸ Common sinusitis pathogens regardless of disease duration include *Streptococcus pneumoniae, Moraxella catarrhalis,* and *Haemophilus influenzae;* anaerobes increase in frequency with protracted disease

▸ Bacterial sinusitis is a clinical diagnosis based on a ≥7- to 10-day history of nasal congestion, cough, ± purulent rhinorrhea

▸ Supportive useful diagnostic modalities include nasal cytology, radiographic imaging, and, in chronically affected adult patients, fiberoptic rhinoscopy

▸ Associated factors include allergic rhinitis, nasal polyps, immunodeficiency, and dysmotile cilia

▸ Antibiotics are primary medical therapy for suspected bacterial sinusitis with choice based on likely microorganisms, response to prior therapy, and disease duration; treatment should be continued at least 1 week after the patient's symptoms have resolved

▸ Useful adjunctive medical therapies include α-adrenergic decongestants, corticosteroids, saline irrigation, and mucolytics

▸ Surgical intervention should be contemplated when aggressive medical approaches fail: in young children this may include maxillary antral lavage and adenoidectomy; in older children and adults functional endoscopic surgery is directed against OMC obstruction

OTITIS MEDIA

Clinical Presentation

Pathophysiology

Otitis media occurs when there is prolonged stasis of secretions within the middle ear. Typically this is an end-point result of persistent, often worsening, eustachian tube dysfunction. Such dysfunction is usually associated with inflammatory disorders such as viral upper respiratory infections, allergic rhinitis, cigarette smoke exposure, or local anatomic impingement such as adenoid hypertrophy, or rarely functional problems with tubal compliance or with tensor veli palatini muscles. Given the relatively close proximity of the eustachian tube to the nasal cavity in children, the smaller anatomy of children, and the fact that adenoid tissue generally involutes by age 10 to 12, it should not be a surprise that otitis media is largely a pediatric disorder.

Bacteriology

The most common pathogens that cause acute otitis media are *Streptococcus pneumoniae,* *Haemophilus influenzae,* and *Moraxella catarrhalis.* Little data exist for subacute or chronic middle ear infections because they rarely occur; either the acute infection resolves completely or with residual fluid (otitis media with effusion) or worsening infection exacerbates middle ear pressure leading to tympanic membrane rupture, drainage, and resolution.

History

Acute otitis media is middle ear fluid accompanied by signs or symptoms of infection, such as a red, bulging tympanic membrane with pain or a perforated tympanic membrane with purulent material. Otitis media with effusion is middle ear fluid without the typical clinical signs or symptoms of ear infection. Occasionally, in addition to pain, patients will complain of plugged ears, decreased hearing (especially lower frequencies), and a sense of their ears popping periodically as the eustachian tube equilibrates middle ear pressure with the ambient air pressure.

Physical Examination

Direct examination of the tympanic membrane is crucial. With acute otitis media, the membrane is typically red and bulging with middle ear purulent secretions or the membrane may be perforated, and the landmarks of the middle ear bones will be obscured. In otitis media with effusion, the tympanic membrane will be retracted with variable amounts of clear middle ear fluid.

The remainder of the examination should search for possible signs of related pathology that might explain the reason(s) for middle ear disease including nasal inflammation secondary to allergy, upper respiratory infection, sinusitis, or signs that often correlate with adenoid hypertrophy like enlarged tonsils and dental malocclusion with overbite. Other clinical problems that heighten the suspicion of underlying allergy include asthma and eczema.

Diagnosis

The diagnosis of otitis media, either acute infectious or with effusion, is largely clinical, documenting the signs and symptoms noted above. In addition, the use of pneumatic otoscopy also can provide supportive information regarding middle ear compliance, which will be reduced in the setting of significant effusion; this technique provides about 80% diagnostic accuracy in experienced hands. Pneumatic otoscopy is inappropriate when the tympanic membrane is bulging or markedly retracted, because this would induce large changes in middle ear pressure and pain.

Audiometry

Although not central to the diagnosis of otitis media, audiometry should be considered as a baseline value when persistent effusion is apparent; such an evaluation should definitely be performed when effusion persists in both middle ears beyond 3 months. Persistent middle ear fluid with pressures in excess of -200 daPA (decapascals) will often lead to lower and/or mid-frequency hearing loss. This hearing loss can be critical, particularly for children between 1 and 4 years of age who are experiencing rapid lexical development. Poor hearing during this span can significantly retard receptive and, thus indirectly, expressive language development. If pure tone testing cannot be adequately performed in a child, an attempt should be made to determine speech reception threshold, and to review the history for appropriate verbal communication developmental milestones.

Tympanometry

When the diagnosis of middle ear effusion is suspected, tympanometry can provide an indirect measure of tympanic membrane compliance and an estimate of middle ear pressure. The positive predictive value of an abnormal tympanogram (flattened tracing or shift of diminished peak to higher negative values) varies between 49% and 99%. The positive predictive value of tympanometry is enhanced when the tympanogram is accompanied by pneumatic otoscopy; this test helps to screen for many abnormalities of the ear canal or ear drum such as excessive cerumen or tympanic membrane perforation that might skew results. The negative predictive value of a tympanogram is generally excellent; virtually all middle ears with normal tympanograms will be normal.

Associated Factors

Allergic Rhinitis

Direct evidence for the possible role of allergic rhinitis in both persistent otitis media with effusion and recurrent acute infectious otitis media comes from demonstrating eustachian tube dysfunction after intranasal allergen (e.g., dust mite) and histamine challenge. This association is further suggested by retrospective studies of patients with chronic middle ear

disease in whom the incidence of significant allergic rhinitis has ranged from 40% to 90%. Although demonstrating allergic rhinitis in patients with middle ear disease does not prove cause and effect, evaluation for allergy seems prudent if the examination and nasal cytology results are suggestive and when more invasive surgical procedures (e.g., tympanostomy tubes and adenoidectomy) are being contemplated.

Adenoid Hypertrophy

In addition to viral upper respiratory infections and allergic rhinitis, a common mechanical factor of eustachian tube dysfunction in children is adenoid hypertrophy. Typically, affected children are constant mouth breathers and often do not have chronic rhinitis. Associated features linked to open mouth and tongue thrusting often include long slender facies, high-arched palate, lower arch dental crowding, and malocclusion with overjet of the upper arch. Invariably, this group of findings necessitates orthodontic therapy in the adolescent years.

Chronic Sinusitis

As discussed previously, chronic sinusitis can be a frustrating clinical problem to resolve, particularly in the setting of severe underlying rhinitis, nasal polyps, or baseline small sinus ostia. When refractory sinusitis occurs with otitis media it is frequently easy to clear the middle ear infection within 10 to 14 days albeit with some residual middle ear effusion. If the sinus component is not aggressively treated for a longer period or is simply not recognized, the result is predictable: the sinusitis will lead to recurrent otitis media either directly from introduction of infected secretions or indirectly as a consequence of heightened upper airway edema and enhanced eustachian tube dysfunction. Unresolved chronic sinusitis, therefore, can be an important and sometimes subtle cause of recurrent otitis media.

Functional Eustachian Tube Obstruction

Rarely, the eustachian tube may be obstructed functionally without interference from underlying rhinitis, sinusitis, or adenoid hypertrophy. This obstruction may occur by means of two mechanisms: poor tensor veli palatini function or increased tubal compliance. Normally, active opening of the eustachian tube is accomplished by contraction of the tensor veli palatini muscle during crying, sneezing, swallowing, or yawning. This process transiently opens the eustachian tube and allows for ventilation of the middle ear and equilibration of air pressure with atmospheric pressure. Inadequate muscle function does not achieve this result, potentially leading to chronic negative middle ear pressures, secretion retention, and acute middle ear infection(s). A related problem, particularly in infants and small children, is increased tubal compliance (less stiffness) owing to inadequate cartilaginous support. This increased compliance leaves the patient with a floppy eustachian tube that cannot be appropriately opened even with normal tensor veli palatini function.

Medical Therapy

The mainstay of medical therapy for acute infectious otitis media is appropriate antibiotic administration. There is no convincing evidence that antihistamines, decongestants, or corticosteroids are useful in treating either acute infection or chronic persistent middle ear effusion.

Antibiotics

Given the similar bacteriology of acute otitis media and sinusitis, the choice of antibiotic should also be similar (see Table 9–5). Particularly over the last 4 to 5 years, with the increasing penicillin resistance observed in *Streptococcus pneumoniae* strains and the increasing incidence of β-lactamase–producing *Haemophilus influenzae* and *Moraxella catarrhalis,* the initial use of amoxicillin has been called into question. With the relative prevalence of these organisms, the likelihood of successful treatment with amoxicillin is now only about 60%. The clinician should consider other factors in individualizing antibiotic therapy: patient age, compliance (frequency and tolerability of suspensions), cost (comparable spectrum, insurance coverage, etc.), side-effect profile, and the presence of associated chronic sinusitis. Some infectious disease experts also advocate the use of tympanocentesis in refractory otitis media so that antibiotic choice can be based directly on culture and sensitivity data to maximize clinical success and avoid risk for inducing antimicrobial resistance.

Surgical Therapy

Recommendations for surgical intervention are based on a consensus report from The Otitis Media Guideline Panel, a conjoint panel of members from the American Academy of Pediatrics, the American Academy of Family Physicians, and the American Academy of Otolaryngology–Head and Neck Surgery. This panel suggests bilateral myringotomy with tube placement (or more aggressive antibiotics) only in patients with persistent otitis media with effusion and at least a 20-dB hearing loss persisting 3 or more months after the initial diagnosis of otitis media with effusion (with or without infection). Insertion of tympanostomy tubes has several potential risks: postoperative tympanosclerosis (51%), postoperative otorrhea (13%), and general anesthesia (1%).

Adenoidectomy in concert with tympanostomy tubes is indicated only with clear cut evidence for significant adenoid pathology (as noted earlier). Potential risks include excessive postoperative bleeding and general anesthesia.

Subspecialty Referral
Allergist/Immunologist

Referral to an allergist/immunologist should be considered with the following clinical patterns:

- Persistent otitis media with effusion with or without recurrent acute infectious otitis media associated with hearing loss, language delay, or both, and evidence for coincident eosinophilic rhinitis
- Recurrent infectious otitis media, particularly with associated patterns of recurrent sinusitis or bronchitis
- Otitis media caused by low pathogenicity organisms
- Multiple antibiotic allergies

Otorhinolaryngologist

Referral to an otorhinolaryngologist should be considered with the following clinical patterns:

- Persistent otitis media with effusion with or without recurrent acute infectious otitis media associated with hearing loss, language delay, or both despite optimal therapy for underlying rhinitis
- Recurrent infectious otitis media with associated chronic sinusitis despite prolonged (8–12 weeks) medical therapy
- Persistent otitis media with effusion and associated clinically significant nasal obstruction (including radiographic adenoid enlargement) despite optimal therapy for underlying rhinitis

KEY POINTS

- ▶ Otitis media occurs after prolonged eustachian tube dysfunction and associated stasis of secretions within the middle ear; common causes include rhinitis, adenoid hypertrophy, and functional tubal or tensor veli palatini problems
- ▶ Common pathogens for acute infectious otitis media include *Streptococcus pneumoniae, Moraxella catarrhalis,* and *Haemophilus influenzae*
- ▶ Acute otitis media is a clinical diagnosis based on examination demonstrating a red, bulging tympanic membrane often with pain or a perforated ear drum and associated purulent discharge
- ▶ Supportive useful diagnostic modalities include pneumatic otoscopy, tympanometry, and audiometry
- ▶ Associated factors include allergic rhinitis, adenoid hypertrophy, chronic sinusitis, and functional eustachian tube obstruction
- ▶ Antibiotics are primary medical therapy for suspected bacterial otitis media with choice based on likely microorganisms and consideration of patient age, compliance, cost, side-effect profile, and the presence of associated chronic sinusitis
- ▶ Surgical intervention (tympanostomy tube placement) should be contemplated when aggressive medical therapy fails to alter a course of ≥3 months of persistent otitis media with effusion and ≥20-dB hearing loss with or without recurrent infection
- ▶ Adenoidectomy is indicated only when hy-

pertrophy is a significant reason for pathology, e.g., eustachian tube dysfunction, difficulty with eating or sleep, or evidence for chronic infection with refractory sinusitis

NASAL POLYPS
Clinical Presentation
Pathophysiology

The most convincing theories regarding the etiology of nasal polyps suggest that eosinophilic rhinitis is an important pathophysiologic mechanism. Nasal eosinophilia may be a consequence of the late phase of allergic rhinitis, or it may be induced in the nonallergic patient secondary to release of epithelial-derived chemokines such as RANTES and eotaxin.

Turbulent airflow on such a preinflamed airway may eventually give rise to ulceration and prolapse of the submucosa with re-epithelialization and new gland formation. All of the cells in the initial micropolyp—epithelia, vascular endothelia, and fibroblasts—can produce granulocyte-monocyte colony-stimulating factor (GM-CSF), which can amplify the inflammatory cascade. Ultimately, as a consequence of inflammatory mediators, the bioelectric integrity of the sodium and chloride epithelial channels can be affected. Altered sodium absorption may result in increased water movement into the cell, accumulation of interstitial fluid, and ultimately enlargement of the nasal polyp.

Why nasal polyps have such a high recurrence rate after surgical removal is open to conjecture. The high recurrence rate is probably because the underlying eosinophilic rhinitis is not directly suppressed by surgical therapy. Failure to medically eliminate nasal eosinophilia for a prolonged period after surgery allows the underlying inflammation to persist and the cycle of polyp reformation occurs. Unfortunately, this happens in many patients despite aggressive postoperative use of corticosteroids.

History

In patients with nasal polyps, the history is often that of progressive nasal obstruction—

congestion that is typically so significant that patients will experience dyspnea with eating and sleeping because of obligate mouth breathing. Frequently, because of associated eosinophilic rhinitis (and the polyps themselves), patients also complain of anosmia and related blunted appetite, and they may experience sneezing, rhinorrhea, or ocular itching. With the proximity of nasal polyps to the sinus ostia, chronic or recurrent sinusitis is a very common finding. A subset of patients also is sensitive to aspirin or other NSAIDs, and will have chronic steroid-dependent asthma.

Most nasal polyp patients are over 40 years old, with men outnumbering women by 2:1. Nasal polyps are very rare in children, particularly under age 10. When nasal polyps do occur in this age group, the possibility of cystic fibrosis should be considered.

As suggested earlier, because underlying eosinophilic rhinitis is often persistent despite surgical polyp removal, the recurrence rate for nasal polyps is very high, in some series approaching 60% to 80%.

Physical Examination

Nasal polyps appear as rounded or pear-shaped translucent mucosal structures. They are normally soft, mobile, gelatinous, insensitive to manipulation, do not readily bleed, and are bilateral, although not necessarily symmetrically equal. The appearance of the surrounding nasal mucosa is variable and dependent on the nature of underlying rhinosinusitis, for example, pale with allergic rhinitis or erythematous with sinusitis.

Diagnosis

The diagnosis of nasal polyps is clinical, based on the examination findings and often supported by the history. The most common condition that is confused with nasal polyps is hypertrophied or polypoid nasal turbinates; ironically this may well be a prepolyp condition for such patients, and fortunately such tissue will usually respond to treatment with corticosteroids.

Tumors, such as squamous cell carcinoma, sarcoma, angiofibroma, encephalocoele, and inverting papilloma may be mistaken for nasal polyps. Clinical features that should heighten suspicion for these conditions include unilateral presentation, friability, firmness, and bleeding spontaneously or with manipulation. When any of these attributes are present with a nasal mass, the patient should be referred to an otolaryngologist for evaluation and probable biopsy.

Associated Factors

Eosinophilic Rhinitis

In nearly all patients with nasal polyposis, eosinophilic rhinitis and eosinophilic infiltration of the polyp tissue are observed. Accordingly, it seems plausible that the eosinophil plays an important role in the pathophysiology of nasal polyps. Ironically, several studies suggest that allergy is rarely the cause for the eosinophilic rhinitis seen with nasal polyps; that is, the vast majority of patients have eosinophilic nonallergic disease (ENAR). The cause of ENAR may be prolonged inflammation of the upper airway epithelia because of chronic sinusitis or irritant rhinitis. At some point this inflammation triggers production of RANTES or eotaxin by the epithelia. Both are potent chemotactic agents for eosinophils. Once eosinophils are present in the airway, they can produce interleukin-5 (IL-5), enhancing their own growth and survival. Eosinophil products such as major basic protein (MBP) may create further epithelial irritation, leading to a vicious circle.

Patients with cystic fibrosis are an exception to the ENAR–nasal polyp link. In these patients, an underlying defect in ion transport appears to provide an adequate milieu for the development of nasal polyps. In patients without cystic fibrosis, it appears that eosinophil and other inflammatory cell products may ultimately alter the bioelectric environment, also creating alterations in sodium and chloride transport.

Aspirin Sensitivity

A subset of patients with nasal polyps, often with associated chronic asthma will demonstrate sensitivity to aspirin and frequently to other nonsteroidal anti-inflammatory drugs (NSAIDs). A retrospective review suggests that these patients initially have chronic rhinorrhea and congestion. The rhinorrhea and congestion are followed by the development of nasal polyps, then asthma, and finally aspirin sensitivity. It has been noted that these patients produce significantly more leukotrienes than patients without asthma or without aspirin sensitivity. Other investigators have pointed out that patients with nasal polyps and asthma demonstrate a significant increase in haplotypes HLA-A1 and HLA-B8. Together these observations suggest that unique abnormalities of the immune response and leukotriene production, may be associated with the pathophysiology of polyps, asthma, and aspirin or NSAID sensitivity in these patients. Given excessive leukotriene production as a baseline problem, and that several leukotrienes are potent triggers of asthma, how does aspirin sensitivity fit in? Aspirin blocks cyclooxygenase, an enzyme that enhances production of mediators of pain and fever such as prostaglandins. Blockade of this enzyme creates more available arachidonic acid as a substrate for 5-lipoxygenase, the enzyme that produces leukotrienes.

Medical Therapy

Corticosteroids

The mainstay of medical treatment for nasal polyps is corticosteroids. Initially, with larger polyps or more diffuse disease, systemic corticosteroids or direct polyp injection may be indicated. For more limited disease or to help prevent recurrence, nasal aqueous or aerosol corticosteroid preparations are used because of a better side-effect profile. Corticosteroids exert efficacy by inhibiting the accumulation of inflammatory cells and the synthesis of pro-inflammatory cytokines. In fact, the observed benefit of steroid treatment supports the underlying inflammatory basis of nasal polyps.

Significant improvement occurs in about 80% of patients treated with corticosteroids for moderate to severe nasal polyps. Corticosteroid treatment failure occurs in some patients with extensive nasal and sinus mechanical obstruction or with resistant infectious sinusitis. Although patients may relate some symptomatic improvement, there is no evidence that antihistamines, decongestants, cromolyn, or nedocromil are of benefit in either active or prophylactic treatment of nasal polyps.

Leukotriene Antagonists

In patients with nasal polyps, asthma, and aspirin sensitivity there does appear to be a useful preventive role for leukotriene antagonists including 5-lipoxygenase inhibitors (zileuton) and leukotriene receptor blockers (zafirlukast, monteleukast, pranlukast). Given the relative importance of leukotrienes in affected patients, the addition of these medications offers hope for better asthma management and breaking a cycle of recurrent polyps requiring endoscopic sinus surgery.

To date, there are no well-controlled long-term studies on the use of these agents either alone or with corticosteroids as prophylactic therapy in patients with nasal polyps but without asthma or without aspirin sensitivity.

Surgical Therapy

When nasal polyp patients have refractory mechanical obstruction, and particularly with associated sinusitis or steroid-dependent asthma, polypectomy and often additional FESS are indicated. The goal of FESS is to remove polyp tissue as completely as possible, restore nasal aeration, and lavage infected sinus cavities.

Postoperative follow-up is crucial in these patients to assure stability and lack of adhesion formation and to re-emphasize the importance of medical prophylaxis with topical steroids (and leukotriene antagonists in select patients).

Subspecialty Referral

Allergist/Immunologist

Referral to an allergist/immunologist should be considered with the following clinical patterns:

- Nasal polyps associated with eosinophilic rhinitis, particularly with a personal and family history of atopic disease
- Nasal polyps and associated refractory sinusitis
- Nasal polyps associated with aspirin or other NSAID sensitivity and asthma

Otorhinolaryngologist

Referral to an otorhinolaryngologist should be considered with the following clinical patterns:

- Nasal polyps refractory to medical therapy with corticosteroids
- Nasal polyps creating OMC obstruction and secondary recurrent or chronic sinusitis

KEY POINTS

▶ Nasal polyps are probably caused by airflow on chronic inflammation; inflammatory mediators disrupt the integrity of the sodium/chloride channels leading to interstitial edema and polyp enlargement

▶ Patients with nasal polyps typically have severe nasal obstruction, decreased sense of smell, and variable rhinorrhea; a subset have aspirin sensitivity and chronic asthma

▶ Nasal polyps are generally bilateral, soft, gelatinous, mobile, insensitive to manipulation, and do not bleed easily

▶ The possibility of underlying allergic rhinitis or cystic fibrosis should be considered in patients with nasal polyps

▶ Corticosteroids are the primary medical therapy for nasal polyps; such therapy may be topical, systemic, or direct injection into the polyps

▶ Leukotriene antagonists should be considered in patients with nasal polyps and aspirin sensitivity and chronic asthma

▶ Surgical intervention is indicated when nasal polyps are refractory to aggressive medical therapy and when associated with OMC compromise, recurrent sinusitis, and severe chronic asthma

Suggested Reading

Sinusitis

Gwaltney JM Jr, Scheld WM, Sande MA, et al: The microbial etiology and antimicrobial therapy of adults with acute community acquired sinusitis: A fifteen year experience at the University of Virginia and review of other selected studies. J Allergy Clin Immunol 90S:457, 1992

Hisamatsu K, Canbo T, Nakazawa T, et al: Cytotoxicity of human eosinophil granule major basic protein to human nasal sinus mucosa in vitro. J Allergy Clin Immunol 86:52, 1990

Kennedy DW: Functional endoscopic sinus surgery: Technique. Arch Otolaryngol Head Neck Surg 111:643, 1985

Siegel SC: Topical corticosteroids in the management of rhinitis. *In* Settipane GA (ed): Rhinitis. Providence, Oceanside Publications, 1991, pp 231–240

Umetsu DT, Ambrosino DM, Quinti I, et al: Recurrent sinopulmonary infections and impaired antibody responses to bacterial capsular polysaccharide antigens in children with selective IgG subclass deficiency. N Engl J Med 313:1247, 1985

Virant FS, Shapiro GG: Sinusitis. *In* Tierney FD (ed): Current Pulmonology, Vol. 15. St. Louis, Mosby, 1994, pp 75–112

Wald ER, Milmoe GJ, Bowen AD, et al: Acute maxillary sinusitis in children. N Engl J Med 304:749, 1981

Williams JW Jr, Simel DI, Roberts L, et al: Clinical evaluation for sinusitis: Making the diagnosis by history and physical examination. Ann Intern Med 117:705, 1992

Zinreich SJ, Kennedy DW, Rosenbaun AE, et al: Paranasal sinuses: CT imaging requirements for endoscopic surgery. Radiology 163:769, 1987

Otitis Media

Berman S, Roark R, Luckey D: Theoretical cost effectiveness of management options for children with persisting middle ear effusions. Pediatrics 93:353, 1994

Bernstein JM, Lee J, Conboy K, et al: The role of IgE mediated hypersensitivity in recurrent otitis media with effusion. Am J Otology 5:66, 1983

Etzel RA, Pattishall EN, Haley NJ, et al: Passive smoking and middle ear effusion among children in day care. Pediatrics 90:228, 1992

Fireman P: Otitis media and eustachian tube dysfunction: Connection to allergic rhinitis. J Allergy Clin Immunol 99:S787, 1997

Kaleida PH, Casselbrant ML, Rockette HE, et al: Amoxicillin or myringotomy or both for acute otitis media: Results of randomized clinical trial. Pediatrics 87:466, 1991

The Otitis Media Guideline Panel: Managing otitis media with effusion in young children. Pediatrics 94:766, 1994

Paradise JL, Bluestone CD, Rogers KD, et al: Efficacy of adenoidectomy for recurrent otitis media in children previously treated with tympanostomy-tube placement. JAMA 263:2066, 1990

Rees T: Tympanometry in middle ear disease. J Family Prac 3:81, 1976

Roberts JE, Sanyal MA, Burchinal MR, et al: Otitis media in early childhood and its relationship to later verbal and academic performance. Pediatrics 78:423, 1986

Nasal Polyps

Bachert C, Wegenmann M, Hauser U, Rudack C: IL-5 synthesis is upregulated in human nasal polyp tissue. J Allergy Clin Immunol 99:837, 1997

Beck LA, Stellato C, Beall LD, et al: Detection of the chemokine RANTES and endothelial adhesion molecules in nasal polyps. J Allergy Clin Immunol 98:766, 1996

Bernstein JM, Gorfein J, Noble B: Role of allergy in nasal polyposis: A review. Otolaryngol Head Neck Surg 113:724, 1995

Bernstein JM, Gorfein J, Noble B, et al: Nasal polyposis: Immunohistochemistry and bioelectric findings (a hypothesis for the development of nasal polyps). J Allergy Clin Immunol 99:165, 1997

Brown BL, Harner SG, Van Dellen RG: Nasal polypectomy in patients with asthma and sensitivity to aspirin. Arch Otolaryngol 105:413, 1979

Drake-Lee AB, Lowe D, Swanston A, et al: Clinical profile and recurrence of nasal polyps. J Laryngol Otol 98:783, 1984

Elovic A, Wong DTW, Weller PF, et al: Expression of transforming growth factors-α and β_1 messenger RNA and product by eosinophils in nasal polyps. J Allergy Clin Immunol 93:864, 1994

Hamilos DL: Nasal polyps as immunoreactive tissue. Allergy Asthma Proc 17:293, 1996

Ruhno J, Andersson B, Denburg J, et al: A double-blind comparison of intranasal budesonide with placebo for nasal polyposis. J Allergy Clin Immunol 86:946, 1990

Chapter 10

Asthma: Pathophysiology and Epidemiology

Wayne A. Sladek

Asthma is a complex clinical syndrome that is difficult to define. In an individual, clinical asthma varies in severity and expression throughout life; in a population it varies in clinical presentation. Each discipline that studies asthma brings a different perspective and emphasis to the definition. This has led to the complicated, all encompassing, definition of asthma used in the Global Initiative for Asthma: "a chronic inflammatory disorder of the airways in which many cells and cellular elements play a role, in particular, mast cells, eosinophils, T lymphocytes, neutrophils, and epithelial cells. In susceptible individuals, this inflammation causes recurrent episodes of wheezing, breathlessness, chest tightness, and cough, particularly at night and in the early morning. These episodes are usually associated with widespread but variable airflow obstruction that is often reversible either spontaneously or with treatment. The inflammation also causes an associated increase in the existing bronchial hyper-responsiveness to a variety of stimuli." The emphasis on chronic inflammation underlying asthma has very significant ramifications in the treatment and possibly in the prevention of asthma. However, there are no well-validated, noninvasive measurements of asthmatic airway inflammation, and no pathognomonic signs or diagnostic tests for asthma. The diagnosis relies on symptoms, symptom pattern, and documentation of reversible airflow obstruction. The symptoms of wheeze, cough, shortness of breath, chest tightness, and sputum production are not unique to asthma; however, the combination of these symptoms with the diurnal, seasonal, or lifetime patterns, precipitated by allergens, irritants, viral respiratory infections, or exercise, gets us closer to the clinical syndrome we call asthma.

PATHOPHYSIOLOGY

Asthma is considered a chronic inflammatory disorder of the airways. In order to understand the treatment, genetics, and even the changing epidemiology of asthma, one must understand the unique type of inflammatory response found in asthma. Recognition of the central importance of inflammation in asthma initially came from autopsy studies and evaluation of sputum, and then from bronchoscopy and bronchoalveolar lavage (BAL) studies. Allergen challenges, in conjunction with pulmonary function testing, bronchoscopy, and BAL studies, have given insight into the changes in airway cell types, mediators and hyper-responsiveness associated with the asthmatic response.

At autopsy, abnormalities are found in all layers of the airway and contribute to the obstructive process. The post-mortem lungs remain hyperinflated. The airways are occluded from tenacious mucoid plugs, which result in

139

areas of hyperinflation and atelectasis. These plugs are a mixture of inflammatory exudate, thick mucus, cells and cellular debris. Extensive areas of epithelium are desquamated which contributes to the plugging. Obstruction is aggravated by the enfolding of the thickened, edematous bronchial walls that encroach on the lumen. The edematous mucosa and submucosa contain a cellular infiltrate of eosinophilis, neutrophils, and lymphocytes. There is hyperplasia of goblet cells and submucosal glands, which are enlarged and dilated. Bronchial blood vessels are dilated. Bronchial smooth muscle is hypertrophied as much as 3- to 4-fold in some airways. Below the normal epithelial basement membrane is the thickened reticular basement membrane. This thickening of the reticular layer is referred to as subepithelial fibrosis. Desquamation of the airway epithelium, thickening of the reticular basement membrane, and the eosinophilic inflammatory cell infiltrate are found in asthma of all levels of severity. Despite these extensive changes in the airway there is no destructive process leading to emphysema.

After an allergen challenge in a sensitized asthmatic there is development of airway obstruction that usually begins within 10 minutes of inhalation challenge and resolves within 1 to 3 hours. This is called the early phase reaction (EPR). It is followed in 30% to 50% of adults and greater than 75% of children by a late phase reaction (LPR), which is maximal in 4 to 12 hours. This late phase reaction is associated with increased airway hyper-responsiveness to histamine or methacholine. Only asthmatic patients who develop this late phase reaction develop increased airway responsiveness. Development of the LPR is dependent on the allergen dose, how sensitive the individual is to that allergen, the level of specific IgE, the baseline forced expiratory volume in 1 second (FEV_1), and baseline bronchial hyper-responsiveness (BHR). Both EPR and LPR to allergens are mediated through IgE.

The mast cell is central to the development of the IgE-mediated EPR. Mast cell numbers are increased in the sub-basement membrane and in BAL fluid of individuals with asthma. Their numbers in BAL fluid correlate with bronchial reactivity. There are multiple triggers of mast cell mediator release, including allergens, opiates, dextran, and radiocontrast material. Allergens cause cross-linking of surface IgE bound to the high-affinity IgE receptors on the mast cell surface. This triggers the release of pre-formed mediators from the 50–200 membrane-bound granules in each cell. These mediators are responsible for the bronchial constriction, increased mucus secretion, and the airway edema found in the EPR. There are a multiplicity of mediators involved with a great redundancy of function. Histamine, prostaglandin D_2 (PGD_2), leukotriene C4 (LTC_4), bradykinin, and platelet-activating factor (PAF) cause smooth muscle contraction. PGD_2, LTC_4, and histamine stimulate goblet and submucosal gland secretion. Histamine, LTC_4, PAF, and bradykinin cause endothelial cell contraction and exudation of plasma.

Human lung tissue is one of the richest sources of histamine, containing 10–12 μg of histamine per gram of tissue. Histamine acts directly on airway smooth muscle through the H1 receptor, causing contraction. Other direct actions of histamine include enhanced mucus secretion and increased vascular permeability that results from endothelial cell constriction. Histamine is relatively more potent than prostaglandins and leukotrienes in promoting vascular leakage, but less potent in causing smooth muscle contraction. Apart from its direct actions, much of histamine's action is indirect through the stimulation of prostaglandin secretion. These effects are all recognized in asthma, but antihistamines have a very limited role in treating asthma. In addition to the preformed mediators such as histamine, triggering of the mast cells also results in the production of newly formed mediators. These include PAF and two groups of arachidonic acid metabolites: the prostaglandins and the leukotrienes. Platelet activating factor has multiple proinflammatory actions. It is a potent eosinophil chemoattractant and activates both eosinophils and neutrophils. It enhances vascular permeability, causes bronchoconstriction, upregulates adhesion molecule expression on eosinophils, and increases the synthesis of prostaglandins and LTC_4.

After release from the cell membrane, arachidonic acid can be metabolized along either the cyclooxygenase or lipoxygenase pathways. This results in two major families of inflammatory mediators, the prostaglandins and the leukotrienes. The most abundant cyclooxygenase product resulting from mast cell activation is PGD_2. It is released in significantly smaller amounts than histamine, but is about 30 times as potent a bronchoconstrictor.

The second group of arachidonic acid metabolites, the leukotrienes, is generated through the lipoxygenase pathway. In conjunction with 5-lipoxygenase-activating protein (FLAP), 5-lipoxygenase oxidizes arachidonic acid to form leukotriene A_4 (LTA_4). LTA_4 is metabolized by LTC_4 synthase to LTC_4, which is followed sequentially by the formation of LTD_4 and then LTE_4. These three leukotrienes, LTC_4, LTD_4, and LTE_4, are known as the cysteinyl leukotrienes, and in the past were known as slow reactive substance of anaphylaxis. Their duration of effect, 15 to 20 minutes, is significantly greater than that of histamine. The cysteinyl leukotrienes all use a common receptor in the human lung. LTC_4 is the major lipoxygenase product of the mast cell, but it is also made by macrophages and eosinophils. It is released in significantly smaller amounts than histamine, but is 1000 times more potent than histamine as a bronchoconstrictor. Cysteinyl leukotrienes also increase mucus secretion, induce eosinophil infiltration, and augment vascular permeability and edema formation. Following allergen challenge, LTC_4 can be detected in the airway within 5 minutes, and an increase in urinary LTE_4 can be found within 2 hours. Plasma LTE_4 levels correlate with chronic asthma severity. The relative importance of leukotrienes is further demonstrated by the effectiveness of leukotriene antagonists in treating asthma.

Three to 6 hours after an allergen challenge there is a second drop in pulmonary function, which can last several hours to days. This LPR is associated with a large increase in the number of inflammatory cells in and around the airway. During the EPR multiple mediators are released that induce specific patterns of cellular adhesion molecule expression. This results in preferential recruitment and accumulation of specific inflammatory cells. The resulting inflammatory response is thought to be responsible for the increase in bronchial hyper-reactivity found in the LPR. Increased bronchial reactivity in the LPR may last over a week after a single antigen challenge. The type of inflammation found during

the LPR in combination with the increase in bronchial hyper-responsiveness is thought to reflect the changes seen in chronic asthma. The LPR is therefore used as a model to study chronic asthma.

Basophils and eosinophils are two important inflammatory cells in the development of the LPR and chronic asthma. Basophils are recruited to the airway after allergen challenge, and their numbers correlate with BHR and severity of the LPR. During the LPR, different releasing factors may contribute to persistent airways inflammation through their action on basophils. The levels of peripheral eosinophilia, airway eosinophilia, and eosinophil major basic protein all correlate with the clinical severity of asthma. During the LPR there is eosinophil activation, an associated drop in the peripheral eosinophil count, and the development of bronchoalveolar eosinophilia as eosinophils migrate to the airway and into the lumen where they cause significant epithelial damage. Inhibition of adhesion molecules important for eosinophil recruitment inhibits airway eosinophilia and the subsequent increase in airway responsiveness after allergen challenge. The loss of the surface epithelium, which is found even in patients with mild asthma, correlates with the degree of BHR.

Eosinophils become part of the material filling the airway lumen, which results in airway obstruction. Sputum from asthmatic patients gives evidence of the underlying eosinophilic processes, which is not seen in patients with bronchitis. The sputum from asthmatic patients contains eosinophils, sloughed clumps of epithelium known as Creola bodies, and crystals of eosinophil granule membrane lysophospholipase known as Charcot-Leyden crystals. The sputum also may contain twists of thickened mucus known as Curschmann's spirals.

The T cell is thought to have a central role in directing and maintaining the inflammatory response that results in airway eosinophilia, BHR, and symptoms. In chronic asthma there are increased numbers of intraepithelial activated T cells, and their numbers correlate with the degree of airway eosinophilia. The number of allergen-specific T cells in blood correlates with the degree of BHR in chronic allergic asthma. In severe, acute asthma there are increased numbers of activated peripheral helper T cells and their numbers correlate with the degree of bronchial obstruction.

Helper T cells are categorized into two distinct subtypes, TH1 and TH2, based on different patterns of cytokine secretion. TH1 cells produce interleukin 2 (IL-2) and interferon gamma (IFN-γ) and promote cell-mediated immunity. The cytokine IFN-γ inhibits the development of TH2 cells. TH2 cells produce IL-3, IL-4, IL-5, IL-6, IL-13, and granulocyte-macrophage colony-stimulating factor (GM-CSF). These cytokines lead to increased IgE synthesis, eosinophilia, and allergic inflammation. The BAL fluid from atopic asthmatic cells encodes for cytokines consistent with the TH2 type. In severe asthma or an allergen-induced LPR there is an increased production of the TH2 cytokines IL-4, IL-5, and GM-CSF. In chronic disease the number of cells producing these cytokines corresponds to airflow obstruction, BHR, and asthma symptom scores.

TH2-derived cytokines are involved in the maturation, activation, and recruitment of other inflammatory cells. IL-3 and IL-9 are involved in growth and differentiation of mast cells, and IL-10 contributes to the survival of mast cells. GM-CSF and IL-5 are important for the differentiation, activation, and survival of eosinophils. Anti-IL-5 inhibits allergen-induced BHR and eosinophilia in a primate model of asthma. The TH2 cells are a major source of IL-4, which induces B cells to switch to IgE synthesis. Mast cells, basophils, and eosinophils are other potential sources of IL-4. IL-4 and IL-10 are both produced by, and favor the expansion of, the TH2 phenotype. These cytokines enhance the differentiation, proliferation, and survival of TH2 cells while inhibiting the differentiation of TH1 cells. This autocrine process could potentially lead to a state of chronic, self-sustaining airway inflammation, in which allergens play an important initiating role but becoming less important as the disease becomes more chronic.

In the normal lung, muscle contraction results in shortening and narrowing of the airway. In asthma, all layers of the airway wall are thickened. Subepithelial airway thickening correlates positively with the severity of asthma, and degree of BHR, and negatively with pulmonary function. The combination of increased airway muscle constrictor force, increased wall thickness, and increased airway stiffness from collagen deposition in the reticular basement membrane results in an exaggerated encroachment on the lumen and marked increase in airway resistance. The thickening of the airway wall has a minimal effect on the lumen of a fully dilated airway; however, with smooth muscle shortening, airway thickening produces an exaggerated increase in airway resistance. Clinically this is seen as an increase in airway responsiveness. This thickening may also result in progressive, severe obstruction. In the normal airway there is a limit to the degree of pharmacologically induced airway narrowing. In the patient with more severe asthma, this plateau does not exist, and there is a continued increase in airway resistance from ongoing, widespread closure of the thick-walled, peripheral airways.

Asthma is considered a disease of reversible airway obstruction. A post-bronchodilator improvement in the FEV_1 by 15% is diagnostic of asthma. However, the degree of obstruction and reversibility is variable over time, and reversibility may not be complete. More limited reversibility may be secondary to airway edema, mucus, or airway remodeling. With acute or chronic worsening of asthma there is increased airway obstruction, which results in premature and possibly persistent closure of the smaller bronchi and bronchioles. The lungs become hyperinflated to overcome the premature airway closure. This results in hyperexpansion of the chest and an increase in the anteroposterior (AP) diameter. With increased residual volumes there is a necessary decrease in the inspiratory capacity. Respiratory rate begins to rise. Breathing at higher lung volumes is less efficient because of the abnormal position of the diaphragm and decreased lung compliance. With worsening obstruction, passive expiration may become insufficient and respiratory muscles become active during both inspiration and expiration. Accessory muscle use is typically seen when FEV_1 approaches 40% of predicted values. Persistent inspiratory muscle activity results in increased work of breathing. At an FEV_1 of 50%, the inspiratory work is increased approximately 11-fold.

In status asthmaticus airway obstruction is not uniform throughout the lung. This leads to a mismatch between perfusion and ventilation. Alterations in gas exchange are determined by relative differences between the ventilated and nonventilated areas. Initially, the increased respiratory drive results in a decrease in CO_2. With increasing obstruction and $\dot{V}/\dot{Q}$ mismatch, there is a rise in CO_2. When FEV_1 or peak expiratory flow rate (PEFR) is $\leq 25\%$ of predicted the CO_2 level is likely to be ≥ 40 mmHg and there is a risk for ventilatory failure. Pulmonary function correlates better with CO_2 level than oxygen level. Presence of hypoxia correlates poorly with measured pulmonary obstruction and may be present with milder degrees of obstruction. Oxygen saturations should be measured in patients with status asthmaticus. Persistent hypoxia after initial treatment significantly increases the risk of hospitalization. $\dot{V}/\dot{Q}$ mismatch is slow to recover. Oxygenation may not return to normal until a week or more after an acute episode.

EPIDEMIOLOGY

Prevalence

According to the National Center for Health Statistics over 13.7 million Americans (5.4%) reported having asthma in 1994, an increase of 75% from the 6.7 million with asthma in 1980. Asthma is one of the most common chronic diseases in the United States. Asthma usually begins in childhood, and the highest incidence occurs during the first four years of life. There is a gradual decrease in the incidence until a low is reached in the mid to late teens; thereafter, the incidence remains steady throughout adulthood. Boys are affected more than girls through age 9. From 10 through 14 years of age, the incidence rates are nearly equal, whereas between 15 and 49 years of age, the incidence rates are somewhat higher in women. Since disease prevalence is dependent on the incidence, the number of persistent cases, the number of remissions, and number of exacerbations, the prevalence rate may differ from the incidence for a given age. Although the incidence is highest in the 0- to 4-year-old age group, the prevalence is highest in the 4- to 15-year-old age group where it is 7.4%. It decreases to 5.2% in 15- to 34 year-olds before decreasing to 4.5% in those older

than 35 years of age. Blacks (5.8%) are affected more than whites (5.1%) and peoples of other races (4.9%). Asthma prevalence is increasing in all ages, races, and regions of the country. The increase is most marked in young people in whom there was a 160% increase in the 0- to 4-year-old age group and a 74% increase among 5- to 14-year-olds since 1980. This increase is not confined to the United States. Serial studies from other countries that use a consistent definition of asthma have demonstrated an increase in wheezy illnesses of childhood and adolescence. Without a clear definition or standardized tools for the study of the epidemiology of asthma, the prevalence of asthma within and among countries cannot be reliably compared. Standardized approaches are now being used in two major international studies: the International Study of Asthma and Allergies in Children (ISAAC) and the European Community Respiratory Health Survey (ECRHS) in young adults. Comparisons are being primarily based on symptoms, as multiple studies have indicated substantial underdiagnosis when a definition of physician-diagnosed asthma is used. Initial findings have been reported on 13- and 14-year-old children from 56 countries who responded to the question, "Have you had wheezing or whistling in the chest in the last 12 months?" There were striking differences in the prevalence of wheezing among different centers throughout the world, with a 20-fold difference between the center with the lowest prevalence (1.6%) and the highest (36.8%) and an 8-fold variation between the 10th and 90th percentiles (3.9%–30.6%). Wide variations were seen among regions, especially in Europe and Asia, and even among centers within some countries. Overall, the highest prevalences were in English-speaking and Western countries. Similarly, the ECRHS report indicated a wide variation in the prevalence of self-reported, asthma-like symptoms and asthma attacks in 20- to 44-year-old adults. There was a higher prevalence of symptoms in English-speaking countries such as England, Australia, New Zealand, and the United States, with a lower prevalence of symptoms in the central part of continental Europe and the Mediterranean countries.

In contrast to the high prevalence of asthma in Western countries there is a striking absence of asthma in rural areas of nonindustrialized countries in which people are living a traditional life-style. Urbanization or westernization of nonindustrialized peoples has been associated with a marked increase in the prevalence of asthma. In Africa, the prevalence of asthma in Xhosa children living a traditional life-style in small communities in homes with mud-brick walls, thatched roofs, and floors of stamped-down cow dung, who sleep on aired mats was 0.14%, whereas Xhosa children living in a densely populated township of Capetown in brick homes who sleep on beds had a 3.17% prevalence of asthma. The low prevalence of asthma in rural Xhosa children was comparable to reports from other parts of Africa, whereas the higher rate in urban children was similar to rates in Western countries. A similar striking increase in asthma prevalence has been seen in other studies that examined the westernization of nonindustrialized peoples. This difference between rural and urban settings is not seen in westernized countries.

Morbidity

Asthma has significant morbidity. It is the most common chronic disease of childhood and the most common cause of school absenteeism; asthmatic children miss three times as many school days as nonasthmatic children. In the United States in 1994 asthma was the sixth most frequent diagnosis for outpatient visits, and the eleventh most frequent cause for emergency department visits. Only hypertension, diabetes, and otitis media have more repeat visits than asthma. The number of hospital discharges for asthma has increased since 1978; however, the overall hospitalization rate has not changed. Young children (0–4 years) are an exception, as hospitalization rates have increased in this group 182% from 1980 to 1993 (35.6 to 64.7/10,000). Black patients are 4.7 times as likely to be seen in the emergency department and 3.3 times as likely to be hospitalized with asthma than white patients. Poor asthmatic children have fewer doctor visits and a greater reliance on the emergency department for management and have more hospital admissions for asthma. Patients hospitalized for asthma tend to have more severe disease and use nebulized medications. They are less

likely to have asthma treatment plans, increase medication use early during an exacerbation, or follow allergen avoidance measures.

There has been a global trend toward increasing asthma morbidity. This trend reflects an increase in the frequency of more severe asthma, increasing numbers of primary care visits, and increasing hospital discharge rates. Most hospitalizations remain preventable despite their increasing frequency. Unfortunately, the burden of morbidity is not restricted to those diagnosed with asthma because prevalence studies indicate asthma is substantially underdiagnosed and inadequately treated. Both recognized and unrecognized childhood asthma results in significant sleep disruption, increased school absenteeism, lack of attendance at physical education classes, increased use of medical services, and increased parental concern over the child's health.

Mortality

In Western countries there has been a gradual increase in mortality from asthma during the last 50 years. Since the mid-1970s there has been an overall increase in mortality between 1.5 and 2 times in many countries throughout the world. Mortality rates are highest in West Germany, Norway, and New Zealand; and rates are lower in the United States, Hong Kong, the Netherlands, and Canada. In the United States, asthma deaths peaked in 1952 at 6,943 deaths (4.5/100,000 people). Asthma deaths then fell sharply in the 1950s, possibly because of the introduction of corticosteroids in 1951, and reached a low in 1977 at 1674 deaths (0.8/100,000 people). Asthma deaths then increased gradually until stabilizing in 1989. After that rates remained fairly steady between 1.9 and 2.1/100,000 until 1994, when there were 5,487 deaths. These rates are lower than mortality rates for other diseases, and asthma is not in the top 10 leading causes of death in the United States. The mortality rate from asthma is just stabilizing, whereas the rates for other chronic diseases amenable to medical intervention are declining.

Asthma mortality is not evenly distributed among populations in the United States. It is greatest in the poor, in minorities, in those living in inner cities, and in patients over 65 years old. Asthma mortality in the elderly (>65 years) is 89.8 per million compared to 3.7 per million among 5- to 14-year-olds. The highest mortality rate and the greatest increase in mortality has been in black Americans, who have a mortality rate 2.5-fold higher than that of white Americans. Asthma mortality varies significantly among states and different geographic areas within the United States. Mortality is highest in Hawaii and lowest in Alaska.

Most deaths are in patients with severe or unstable asthma that suddenly deteriorates. There is a much smaller group of patients who have sudden asphyxic asthma. These patients deteriorate rapidly over a short period, and are more likely to be in respiratory failure or to have respiratory arrest on presentation. These may be young people who have had an overwhelming allergen exposure or emotional upset.

Many risk factors for severe life-threatening asthma attacks or death have been identified. These can be categorized into factors that identify severe disease, previous severe exacerbations, inadequate care, and psychosocial factors. Factors that identify severe disease include a high degree of reversibility on initial FEV_1, a blunted perception of dyspnea or hypoxia, and previous severe attacks in chronic unstable patients. Previous severe exacerbations are identified by a history of prior intubation, respiratory acidosis, hospitalizations for status asthmaticus while taking long-term steroids, and episodes of pneumomediastinum, pneumothorax, or seizures during status asthmaticus. Inadequate or improper care is identified by gross underuse of anti-inflammatory asthma medications, overuse of beta-agonists, inadequate and inappropriate drug regimens, lack of continuity of care, lack of environmental control, and delays in seeking medical attention. Psychosocial factors include poor patient cooperation with asthma management, poor cooperation within the family and with medical staff, problems with self-care, depressive symptoms, disregard for symptoms and the use of illicit drugs, alcohol, or tranquilizers. Patients who are identified as having any of these factors should be considered at high risk. They should be monitored closely and have more frequent follow-up. Most importantly, the reduction in morbidity and mortality from asthma starts with appreciating the potential severity of the disease.

This paradoxical increase in the mortality and morbidity of asthma at a time when scientific advances are improving our understanding of asthma and providing new therapies has been the major impetus driving the development of multiple guidelines for the care of patients with asthma. The differences in the epidemiology of the morbidity and mortality of asthma indicate that both have the potential to be greatly reduced. Preventable factors contribute to 70% to 86% of asthma deaths. Those patients who receive follow-up outpatient visits are less likely to be hospitalized. Use of inhaled steroids decreases the risk of fatal asthma, asthma hospitalization, emergency department visits, missed work, and missed school days. Both the morbidity and mortality can be greatly reduced by the use of the four components of effective asthma management: the use of objective measures, environmental control, comprehensive pharmacologic therapy, and patient education. To do this, the provider must determine the course and severity of disease and must understand the patient's triggers, living situation, knowledge level, management skills, and the impact of disease on the individual and family. Recently the increase in worldwide mortality seems to be falling, with the glaring exception of the United States where it has remained steady.

New guidelines also are trying to address the high cost of asthma, which is estimated at 13% of the total cost of care for all respiratory disease. The economic impact of asthma to the United States in 1990 was estimated to be 6.2 billion dollars, with 3.6 billion dollars of direct costs and 2.6 billion dollars of indirect costs. Cost continues to rise with the increasing prevalence of asthma. The largest single direct medical expenditure was for hospitalization, which consumed 43% of all direct costs, whereas pharmacy costs were 30.2% and outpatient physician costs were 9.5% of direct costs. Indirect costs include loss of work ($\sim$15.4 $\times$ 10^6 days/year), caring for a sick child, not working at full capacity, and premature mortality. In contrast, in an HMO study of childhood asthma, hospitalization costs were 26% and urgent care costs were 11% of all asthma-related direct costs. The cost of outpatient care was considerably higher than in the previously mentioned study, consuming 41% of total asthma-related direct costs. The total cost of care of affected children was twice that of nonasthmatic children.

In most systems, 20% of patients accounted for 80% of all direct costs. Studies showing the greatest savings in asthmatic care most often evaluate the sickest patients, who are significantly undertreated and have the most disjointed care. Comprehensive interventions to targeted populations can result in large cost savings with improved asthma care. However, cost distribution, and therefore, areas targeted for cost savings, may be different in different populations and in different health care delivery systems. This finding implies that different strategies will be required for different populations and systems. In health care systems that have already achieved low hospitalization rates, costs of direct asthma care may actually increase as underlying morbidity is reduced with effective care. Use of the anti-inflammatory medications cromolyn sodium and inhaled steroids have been shown to be cost-effective. A dollar amount cannot be placed on a diminished quality of life.

Risk Factors

Changes in the epidemiology of asthma—its increasing prevalence, the large differences in prevalence among developed countries, and the large increases in prevalence with urbanization of rural, Third-World populations—all strongly suggest an environmental influence on the prevalence in asthma. These changes have been far too rapid, large, and generalized to be interpreted as genetic changes, and must be related to some environmental risk. These findings imply that asthma is a potentially preventable disease.

When one compares different populations, it becomes apparent that there is something about the Western life-style that increases the risk of developing asthma. The risk factors involved with this life-style need to be identified so effective strategies for primary prevention can be developed. This task is very complex because it involves isolating the effects of complex, often inter-related, environmental exposures. At the same time, risk factors for the development of wheezy respiratory

disease or asthma may be different at different ages, with different populations, or with different clinical asthma syndromes.

In recent epidemiologic studies, odds ratios (OR) have been calculated giving the relative risk of different factors for the development of asthma. As part of the ISAAC study in 7- and 8-year-old Swedish children, the main risk factors for asthma were a family history of asthma (OR = 3.2), followed by past or present house dampness (OR = 1.9), male sex (OR = 1.7), and a smoking mother (OR = 1.6). When none of these risk factors was present, the children did not develop asthma, but when three factors were present, 38% of these children were using asthma medications. Two of these factors, smoking and dampness in the home, are alterable, and intervention could potentially decrease the risk of asthma in those homes.

Allergy

Atopy, a genetic predisposition toward the development of allergy, is one of the strongest risk factors associated with asthma. This is reaffirmed in the ECRHS. In Spain, atopy to perennial allergens (OR = 10.2) and seasonal allergens (OR = 11.5) were both associated with current asthma. Past asthma was also associated with atopy (OR = 3.5). In Australia, wheezing when exposed to indoor allergens (OR = 15.1) and pollens (OR = 9.6) had a significant association with current asthma. Atopy was present in 86.3% of those patients with current asthma (OR = 6.4). Allergen sensitization is important in the persistence of asthmatic symptoms. In children, those who develop persistent wheeze after 3 years of age develop positive skin test results, have elevated serum IgE levels, and have a maternal history of asthma. In contrast, transient wheezers do not have this atopic history. With little skin test reactivity or low IgE, asthma present in early childhood tends to disappear, and patients in this group tend to outgrow asthma. Atopy is one of the most consistent and strongest risk factors for the persistence or development of asthma during adolescence. In a study of 13-year-old children from New Zealand, the prevalence of asthma correlated with the degree of atopy. Only 4.4% of those with negative skin test results reported asthma, but if there were four or more positive test results 40.5% reported current asthma symptoms. In 15- to 54-year-olds a progressive increase in the frequency of asthma was seen with increasing skin-test reactivity, but this was not seen in those older than 55 years of age, as the association between asthma and atopy diminishes with advancing age. Despite the strong association of asthma with atopy, atopy does not always lead to clinical disease, as is evident by the finding that 24% of children with four or more positive skin tests results did not report asthma.

Exposure to certain allergens has been associated with an increased risk of developing asthma. These include mites, cats, dogs, *Alternaria,* and cockroaches. In an inner city environment, cockroaches are the major risk factor for the development of asthma. Pet allergens are ubiquitous, and exposure great enough for sensitization can occur in public places, even without a pet at home. The higher the level of exposure in an environment, the greater the risk of sensitization and the development of symptoms. There appear to be threshold levels for sensitization, with higher levels for the development of symptoms. The thresholds vary for each allergen and the genetic predisposition of the host. Environmental control measures that keep exposure below these thresholds can reduce symptoms and theoretically prevent sensitization.

Allergy is common in asthma, and is likely a causative factor. Dust mite sensitivity is found in up to 85% of patients with asthma. Increased exposure to dust mites preceded a 39-fold increase in the prevalence of asthma in New Guinea Highlanders over a 10-year period. Children exposed to high levels of dust mites in their first year of life have an increased risk of developing asthma. Australian studies show a doubling of the risk for current asthma in children for every doubling of *Dermatophagoides pteronyssinus* antigen 1 (Der p1) level, and a quadrupling of the risk with an exposure level above 10 μg/g dust. Dust mite levels, especially those in the bed, are also correlated with the severity of disease. Studies of home dust mite avoidance measures show a decrease in severity of asthma, medication use, and BHR. Although it takes months of allergen avoidance to decrease BHR, there is a return to baseline reactivity within a couple of weeks of re-exposure.

Bronchial Hyper-responsiveness

In asthma the airway is hyper-responsive. Clinically this hyper-responsiveness results in airways that narrow too easily to a variety of direct and indirect stimuli. The more hyper-responsive the airways, the more readily cold air, laughter, or exercise will precipitate symptoms, and the more night time awakening, morning dipping, and variability in peak flow will occur. BHR can be measured by graded bronchoprovocation, most commonly using methacholine or histamine. The occurrence of bronchial airway hyper-responsiveness is often used as a marker for asthma. In general, the greater the bronchial reactivity, the more severe the asthma, and the more difficult it is to control. Medication requirements are roughly related to airway reactivity.

This increased airway responsiveness is thought to be fundamental to the pathogenesis of asthma. BHR may precede the development of asthma and is a risk factor for the development of asthma in the future. Patients with current asthma have a 9- to 20-fold increase in the risk of BHR compared to nonasthmatics, whereas patients with a past history of asthma have a 3- to 6-fold higher risk of BHR. This finding suggests that the effect of asthma on BHR decreases with passage of time from the last attack, but does not disappear. Other observations also indicate that BHR is not static in asthma. BHR will increase after a viral infection or during the LPR after an allergen exposure. It can decrease with allergen avoidance and immunotherapy. Long-term treatment with inhaled steroids, nedocromil, and cromolyn also may decrease BHR. Unfortunately BHR is not specific for asthma, but it is sensitive. BHR is about twice as common as asthma. Other respiratory diseases such as allergic rhinitis without asthma, cystic fibrosis, bronchiectasis, and chronic obstructive pulmonary disease also may be associated with BHR. BHR is closely associated with the development of chronic obstructive pulmonary disease in smokers. Even nonrespiratory diseases such as congestive heart failure may be associated with BHR.

In children, BHR increases from early to mid-childhood before it begins to decline in late childhood and adolescence. Male children are more likely to have elevated rates of BHR than females, but there is a more rapid decrease in reactivity in males, so that by 15 years of age BHR is the same in both sexes. The tendency to retain BHR is closely related to elevated serum IgE levels and positive allergy skin test results. In the group with the highest IgE levels or the most positive skin test results there was no tendency for BHR to decline, but BHR almost completely disappeared by age 15 years in those with low IgE levels or little skin test reactivity. Elevated total IgE and specific IgE levels are independent risks, but taken together are the main determinants of BHR. In adults, BHR decreases with advancing age.

Genetics

It is a common clinical observation that allergic diseases such as allergic rhinitis, eczema, and asthma run in families. Family studies indicate that children are more likely to develop the same allergic condition as their parents. Data from the ECRHS verify family history of parental asthma as a strong risk factor for asthma. The mean risk for a child developing asthma was 2.9 (2.4–3.5) if a father had asthma, 3.2 (2.6–3.9) if a mother had asthma, and increased to 7.0 (3.9–12.7) if both parents had asthma. Extrinsic asthma in any parent was a greater risk factor (4.9–6.0, 3.9–6.0) than intrinsic asthma of a parent (1.5–2.6, 0.8–2.6) for a child developing extrinsic asthma. This increased risk for the development of asthma from parental atopy or asthma extends into adulthood.

Parents are most interested in what their child's empiric risk is for developing asthma. Empiric risk, however, must be derived from the population of which the parents are members. In England the risk of a nonatopic asthmatic parent having an affected child is low, only slightly different from the population at large, which is 5% to 10%. The probability of an atopic asthmatic parent having a child who develops asthma is 14% if one parent is affected, and 29% if both parents are affected. The risk of asthma is 2- to 3-fold higher when a family history of asthma is accompanied by

one of atopy. Despite this, over one-half of all children who develop asthma will be from a family in which neither parent is affected. Family studies show that the risk of asthma increases with increasing atopy, defined as either IgE level or number of positive skin test results. Either genetic or environmental factors, or the interplay between them can explain the family clustering of asthma and the association of asthma with atopy.

Twin studies can help estimate the relative magnitude of the genetic and environmental effects by comparing concordance between monozygotic (MZ) twins, who are genetically identical, and dizygotic (DZ) twins, who share only 50% of their genes. Concordance rates for asthma range from 4.8% to 33% in DZ twins and 12% to 89% in MZ twins. These rates have varied among different populations and over time. In population-based twin studies, the estimated effect of genetic factors has ranged from 35% to 70%. In a recent twin family study, asthma was reported in 11% of children of asthmatic mothers, 10% of children of asthmatic fathers, and only 3% of children of nonasthmatic parents. There was an 11-fold higher risk of an MZ twin and a 5-fold higher risk of a DZ twin having asthma if their cotwin had asthma compared with the general population. In this and other twin studies, the concordance rate for MZ:DZ twin was 2:1. Despite this high genetic effect, only one-third of MZ pairs were concordant.

Despite the close relationship between asthma, total IgE serum levels, BHR, and atopy, these traits are not interchangeable. Each is under strong genetic control. Genetic factors that govern the specific IgE immune response are different from those that govern total serum IgE. Specific IgE responses are correlated with specific HLA alleles and haplotypes, and therefore, are linked to the HLA complex on chromosome 6. Serum IgE levels, which have heritability in the range of 50% to 84%, are regulated by a major genetic locus found on chromosome 5, location q31-q33. BHR is also under strong genetic control, with an estimated heritability of 66%. A family study has found there is cohinheritance and colocalization of BHR to the high IgE phenotype on chromosome 5. The presence of a set of genes that is coinherited and colocalized and that determines both elevated IgE and BHR could explain the genetic relationship between atopy and BHR. Analysis of this chromosome region reveals that it is the location for the genes of many of the cytokines involved in allergic inflammation and IgE regulation, and the beta$_2$-adrenergic receptor gene. This gene cluster includes 1L-4, IL-5, IL-6, IL-10, and IL-13. These cytokines are involved in the TH2 response.

There are likely several major genes and multiple different modes of inheritance associated with asthma. Family studies also have identified loci on chromosomes 6, 12, and 14. Research to date indicates asthma genes may vary with ethnic groups, as linkages to different chromosomal regions have been found for African Americans, Afro-Caribbeans, Caucasians, and Hispanics.

Tobacco Smoke

Tobacco smoke affects the development of asthma differently at different ages. There is an increased risk of asthma with all age groups by either passive or active exposure to tobacco smoke. The effect of tobacco smoke is much smaller than atopy, but of similar magnitude to the genetic effect. It is potentially one of the most preventable of risk factors.

Maternal smoking during pregnancy is associated with preterm delivery, low birth weight, and smaller initial lung function. Infants who have lower levels of lung function are more likely to wheeze with viral respiratory infections. After birth affected children also have increased airway hyper-responsiveness. Young children of smoking mothers are 1.5 times as likely to develop significant lower respiratory infection (LRI) and are twice as likely to be hospitalized with an LRI compared with children of nonsmoking mothers. There is an increased risk of wheezing with LRI and for the development of asthma in children exposed to environmental tobacco smoke. The risk of environmental tobacco smoke causing significant LRI, wheeze with LRI, and development of asthma decreases with increasing age. Tobacco smoke imparts a higher risk for the development of asthma on low birth weight infants, children of mothers with less education, and males. In children who have asthma, maternal smoking increases the severity of asthma. These children have more asthmatic symptoms, emergency room visits, and hospitalizations. Active smoking is a cause of asthma in all age groups. In young adults, current smokers are 1.7 times more likely to have current asthma.

Pollution

Pollutants can act directly or indirectly as adjuvants increasing the risk of sensitization or augmenting allergic inflammation already present. Pollution as a factor in explaining worldwide differences in asthma prevalence was examined in both the ISAAC and ECRHS. The patterns of asthma prevalence indicate that air pollution is not a major risk factor for development of asthma in populations. China and Eastern Europe had low rates of asthma prevalence despite some of the highest levels of air pollutants, especially with particulate matter and sulfur dioxide. Europe and the United States had intermediate prevalence of asthma but high degrees of ozone. New Zealand had a high prevalence of asthma but the lowest degree of air pollution. Life prevalence of asthma is lower in the more heavily polluted former East Germany compared with the former West Germany. Studies of German children indicated that the type of environmental pollution might be important. These children had less risk of developing asthma if they were exposed to indoor exposures from wood or coal heating and greater risk of developing asthma if they were exposed to tobacco smoke or truck traffic on residential streets. Diesel engines release large numbers of particles, which may cause increased airway inflammation, enhanced IgE production, and preferentially deliver specific allergens to the lower airway.

Although there is not much evidence that air pollution causes asthma, there is considerable evidence that it has adverse health effects on people with asthma. High ozone levels are associated with an increased number of asthma attacks, as well as increased emergency room visits and hospital admissions for respiratory diseases including asthma. Asthmatic patients have an exaggerated inflammatory response to ozone that can last for days. Both ozone and nitrogen dioxide may result in an exaggerated response to aeroallergens. Asthmatic patients are very sensitive to sulfur dioxide, which can exacerbate asthma at low concentrations, especially if the subject is mouth breathing or exercising. On days when particulate pollution is elevated, patients with asthma have lower peak flows, increased symptoms, increased medication use, and increased acute care medical visits.

Infection

Respiratory infections are a known trigger for asthma, especially in young children. In different age groups the epidemiology, the respiratory pathogen, the associated risk factors, and the mechanisms of airway obstruction are different. The existence of a small, underdeveloped airway is thought to predispose some infants to wheeze from airway obstruction. This smaller airway becomes less of a problem as the child grows older. In emergency department studies in children younger than 2 years, respiratory syncytial virus (RSV) is the most frequent infection associated with wheezing, and passive smoke exposure is the major associated risk factor. In wheezing children older than 2 years, rhinovirus is the major virus detected, and the coexistence of allergic disease is the major associated risk factor. In older children up to 80% of wheezing episodes are associated with viral infections, with rhinovirus being noted in 60% of these episodes. Nonviral infections such as *Chlamydia pneumoniae* also may be important in older children. In patients with asthma, viral infections increase BHR, enhance the immediate airway response to inhaled allergens, and increase the frequency of LPR to allergen challenge. Respiratory viruses are thought to up-regulate existing asthmatic airway inflammation.

The ability of respiratory infections to cause asthma is debated. Epidemiologic studies indicate that a serious respiratory infection before 5 years of age increases the risk of current asthma in young adults by 2.3-fold. This increased risk may be more important in asthma that starts before the age of 15 years, but not after. Observational studies have shown that 50% of infants who wheeze with bronchiolitis have subsequent wheezing, and young children hospitalized for croup, bron-

chiolitis, or pulmonary RSV infection have increased BHR 9 to 10 years later. These studies have not clearly resolved the debate over whether these viruses actually cause asthma or precipitate wheeze in a predisposed host. Complicating the picture are family studies that have shown a decrease in allergen sensitization and asthma prevalence with increasing numbers of older siblings, implying that an increased number of early respiratory infections protects against sensitization and the development of asthma. After severe infections such as measles or tuberculosis, the development of atopy is significantly reduced. With tuberculosis, there is a marked increase in the remission of asthma. Tuberculin responders have higher levels of the TH1 cytokine IFN-γ. Infections, which strongly promote a TH1 response, could potentially protect against the development of atopy or cause its remission by repressing the TH2 response. Infections, which promote a TH2 response, may positively influence the development of atopy. People in developing countries that still have high rates of infectious disease and lower immunization rates may be protected against the development of atopy, whereas those in countries that have better immunization, more access to antibiotics, and better housing may actually increase their risk for the development of allergic disease.

Diet

A diet high in salt, saturated fat, and processed foods and low in fresh fruits, vegetables and whole grains is associated with a Western lifestyle. Epidemiologic studies indicate that a diet low in fresh fruits and vegetables is a risk factor for decreased lung function. Population studies have shown decreased lung function with low vitamin A and C intake, and higher lung function with higher vitamin E intake. Several studies show low plasma levels of vitamin C in asthmatic subjects. In population studies, those with the highest vitamin C levels were 30% less likely to wheeze than those with the lowest levels. Unfortunately, vitamin C supplementation studies show questionable benefit in the treatment of asthma. Epidemiologic studies show that adults who regularly eat fish have better lung function. Children who eat fish more than once per week were 30% to 70% less likely to have asthma. Short-term trials of dietary fish oil supplements have not resulted in improved lung function, BHR, or reduced asthma symptoms. Western diets also are high in sodium and low in potassium. Short-term studies of low salt diets in patients with asthma have resulted in a reduction in BHR, peak flow variability, and symptoms. A population-based study of dietary magnesium intake showed a significant association of greater than 100 mg of dietary magnesium per day with higher FEV_1, decreased wheeze, and lower risk of having BHR. Unfortunately, supplement studies have shown no conclusive benefit of magnesium in acute asthma.

Infants who are breast-fed have lower IgE levels, less sensitization to house-dust mites at 1 year, fewer respiratory infections, and overall less allergic disease in early childhood. Clinical trials have shown no reduction in incidence of asthma.

NATURAL HISTORY

Recent research suggests that asthma is a clinical syndrome with different phenotypes. The natural history of asthma may differ with each phenotype. Young children who wheeze can be categorized into two broad groups, those who wheeze only with respiratory infections and those who wheeze with or without respiratory infections. Almost 50% of all children wheeze at sometime before 6 years of age. Of those who have wheezed before 3 years of age, about 60% are categorized as transient early wheezers, as they no longer wheeze at 6 years of age. Transient wheezers are more likely to wheeze with common viral respiratory illnesses, have lower levels of lung function, and have mothers who smoke. In those who have persistent wheezing at 6 years or have the onset of wheezing after 3 years, the major risk factors are atopy and more severe disease. Maternal smoking was the only factor associated with all groups. Asthma is not a fixed phenotype. In 14- to 15-year-olds who wheeze, only 55% had wheezed at 7 to 8 years of age; the rest developed wheeze in the interim. In older children, the prevalence of wheeze is more stable in males but increases in females. Remission rates for childhood asthma vary from 20%

to 75%. In those who wheeze before 7 years of age, 50% will outgrow asthma by adulthood. Remission rates are different in different age groups. Readmission is highest in the adolescent group from 10 to 19 years of age in which it is 65%, and lowest in the 40- to 49-year-old category in which it is only 6%. The overall remission rate in asthmatics between 30 and 60 years is around 1% per year. After age 60 remission rates again increase.

Various risk factors have been identified that affect the persistence of asthma versus its remission. The main risk factor is severity of disease—the milder the disease the more likely it is to remit. If there are frequent symptoms, more severe attacks, or lower baseline lung function remission is less likely. Age of onset affects remission, as those with severe disease before age 3 are less likely to experience remission. Comorbid states such as the presence of persistent eczema, coexistence of allergic rhinitis, chronic bronchitis or emphysema, all negatively impact the rate of remission. Gender is not a factor in most studies. Allergy is a major risk factor for the persistence of disease in those younger than 55 years of age. Current smokers have the lowest remission rate and the highest relapse rate.

Disappearance of asthma before adulthood does not indicate cure of disease, because asthma may recur. The longer patients are followed into adulthood, the less favorable the prognosis. About one third of those who were thought to have outgrown asthma will have a recurrence of wheezing. Relapse is not rare at any age, but reaches a high of 67% in subjects aged 60 to 69 years. Relapses are so frequent with advancing age that this feature may be part of the long-term natural history of asthma. Risk of relapse is higher in patients who continue to have any symptoms and those who smoke. It is unrelated to IgE level, gender, or symptoms of rhinitis.

Aspirin intolerance varies between 9% and 20% in asthmatic patients depending on the population evaluated. The more severe the asthma, the greater the risk of aspirin intolerance. This subset of patients with aspirin-sensitive asthma may have a different form of asthma, as risk of aspirin intolerance is greater in those with pansinusitis and nasal polyposis. Clinically it often begins with a chronic, nonallergic rhinitis with nasal eosinophilia. There may be progression to hyperplastic rhinosinus-itis and nasal polyps complicated with bouts of sinusitis. In about one-third of these patients there is the appearance of intrinsic asthma, which may progress to steroid dependence. Symptoms can occur immediately to a few hours after ingestion, most commonly within 20 to 60 minutes. Classically, aspirin ingestion is followed by the appearance of facial or gen-eralized flushing, ocular or nasal congestion or both, and rhinorrhea, followed by an acute, often-severe asthma attack. In the aspirin-sensi-tive asthmatic patient, monocytes are found to be very sensitive to inhibition of cyclooxygen-ase 1 by aspirin. This inhibition results in an increase in the synthesis of leukotrienes through the lipoxygenase pathway. Baseline urinary levels of LTE_4 are six-fold greater than in nonaspirin-sensitive asthmatic patients, and there is a four-fold greater increase in LTE_4 levels after challenge. Despite this defect, there are no HLA associations with this disease and family aspirin intolerance is rare. The nat-ural history of this form of asthma is unknown.

IMMUNOLOGIC SUSCEPTIBILITY

Epidemiologic data suggest that events that occur during pregnancy and early infancy can influence the development of asthma. Prenatal and postnatal developmental pathways affect the structure and function of the immune sys-tem and the airway. Maternal age, smoking, allergies, and nutrition all may influence the risk of developing asthma and asthma-like symptoms. Infants born to young mothers are at increased risk of having wheezing with lower respiratory infections during their first year of life and of developing asthma in later child-hood. Younger mothers have smaller babies and babies with lower expiratory flow levels. The effects of maternal age and smoking are independent, and therefore, additive. Being born prematurely and requiring ventilation in-crease the risk of asthma later in childhood. Maternal asthma is strongly associated with childhood asthma. Maternal nutrition or pla-cental function may alter fetal immune func-tion, as children with low birth weights are less likely to develop persistent atopic asthma and

those with large head circumferences are more likely to develop adult asthma.

During pregnancy the maternal immune response is heavily biased toward the TH2 type. This may influence the development of the allergic phenotype in the child. TH2 cyto-kines seem to protect the pregnancy, and IL-4 production is increased in both maternal and placental monocytes. In contrast the TH1-type cell-mediated immune response is thought to be undesirable for the maintenance of preg-nancy because IFN-γ is an abortifacient. Pro-duction of IFN-γ and IL-2 by maternal and placental monocytes remains low during preg-nancy. During the second and third trimesters the fetus begins to spontaneously release IFN-γ. This action is hypothesized to counteract the effects of IL-4 and IL-10 in order to pre-vent the TH2, allergic phenotype in the new-borns. Failure of this mechanism may lead to the development of atopy as IFN-γ inhibits transformation to the IgE isotype. Fetal pro-duction of IFN-γ increases with gestational age, but some infants produce little or no IFN-γ. Infants of allergic families are found to have reduced IFN-γ production and a slower rate of postnatal T cell maturation increasing their risk for persistence of a TH2 profile. The in-fants of atopic mothers also are exposed to a different cytokine profile *in utero*. In atopic mothers, the concentration of IL-10 in amni-otic fluid is higher than that of nonatopic mothers. IL-10 inhibits IFN-γ production, which results in T cells differentiating into a TH2 type.

There seems to be a critical period in infancy and early childhood for exposure to allergens and the later development of allergy. This critical early exposure occurs when the infant is immunologically predisposed to de-velop allergy. Early life exposure to pollen, animals, and dust mites increases the risk of sensitization that persists through adolescence. Early childhood sensitization imparts a higher risk for developing asthma than later sensitiza-tion. However, T cell sensitization may also occur *in utero*. Beginning at 22 weeks' gesta-tion, fetal T cells have been found to respond to a range of allergens including dust mite, cat, birch tree pollen, β-lactoglobulin, and ovalbumin. This response strongly suggests that maternal allergen exposure is important in the priming of fetal T cells. These infants are already capable of responding to environmental allergens at birth. This may not be seen immediately as clinical allergy since the maturation of the ensuing immune response may take as long as 2 years before allergen-specific IgE is produced.

KEY POINTS

▶ Asthma is increasing in prevalence, morbidity, and mortality despite better understanding of its pathophysiology and better drugs for its treatment.

▶ Asthma incurs a high cost to society with its low mortality, chronicity, and high morbidity.

▶ Desquamation of airway epithelium, thickening of the reticular basement membrane, and the eosinophilic inflammatory cell infiltrate are found in asthma of all levels of severity.

▶ TH2 cells and their cytokines are of central importance in asthmatic inflammation. Processes that promote TH2 responses may increase the risk for the development of asthma.

▶ Atopy is one of the strongest risk factors associated with asthma, and exposure to certain allergens has been associated with an increased risk for the development of asthma.

▶ With the increased understanding of the genetics and epidemiology of asthma, primary and secondary prevention may be possible.

Suggested Reading

Barnes PJ, Grunstein MM, Leff AR, Woolcock AJ (eds): Asthma, Vols 1 and 2. Philadelphia, Lippincott-Raven Publishers, 1997

Chadwick DJ, Cardew G (eds): The rising trends in asthma. CIBA Found Symposium 206, 1997

European Community Respiratory Health Survey: Variations in the prevalence of respiratory symptoms, self-reported asthma attacks, and use of asthma medication in the European Community Respiratory Health Survey. Eur Respir J 9:687–695, 1996

European Community Respiratory Health Survey: Italy, Determinants of bronchial responsiveness in the European Community Respiratory Health Survey in Italy: Evidence of an independent role of atopy, total serum IgE levels, and asthma symptoms. Allergy 53:673–681, 1998

International Study of Asthma and Allergies in Childhood (ISAAC) Steering Committee: Worldwide variation in prevalence of symptoms of asthma, allergic rhinoconjunctivitis, and atopic eczema: ISAAC. Lancet 351:1225–1232, 1998

Kay AB (ed): Allergy and Allergic Diseases. Oxford, Blackwell Science, 1997

Mannino DM, Homa DM, Pertowski CA, et al: Surveillance for asthma—United States, 1960–1995. In CDC Surveillance Summaries, April 24, 1998. MMWR 47 (No. SS-1):B1–27, 1998

Martinez FD, Wright AL, Taussig LM, et al: Asthma and wheezing in the first six years of life. N Engl J Med 332:133–138, 1995

Middleton E Jr, Reed CE, Ellis EF, et al (eds): Allergy: Principles and Practice. St. Louis, Mosby-Year Book, 1998

Pearce N, Beasley R, Burgess C, Crane J: Asthma Epidemiology: Principles and Methods. New York, Oxford University Press, 1998

Chapter 11

Asthma: Diagnosis and Management

Golda Hudes, Ashok Vaghjimal, and David L. Rosenstreich

Asthma is one of the most common problems with which primary care physicians have to deal and is one that is growing in frequency and severity. All physicians should therefore be familiar with its diagnosis and treatment. A thorough understanding of its pathophysiology is essential for optimal management of this disease.

Asthma is a chronic inflammatory disorder of the airways that causes recurrent episodes of wheezing, breathlessness, chest tightness, and cough, particularly at night and in the early morning. These episodes are usually associated with widespread, but variable, airflow obstruction, which is often reversible either spontaneously or with treatment. The inflammation also causes an associated increase in the existing bronchial hyper-responsiveness to a variety of stimuli.

Asthma is a very common disease. In the United States, it affects 14 to 15 million people, about 5% of the population, and it has a significant economic and social impact. In 1990, it was estimated that costs associated with asthma amounted to $6.2 billion or nearly 1% of total U.S. health care costs. Approximately 59%, or $3.6 billion, was related to direct medical care, of which half was spent for in-patient hospital care and emergency room use. The remaining 41% resulted from indirect costs such as lost productivity at work.

EPIDEMIOLOGY

Until the beginning of this century, the frequency of asthma, and especially death from it, were considered to be rare. According to a French physician of the early 20th century, Armand Trousseau, "asthma n'est fatale" (asthma is not fatal). Deaths from asthma in the United States decreased by 7.8% per year from 1965 through 1978, perhaps because of better understanding of its cause and the introduction of new and better therapies.

For unknown reasons, this trend underwent a marked reversal; since 1978, asthma prevalence and deaths have increased dramatically throughout most of the developed world. A recent editorial in the *Annals of Allergy, Asthma and Immunology* states: "Asthma has become more prevalent, more severe and more deadly." This change has manifested itself as increased office and emergency room visits, hospitalization rates, and mortality. Asthma rates have increased in every age group, most especially in children (Fig. 11–1). According to the Centers for Disease Control and Prevention, asthma is the most common chronic disease of childhood, affecting approximately 4.8 million children.

More worrisome than the increased prevalence, is the fact that asthma mortality has also been increasing throughout the world since 1977. As shown in Fig. 11–2, over a 9-year period (from 1979 to 1987), asthma-related mortality increased for persons aged 5 to 34 years. This increase differed by ethnicity, being significantly higher in nonwhite individuals. For the last decade, asthma-related morbidity and mortality have been consistently greater in African Americans than in whites nationwide, with males being affected the most. Al-

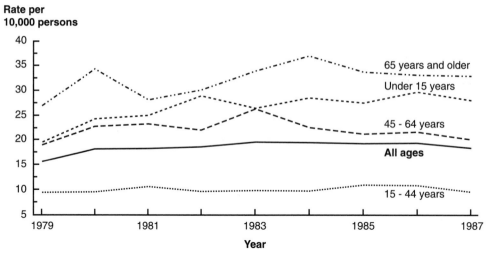

Figure 11–1. Trends in U.S. asthma hospitalizations for selected age groups, 1979–1987. (From Weiss K, Wagener DK: Asthma surveillance in the United States. A review of current trends and knowledge gaps. Chest 98 (Suppl):179s–184s, 1990. Source: NCHS, National Hospital Discharge survey, first listed diagnosis; reprinted with permission.)

though overall numbers of asthma-related deaths have remained stable since 1988, the death rate has not stabilized among 5- to 34-year-olds and continues to increase in African Americans. Mortality in the nonwhite United States population has continued to increase about 5% per year since that time.

Although the prevalence of asthma has increased nationwide, geographic location plays a significant role in asthma morbidity and mortality. According to the National Health and Nutrition Examination Survey (NHANES), asthma prevalence is higher in urban than in rural areas. The disease is more

common in the South and West than in the Midwest or the Northeast. Among urban areas, places such as New York City and Cook County, Illinois lead in asthma mortality and morbidity, and accounted for 21% of all the asthma-related deaths occurring in 1985. These areas are followed by Maricopa County, Arizona and Fresno, California. In addition, a study in New York City revealed that the highest rates of asthma hospitalization and asthma-related deaths occurred in the city's poorest neighborhoods.

These statistics suggest that living in overcrowded, polluted, urban environments and

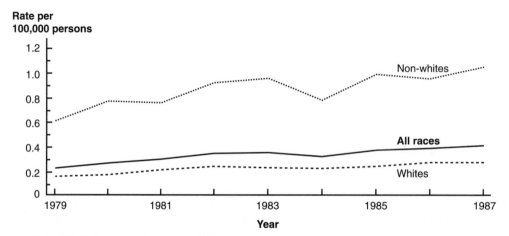

Figure 11–2. U.S. asthma mortality by race for persons aged 5 to 34 years, 1979–1987. (From Weiss K, Wagener DK: Asthma surveillance in the United States. A review of current trends and knowledge gaps. Chest 98 (Suppl):179s–184s, 1990. Source: NCHS, National Vital Statistics System, underlying cause of death. Reprinted with permission.)

poverty contribute to asthma morbidity and mortality. Socioeconomic status is probably a more significant determinant of asthma mortality and morbidity than race, ethnicity, or living in certain geographic locations. Sixtyone percent of asthma deaths in North Carolina in 1990 occurred in largely rural counties. The link between rural North Carolina and urban New York City or Chicago is probably the socioeconomic problems common in all these areas.

The rising prevalence of asthma and increasing mortality is not only a phenomenon in the United States, also having been reported in France, Sweden, Norway, Switzerland, Israel, Denmark, Germany, Australia, the Netherlands, United Kingdom, New Zealand, and Canada. Increased asthma deaths in the latter three countries have been attributed to β-agonist use.

Although the causes of the increase in asthma deaths in most Western countries are not completely understood, Lang has suggested a profile of high risk for fatal and near-fatal asthma based on case-controlled studies done in New Zealand, Canada, and the United States. He proposed three major risk factors. The first is severe asthma (meaning frequent hospitalizations and emergency room visits, corticosteroid use, past requirement for mechanical ventilation, and use of more than three medications for treatment) coupled with complicating factors such as exposure to allergens, pollutants, or tobacco smoke and recent symptom worsening. The second is psychological comorbidity resulting in nonadherence to treatment regimens and delay in seeking medical care. The third is African-American or Hispanic-American ethnicity and residing in an area in which the poverty rate is high. The risk factors related to ethnicity do not hold for the rest of the world. Asthma is rare in the tropics and in underdeveloped countries. Studies conducted in Peru, Gambia, Nigeria, Ethiopia, Kenya, and Zimbabwe confirm the low prevalence of asthma in economically poorer developing countries.

It has been postulated that parasitic infection may provide immunologic protection against asthma. High IgE levels characteristic of parasitization might prevent the development of asthma either by inhibiting the production of specific IgE, or by blocking IgE receptors. Consistent with this hypothesis, the IgE levels in patients with asthma in African countries was lower than those in controls unlike the pattern seen in western countries, where asthma is associated with increased IgE levels. The low rates of asthma in third-world nations also have been attributed to factors such as the lack of air pollution and the high level of physical activity in these areas.

Although asthma appears to be worse among segments of the population and in certain areas, it is nevertheless extremely widespread, sparing no socioeconomic or ethnic group. As a result, it is reasonable to assume that virtually every primary care practitioner will have to take care of one or more patients with asthma at some time during the average week.

PATHOPHYSIOLOGY OF BRONCHIAL ASTHMA

A tremendous amount has been learned about the pathophysiology of asthma over the past 25 years. A good working understanding of the pathophysiology of asthma is essential for logical management of this disease. Time spent in learning the essentials of this area is a valuable investment that will translate into better and more effective patient care.

Pathology

Airway inflammation is the major feature of the histopathologic findings in asthma. The understanding that asthma is an inflammatory disease is fundamental to the successful management of this disorder.

Autopsies of patients who die of asthma reveal lung hyperinflation, edema of airway mucosa with thick basement membranes, mucous plugging, collagen deposition beneath the basement membrane, denudation of the airway epithelium, creola bodies (sloughed epithelial cells), and infiltration by different cells, predominantly eosinophils and plasma cells. Another study found similar bronchial changes, such as goblet cell hyperplasia, mucous plugging, and collagen deposition beneath the epithelial basement membrane in lung biopsy specimens from two children with bronchial asthma in remission and from two children who died in status asthmaticus. The only differences were the presence of a larger number of submucosal eosinophils and more extensive denudation of the epithelium in fatal asthma. Thus, significant degrees of airway inflammation are present even in patients with asymptomatic asthma.

Bronchoalveolar lavage fluid from patients with asthma contains increased numbers of activated T cells, mast cells, eosinophils, shed epithelial cells, and the messenger RNA or protein of various cytokines such as tumor necrosis factor, interleukin 5 (IL-5), IL-6, IL-18, granulocyte macrophage colony stimulating factor, and endothelin. Also the allergic mediator, tryptase, which is released in asthma, has been found to induce human lung fibroblast proliferation and an increase in synthesis of predominantly type I collagen, which may contribute to fibrosis in areas of mast cell activation and may be important in the subepithelial fibrosis seen in asthma.

These studies have direct clinical relevance because they provide evidence for airway inflammation in patients with fatal asthma, in those with mild and moderate asthma, and even in patients in remission, supporting the recommendations for early treatment with anti-inflammatory medications.

Immunological Mechanisms

For the majority of patients with asthma, there is good evidence that the underlying inflammation is caused by one or more immunological mechanisms. Type I allergic reactions have been implicated in the pathophysiology of extrinsic asthma, at least in its early stages. This mechanism involves the inhalation of a specific allergen, which results in cross-linking of at least two similar IgE molecules on the surface of mast cells, basophils, or both. This cross-linking produces mast cell or basophil activation, degranulation, and mediator release. These mediators then induce defined biologic effects on the bronchial airways. Histamine is the major mediator of this initial reaction, which is often referred to as the early phase response.

In most patients with asthma and in most forms of asthma, prolonged allergen or irritant exposure produces the characteristic inflammation that is mediated by eosinophils and T lymphocytes. Mediators of this late phase response include a group of sulfidopeptides called leukotrienes. Leukotrienes are potent biochemical mediators released from mast cells, eosinophils, and basophils that contract airway smooth muscle, increase vascular permeability, increase mucous secretion, and attract and activate inflammatory cells in the airways. On a molar basis, leukotrienes are much more potent bronchoconstrictors than histamine (about 100 times), and unlike histamine, whose effects wear off after about 20 minutes, their actions are very prolonged.

In allergic individuals, specific CD4 T lymphocytes called helper type II (TH2) cells are dominant. These cells produce IL-4 and IL-13, which promote IgE production. In people who are not allergic TH1 CD4 T cells predominate. These cells produce gamma-interferon (IFN-γ), IL-2, and IL-10, which inhibit IL-4 action and subsequent IgE synthesis. Even in individuals who are not atopic, but who have significantly elevated IgE levels there is increased IL-4 and reduced IFN-γ, IL-2, and IL-10. TH2 lymphocytes also secrete cytokines such as IL-5, which promotes eosinophil survival and activity, and chemotactic factors such as eotaxin that attract neutrophils, eosinophils, and macrophages to the site of the inflammatory reaction, thereby perpetuating the chronic inflammation characteristic of asthma.

Eosinophils are the most important inflammatory cells in bronchial asthma, and a more accurate name for asthma would be eosinophilic bronchitis. Eosinophils produce two types of products that account for their important role in this disease. On a per cell basis, they are the most active producers of leukotrienes in the body. In addition, after degranulation, they release a number of highly potent cytotoxic substances, including major basic protein and eosinophil cationic protein, that damage airway epithelium and cause the epithelial destruction and shedding that are characteristic of the disease. The combined activities of eosinophil products are sufficient to account for most of the pathology and pathophysiology of asthma.

Other inflammatory cells such as macro-

Table 11–1. **Cells and Cytokines in Asthma**

Cells	Cytokines	Activity
TH2	IL-4, IL-5, IL-13, eotaxin	IgE isotype switch, airway inflammation
TH1	IFN	Inhibits IL-4 action and IgE production
Eosinophils	IL-3, GM-CSF, IL-1, IL-5 PAF, LTC4, MBP	Airway inflammation
Mast cells	IL-3, IL-9, IL-10	Mast cell growth, enhancement of IgE production through IgE inhibition
Macrophages	IL-1, TNF, IL-6, PAF	Express low-affinity IgE Fc receptor (CD23)

IL, interleukin; IFN, interferon; GM-CSF, granulocyte macrophage colony stimulating factor; PAF, platelet activating factor; MBP, major basic protein; TNF, tumor necrosis factor; LT, leukotriene.

phages, basophils, and neutrophils are also found in airways of patients with asthma. They are also capable of producing leukotrienes and cytokines, but their importance and exact role are not clear. The relationships between various cells, cytokines and asthma are summarized in Table 11–1.

Airway Hyper-responsiveness

The end result of chronic airway inflammation is the bronchial hyper-reactivity that is one of the characteristic and universal features of asthma. Virtually all patients with asthma, whether allergic or nonallergic, have increased responsiveness of the lower airway to non-antigen-specific triggers such as cold, exercise, inhaled methacholine, and histamine. Moreover, this hyper-responsiveness exists in individuals with asymptomatic asthma. Airway hyper-responsiveness expressed as a concentration of the challenge agent required to produce a 20% fall in FEV_1 is therefore often used as a clinical test for asthma. Asthma treatment with inhaled corticosteroids and cromolyn sodium reduces bronchial hyper-responsiveness.

It is this bronchial hyper-reactivity that produces the symptomatic bronchoconstriction that patients and physicians recognize as an asthma attack. Episodic bronchoconstriction can therefore be thought of as the tip of the iceberg, that is, the clinically apparent manifestation of the disease, whereas the chronic inflammation that is always there is its underlying cause.

Genetics

A genetic predisposition and a family history of asthma are known risk factors for devel-

oping the disease. As mentioned earlier, racial and ethnic differences have been noted in many studies. Thus, in the United States, asthma-related deaths in nonwhite males ages 5 to 34 years old are five times higher than in whites. The mortality rate in Maoris, a Polynesian population in New Zealand, is also five times higher than for whites. On the other hand, a hospital-based case-control study of white patients suggested that the British are more likely than North Eastern Europeans to develop chronic airflow limitation and that Scandinavians are prone to develop asthma.

With the rapid growth of genetic research in recent years, it was hoped that a single asthma gene could be identified. It has become clear, however, that asthma is a complex genetic disorder with several genetic loci associated with this disease. Not surprisingly, given our understanding of the role of immunologic mechanisms in generating the inflammatory asthmatic state, most of the candidate asthma genes are involved in regulating the immune system in some fashion. These include 14q, which is linked with the T cell antigen receptor, 11q13, which is linked with the high-affinity IgE receptor, and the 5q33 cytokine gene cluster. IL-4 and IL-10 promoter polymorphisms provide potential mechanisms for dysregulation of these cytokine genes in asthma. Understanding the genetics of asthma is complicated by the fact that environmental factors are almost certainly necessary for complete expression of the disease phenotype.

For the present, increased understanding of the genetics of asthma has not yet led to breakthroughs in either our understanding of the cause or the management of this disease. This is an area of active research that holds great promise for the future and that merits careful attention.

Autonomic Dysfunction

Starting in the 1950s, β-adrenergic hyporesponsiveness and deficiency were suggested as potential molecular mechanisms of asthma development. Subsequently, many *in vivo* and *in vitro* studies confirmed the existence of abnormalities in autonomic nervous system function in relation to the pathophysiology of asthma. Since the β_2-adrenergic receptor gene was identified, attempts have been made to connect variants of the gene with the development of asthma. Although no variant has been specifically associated with asthma, substitution of glycine for arginine at position 16 has been associated with more severe disease. Unlike the situation with genetics, this does not seem to be an active research area, and it is not clear if it will prove to be important in the pathogenesis of asthma.

PRECIPITATING FACTORS

There are two types of substances, primarily inhaled, that are involved in the pathogenesis of asthma: those that are inhaled chronically and are responsible for the underlying inflammation and those that are responsible for triggering acute bronchospasm. Some, like allergens, can do both, whereas others, such as irritating fumes, only induce acute symptoms.

Allergens

Allergens are probably the most important inducers of chronic asthmatic inflammation in both children and adults, although formation of antigen-specific IgE antibody to aeroallergens like mites or pollen usually does not occur until 2 to 3 years of life. Table 11–2 presents the most common allergens responsible for the development of asthmatic symptoms. Sensitization to indoor and outdoor aeroallergens is the most common cause of extrinsic asthma.

Dust mites were clearly identified as a cause of asthma more than 20 years ago and are the most important indoor allergens in many areas of the world. Ideal growing conditions for mites are high relative humidity, temperatures around 70°F, and the presence of

Table 11–2. Allergens Responsible for Precipitating Asthma Symptoms

Environmental allergens
Indoor
Dust mites
Furry or feathered pets
Feathers/down
Cockroaches
Rodents
Outdoor
Pollen
Mold spores
Food allergens
Drug allergens
Occupational allergens

shed human skin, which is the mites' major food source. Almost all of the allergen is contained in the mite fecal pellets. Because of these growth requirements, bedding has the highest concentration of mite allergen in the home. It has been estimated that there are about 250,000 mite fecal pellets in every ounce of dust in a mattress. Most individuals in the developed world spend about 8 hours every night of their entire lives breathing in mite feces; therefore it is not surprising that dust allergy is so prevalent. Most patients with asthma throughout the world are allergic to dust mites.

Although animal dander of any mammalian pets can trigger asthma symptoms, cat allergen is probably most common and best studied.

Though dust mites remain important allergens in the pathogenesis of bronchial asthma, recent studies clearly demonstrate that sensitization is determined by the most prevalent allergen in a certain geographic area. Thus, cockroaches are a very important cause of asthma among impoverished inner-city populations. In Northern Scandinavia and the Mountain States of the United States, cats and dogs are the most common source of allergens, and *Alternaria* has been reported to be the dominant asthma-related allergen in Arizona and Australia. Recent data from the National Cooperative Inner City Asthma Study indicate that the bedroom is the most important room in the home in terms of allergen exposure and resultant sensitization.

Interestingly, sensitization with different allergens may determine the severity of asthma symptoms. Thus, pollen-induced asthma usually has a well-defined seasonal incidence and is mild to moderate in severity. On the other hand, hypersensitivity to *Alternaria* has been reported as a risk factor for sudden respiratory arrest in adolescents and young adults with asthma.

Although food and drug allergies are a common cause of allergic skin, gastrointestinal, and systemic reactions, isolated respiratory reactions caused by food and drug allergy are rare. However, there are possible cross-reactions between shrimp and the inhalant or ingested allergens in insect materials such as cockroach, grasshopper and fruit flies. Patients with aspirin or nonsteroidal anti-inflammatory drug (NSAID) intolerance may have exacerbations after ingesting mite-contaminated wheat products.

Environmental Pollutants

Environmental irritants, such as nitrogen dioxide, ozone and paint and varnish fumes, are known triggers of asthma symptoms.

Airway hyper-responsiveness to ozone exposure is well documented. This is postulated to be caused, in part, by increased stimulation of muscarinic receptors on smooth muscles and, in part, by ozone-induced inflammation with an influx of neutrophils in bronchoalveolar lavage fluid and the subsequent development of hyper-responsiveness.

Smoking is a very important nonspecific irritant for all patients with asthma. Studies demonstrate an association of higher rates of asthma with even second-hand tobacco smoke exposure.

Infections

Viral infections are known powerful triggers of asthma symptoms in susceptible individuals. Although viral infections, especially respiratory syncytial virus (RSV), often lead to wheezing in infants, asthma develops infrequently in these individuals. In older children and adults with established bronchial asthma, viral respiratory infections (rhinovirus rather than RSV) contribute to wheezing and are responsible for up to 80% of asthma exacerbations.

Although the mechanisms of these phenomena are poorly understood, experimental studies suggest that viral-induced damage of airway epithelium, virus-specific IgE antibody production, enhancement of eosinophilic recruitment and airway infiltration, and stimulation of cytokines such as IL-1β, tumor necrosis factor a and IL-11 may be important.

Bacterial infection has not been shown to be a trigger of bronchial asthma, with the exception of bacterial sinusitis. This relationship is poorly understood, but explanations include a secondary bronchitis caused by postnasal drip and neural mechanisms such as the nasosinobronchial reflex.

Physical Factors

Physical factors such as high humidity, laughter, breathing cold air, or overheating may precipitate bronchial asthma. One of the most common and best studied physical precipitants of asthma is exercise. Exercise-induced asthma or bronchospasm affects 50% to 80% of patients with asthma and 40% of patients with allergic rhinitis. McFadden and Gilbert believe that practically all individuals with asthma suffer from some exercise-induced symptoms.

Pharmacological Agents

Patients with allergies to drugs, such as penicillin, can develop asthma as a part of a systemic reaction. Other drugs and chemicals also can cause asthma symptoms by a nonallergic mechanism. Aspirin and other NSAIDs are probably the most common and best studied agents. According to various data, 5% to 10% of patients with asthma are at risk of developing asthma symptoms after administration of aspirin or other NSAIDs. There is strong cross-reactivity among various NSAIDs. Reports have suggested that some aspirin-sensitive patients also may react to tartrazine (yellow dye #5), a dye found in various foods and drugs. Other medications known to exacerbate bronchial asthma include angiotensin converting enzyme inhibitors and beta-blockers. Sulfites and metabisulfates may also precipitate or aggravate asthma. These agents are commonly added to various food products to prevent discoloration.

DIAGNOSIS

As in most other diseases, the diagnosis of asthma depends on a combination of history, physical examination, and certain laboratory tests. Asthma is characterized by complaints of dyspnea, wheezing, or cough, or any combination of these. Attacks often occur at night or early in the morning, correlating with periods of low endogenous corticosteroid production. An attempt should be made to identify the relevant triggers such as viral illness, environmental allergens, or even certain drugs. Physical examination usually reveals wheezing and a prolonged expiratory phase on lung auscultation during an attack. However, physical examination can be completely normal in patients who are asymptomatic or even markedly symptomatic.

The most important laboratory test to perform on patients who are suspected of having asthma is a measurement of lung function by spirometry or peak expiratory flow rate, both before and after bronchodilator treatment. Airway obstruction that is responsive to bronchodilator treatment along with a compatible history makes the diagnosis of asthma almost certain. In patients with normal spirometry results, provocative tests with methacholine or histamine may be required. In the case of exercise-induced asthma, exercise challenge is used in place of chemical provocation. Other laboratory tests that may prove useful are a complete blood count (CBC) with eosinophil count, chest radiograph, and aeroallergen skin testing.

Differential Diagnosis of Asthma

A number of disorders can mimic asthma. A partial list follows:

1. Chronic obstructive pulmonary disease can be differentiated from asthma based on history of smoking, irreversible airway obstruction, and abnormal diffusing capacity on pulmonary function testing (PFT).
2. Congestive heart failure can present with wheezing and nocturnal tachypnea. Those symptoms usually are associated with basilar rales and peripheral edema. A chest radiograph is helpful and shows cardiac enlargement and Kerley B lines in patients with cardiac failure.
3. Pulmonary embolism can present as an acute asthma attack. In the absence of wheezing and history of asthma and allergies it is helpful to consider other diagnoses. When asthma and pulmonary embolism coexist, a ventilation–perfusion scan helps to make a diagnosis.
4. Laryngeal or vocal cord dysfunction is a functional disorder of the larynx that occurs in patients without asthma but with somatiform-conversion, factitious, or other mental disorders. This can mimic asthma and be refractory to therapy. During the attack, spirometry may show extrathoracic obstruction; nasopharyngoscopy allows visualization of the laryngeal obstruction.
5. Benign and malignant tumors of the airway occasionally produce wheezing and mimic asthma. The progressive course of the disease and a fixed airway obstruction on PFT help to rule out asthma. Bronchoscopy with biopsy provides a definite diagnosis.
6. Allergic bronchopulmonary aspergillosis and Churg-Strauss syndrome present with wheezing, severe steroid-dependent asthma, and eosinophilia. The findings of recurrent or persistent infiltrates on chest radiograph are indications that the patient does not have uncomplicated asthma.
7. Wegener's granulomatosus is characterized by paranasal sinus pain, nasal discharge with or without nasal mucosal ulceration, and kidney and eye involvement. Pulmonary symptoms (dyspnea, cough, and hemoptysis) are almost always associated with the above-mentioned manifestations. Patients can occasionally present with localized tracheal or bronchial forms of this disease that can mimic asthma. Tissue biopsy is diagnostic.

TREATMENT

Effective treatment of asthma involves a combination of environmental control and pharmacotherapy.

Environmental Control

Environmental control is the single most useful method of reducing asthma severity in most patients and should be instituted in all patients with asthma. All surroundings of the patient, particularly the bedroom, should be as free as possible from known and potential asthma triggers. The most common environmental triggers of asthma exacerbations or attacks and measures for their elimination are discussed in the following paragraphs.

Dust Mites

Most people cannot control outdoor pollutants and the dust conditions under which they work or spend daylight hours, but everyone can to a large extent eliminate dust from the bedroom. Recent data from the National Cooperative Inner City Asthma Study indicate that the bedroom is the most important room in the home in terms of allergen exposure and resultant sensitization. Elimination measures include the following:

Allergen-proof Bedding Covers. The patient's bed must have mite-impermeable covers that completely encase the mattress, box spring, and any pillows on the bed. These can be obtained from local stores that sell bedding or from specialized allergy control supply mail order companies. Costs vary with the quality of the product. Inexpensive ones work well but are less comfortable and usually crack after about a year and require frequent replacement. More expensive ones are more cloth-like and are usually guaranteed for 5 to 10 years. Probably the single most important and most cost-effective control measure is a pillow cover.

Patients are often resistant to using plastic bedding covers because of concerns about lack of comfort ("they are hot," "make me sweat," or "are noisy"). These problems can be greatly reduced by covering the pillow cover with two layers of cotton: a zippered pillow ticking and the regular pillow case. The plastic mattress cover should be covered with a quilted mattress pad and then the sheets. Once a week, anything cotton should be washed to remove any dust or mites that have accumulated. The plastic covers do not require regular washing.

Remove Rugs or Carpets. All rugs trap dust whether they are wool or synthetic. Hardwood or vinyl floors are preferable, but a washable throw rug can be used. If it is impossible to remove carpeting, vigorous vacuuming must be performed daily.

Vacuum Cleaners. Vacuum cleaners blow small dust particles out the back when in use (e.g., mite fecal pellets, which have a diameter of 10–30 microns), which can make asthma worse. Special allergen-proof vacuum cleaner bags that retain fine dust particles and mite feces are available from allergy supply companies (Micro-clean or Vacu-filt). Alternatively, patients should use HEPA vacuum cleaners. These work well, but are much more expensive than the special bags.

Dust Collectors. All upholstered furniture, drapes, old books, and stuffed animals should be removed from the bedroom. Light curtains can be used. Soft toys should be stored in plastic bags or sealed boxes. They must be washed in hot water (130°F); if washing is not possible, they should be placed in a deep freezer once a month to kill dust mites.

General Cleaning. The room must be cleaned daily and given a thorough and complete cleaning once a week. The floors, furniture, tops of doors, window frames, and walls should be cleaned with a damp cloth. Air the room thoroughly but keep the door of the bedroom closed as much as possible. Woodwork and floors must be thoroughly cleaned and scrubbed to remove all traces of dust.

Furry or Feathered Pets

Furry or feathered pets are common and avoidable causes of asthma. Elimination includes:

- Complete removal (the best).
- If removal is not feasible, then keep ani-

mals out of the bedroom permanently. No pets should ever be in the bedroom even when the patient is not there.

- Wash dogs frequently. Cats can also be washed, but this requires special training of the pet. Whether pet washing is effective in reducing home allergen levels is controversial.
- Place the litter box outside of the residence if possible.

Feathers or Down

Discard any feather (or down) pillows or quilts (or at least cover them with special allergy-proof encasings as described earlier). Use hypoallergenic pillows (polyester is the best) and washable blankets. The latter should be washed in hot water (above 130°F) when purchased and at least four times a year.

Cockroaches

Cockroaches are a very important cause of asthma, especially among impoverished inner-city populations. Efforts to decrease cockroach exposure include the following.

Intensive Cleaning.   Patients and their families should be informed about the importance of daily housekeeping, including giving everything a good soapy wash. Vacuum under all furniture, eliminate sources of food and water, and get rid of clutter. Food should be kept in glass jars and plastic tubs with tight lids. Used dishes should be washed immediately after use, and not left in the sink. Food should not be left in pets' bowls all day, and cat litter should be changed every few days.

Eliminate Holes, Cracks and Gaps.   Caulk and seal up all holes and cracks with steel wool and sealing caulk or even duct tape. Place screens over the bathroom vents.

Repair Leaks.   Any leaky faucets or plumbing should be repaired.

Mechanical Barriers.   Doors should have weather-stripping and windows should have screens. Screening should be placed over any ventilation ducts.

Trash.   Trash must be emptied daily. Garbage cans should have lids and plastic bags should tie on top.

Pesticides and Traps.   Use nontoxic insecticides or bait stations placed out of the reach of children and pets. Avoid insect sprays or pesticide bombs, which can exacerbate asthma and inactivate the bait stations.

Mold Spores

Mold spores can be effectively eliminated by:

1. Regular ventilation.
2. Washing affected areas with various products. Generally, household bleach is effective. Commercial companies sell mildew remover and mold and mildew control spray. Although mold removal products with strong odors can exacerbate asthma, this cleaning does not need to be done daily.
3. Elimination of any source of moisture. Do not use humidifiers of any kind continuously in the bedroom. Increased humidity increases growth of molds and dust mites and will make asthma worse. The most effective way to keep nasal air passages comfortable during the night in the winter is to keep the bedroom very cold (55–60° F).

Tobacco Smoke

Avoidance of cigarette smoke is very important. This can be achieved by:

1. Smoking cessation. Smoking cessation is ideal, but unfortunately, there is no totally effective smoking cessation protocol.
2. Elimination of tobacco smoke from the household. Smoking must be completely eliminated from the home of each patient with asthma. Such elimination can be easily done, and compliance will be much higher than for smoking cessation. Avoidance of cigarette smoke in the households of pre-schoolers and school-aged children

must be especially stressed, because there are studies showing an association of higher rates of asthma with second-hand smoke exposure.

Nitrogen Dioxide

Patients should be advised to ventilate their homes regularly and not to use gas stoves for heating, because such stoves are the major source of indoor nitrogen dioxide.

Miscellaneous Measures

Heating Sources. Forced air ventilation is very bad for patients. Install filter material (Venti-gard or equivalent) in the bedroom air inlet vent, so that all the air that enters the room is filtered. Wash or change this filter every month.

Fumes. Avoid paint and varnish fumes and unnecessary sprays (e.g., deodorant or hair spray). Use odor-free products whenever possible. Minimize the use of cosmetics with a strong odor.

Air Filters

High efficiency particulate air (HEPA) filters may be of value, especially in removal of ani-

mal dander, although proof of their effectiveness is lacking.

Drug Therapy

An assessment of the severity of asthma is essential before embarking on pharmacotherapy. The recently published guidelines divide asthma into four categories: mild intermittent, mild persistent, moderate, and severe (Table 11–3). These categories are a useful framework for making decisions about asthma pharmacotherapy. The National Institutes of Health (NIH) published guidelines for the long-term pharmacologic management of asthma in May, 1997, that are familiar to most practitioners (Table 11–4).

Overview of Asthma Medications

Corticosteroids

Corticosteroids are the most potent long-term control medications for asthma. They suppress the generation of cytokines, recruitment of airway eosinophils, and release of inflammatory mediators. When inhaled corticosteroids are used in high doses, systemic effects may

Table 11–3. **Severity of Asthma**

	Night Symptoms	Lung Function
Step 1 **Mild intermittent** Symptoms <2x/wk Asymptomatic and normal PEF between exacerbations	<2x/mo	FEV$_1$ or PEF >80% PEF variability <20%
Step 2 **Mild persistent** Symptoms >2x/wk but <1x/d	>2x/mo	FEV$_1$ or PEF >80% PEF variability 20%–30%
Step 3 **Moderate persistent** Daily symptoms Daily use of inhaled short-acting beta-2 agonist Exacerbations >2/week	>1 x/wk	FEV$_1$ or PEF >60%–<80% PEF variability >30%
Step 4 **Severe persistent** Continuous symptoms Limited physical activity Frequent exacerbations	Frequent	FEV$_1$ or PEF <60% predict. PEF variability >30%

Table 11–4. **Long-Term Control Medications**

Step 1
Mild intermittent asthma
  No daily medication needed
  Short-acting beta-2 agonist as needed for symptoms

Step 2
Mild persistent asthma
  Anti-inflammatory (either low dose of inhaled
    corticosteroid or cromolyn or nedocromil)
               OR
  Sustained-release theophylline to serum concentration
    5 to 15 mg/dL is an alternative
  Leukotriene modifiers (zafirlukist, Montelukast, or
    zileuton) may be considered. Position not yet
    established
  Short-acting beta-2 agonist as needed for symptoms

Step 3
Moderate persistent asthma
  Medium dose of inhaled corticosteroid
               OR
  Low to medium dose of inhaled corticosteroid and
    long-acting brochodilator (either long-acting inhaled
    beta-2 agonist or sustained-release theophylline)
  Short-acting beta-2 agonists as needed for symptoms

Step 4
Severe persistent asthma
  Anti-inflammatory medications (high dose of inhaled
    corticosteroids) along with long acting
    bronchodilator (either long acting beta-2 agonist or
    sustained-release theophylline)
  Systemic corticosteroids in some cases
  Short-acting beta-2 agonist as needed for symptoms

occur. A number of potent inhaled corticosteroid preparations are available. Usual side-effects include cough, dysphonia, and oral thrush. Concern about systemic side-effects such as bone loss, cataract formation, and delayed long bone growth in children have been raised with inhaled corticosteroids. Spacer or holding chamber devices and mouth washing after inhalation decrease local side-effects and systemic absorption and are highly recommended. When inhaled agents are not sufficient to control the asthma, daily administration of oral corticosteroids is needed. Prednisone or prednisolone are commonly used for this purpose; however, efforts should be made to avoid regular or frequent use of oral corticosteroids.

Cromolyn Sodium and Nedocromil

Cromolyn and nedocromil both have anti-inflammatory actions. Their mechanism of ac-

tion appears to involve the blocking of chloride channels, modulation of mast cell mediator release, and eosinophil recruitment. Both compounds are equally effective against allergen challenge.

These drugs should be administered four times a day, and a trial of 4 to 6 weeks may be needed to determine the maximal benefit. Both the agents are available in metered-dose inhalers and have excellent safety records. In addition, cromolyn is also available as a nebulizer solution (20 mg/ampoule)

Long-acting β_2-Agonists

The principal action of β_2-agonists is to relax airway smooth muscle by stimulating β_2 receptors, which increase cyclic AMP and produce functional antagonism to bronchospasm. Salmeterol and formoterol are the two agents currently available in this class of drugs. [Only salmeterol (Serevent) is available in the United States at the time of writing]. They are useful agents to control night-time symptoms and to prevent exercise-induced asthma.

Theophylline

The mechanism of theophylline's action in asthma remains unknown. Theophylline is a phosphodiesterase inhibitor and therefore increases intracellular cyclic AMP levels, which in turn may relax smooth muscles. Theophylline may also have anti-inflammatory activity. The main role of this agent is in nocturnal asthma. Several long-acting preparations of theophylline are available. Monitoring of the serum theophylline level is important to prevent the toxic effects of nausea and vomiting and central nervous system stimulation. A number of factors, including several commonly prescribed drugs (e.g., cimetidine, erythromycin, allopurinol, and several quinolones), can affect the serum level of theophylline.

Leukotriene Receptor Antagonists and Synthesis Inhibitors

Leukotrienes are potent biochemical mediators released from mast cells, eosinophils, and basophils that contract airway smooth muscle, increase vascular permeability, increase mucous secretion, and attract and activate inflammatory cells in the airways. Antileukotrienes are an important novel therapy for patients with mild and moderate persistent asthma, but their precise role in the management of this disease is currently being investigated. If one of these agents is chosen for treatment, a 6- to 8-week therapeutic trial should be used to make a decision about efficacy of the treatment. If the treatment is not effective, the medicine should not be continued beyond 8 weeks. Some clinicians are using these agents to decrease the dose of inhaled corticosteroids. Three leukotriene modifiers, zafirlukast, zileuton, and montelukast, are now available.

Zafirlukast (Accolate) (Astro Zereca, Wilmington, DE) is a leukotriene receptor antagonist that is effective in patients with mild-to-moderate asthma and exercise-induced bronchospasm. Its usual dose is 20 mg twice a day. The drug is well tolerated, and the patient does not require laboratory monitoring. There were reports regarding an association between zafirlukast therapy and development of Churg-Strauss syndrome. All reported patients had severe asthma and had been taking oral corticosteroids prior to zafirlukast therapy, which suggests the possibility that pre-existing Churg-Strauss syndrome became manifest when the dose of oral corticosteroids was decreased.

Montelukast (Singulair) (Merck, West Point, PA) recently came on the market and also is a leukotriene receptor antagonist with good efficacy in patients with mild-to-moderate asthma. This agent is a once-a-day medication (10 mg in adults and 5 mg in children age 6–13); it is approved for use in children. Montelukast has no clinically significant side-effects and does not induce any laboratory abnormalities.

Zileuton (Zyflo) (Abbott, North Chicago, IL) is a 5-lipoxygenase inhibitor that blocks the production of leukotrienes, whereas the two other agents are leukotriene receptor antagonists that prevent the binding of leukotrienes. Its dose is 600 mg four times per day. Some patients receiving zileuton have reversible elevations in hepatic aminotransferase levels. One noteworthy feature of this agent is its clear effectiveness in aspirin-sensitive asthma.

Although all antileukotrienes are recommended for use in the latter condition, only zileuton has been shown to block effectively the pulmonary and systemic manifestations of aspirin challenge in patients who are aspirin sensitive.

Quick Relief Medications

Short-Acting Inhaled Beta-2 Agonists.
Short-acting beta-2 agonists (e.g., albuterol, bitolterol, pirbuterol, terbutaline) have been the mainstay of asthma treatment for many years. They provide quick relief in an acute attack of asthma and also are effective in exercise-induced bronchospasm. All products are equipotent on a per puff basis. Potential side-effects of these agents include tachycardia, skeletal muscle tremor, hypokalemia, increased lactic acid secretion, headache, and hyperglycemia.

Anticholinergic Agents.
The anticholinergic agent ipratropium reverses only cholinergically mediated bronchospasm and has no effect on exercise-induced asthma. It is an alternative agent for patients with intolerance to beta-2 agonists and is the treatment of choice for bronchospasm caused by beta-2 blocker medication.

Allergen Immunotherapy

Despite years of use and numerous studies, the exact value of allergen immunotherapy (allergy shots) in asthma remains controversial. We think it should be considered for patients with asthma when there is clear evidence of a relationship between symptoms and exposure to an unavoidable allergen to which the patient is sensitive. As an ascending dose of allergen extract is given, increased tolerance develops to the injected allergen. Although the exact mechanism of immunotherapy is not known, allergen-specific IgE drops over many years and there is a rise in specific IgG blocking antibody. A meta-analysis of 20 randomized placebo-controlled studies confirmed the effectiveness of immunotherapy in asthma. Two recently conducted studies have generated some controversy regarding the benefits of immunotherapy. One, involving 90 patients with asthma, showed symptomatic improvement only in the first year of immunotherapy. The second study comprised 121 children with moderate to severe allergic asthma who were randomized to either placebo or injections of multiple allergens and observed for over 30 months. Both groups improved, and ultimately there were no statistical differences between the placebo and active groups for decline in medication use, remission of asthma, need for medical care, symptoms, or peak flow rates.

ASTHMA IN PREGNANCY

Poorly controlled asthma in pregnancy may result in increased perinatal mortality, prematurity, and low birth-weight. Beta-2 agonists have been widely used during pregnancy; the largest experience is with terbutaline. Long-acting beta-2 agonists are not recommended because of lack of experience with these agents in pregnancy. Cromolyn, theophylline, and inhaled, oral, and parenteral corticosteroids are considered to be safe. Of the inhaled corticosteroid preparations, beclamethasone has had the largest experience during pregnancy and is used almost exclusively.

SURGERY AND ASTHMA

Patients with asthma should have an evaluation before surgery because these patients are at an increased risk for certain complications such as bronchospasm, hypoxemia, and possible hypercapnia. An attempt should be made to improve lung function by maximizing the drug therapy. Prior to surgery, patients who have received systemic corticosteroids during the past 6 months should be given 100 mg of hydrocortisone every 8 hours intravenously during the surgery, and the dose should be rapidly tapered within 24 hours after the surgery.

REFERRAL TO AN SPECIALIST

Although most patients with asthma can be treated satisfactorily by primary care physi-

cians, a referral to an specialist should be made when they

- have difficulty achieving or maintaining control of their condition
- following a life-threatening asthma attack
- are not responding to current therapy
- have other allergic conditions such as hay fever
- need additional diagnostic tests to determine the severity of asthma
- are candidates for immunotherapy
- have persistent asthma
- require continuous oral corticosteroids or high dose inhaled corticosteroid

SUMMARY

Asthma is a very common disease that is increasing both in frequency and severity. Proper knowledge of its pathogenesis and underlying immune mechanism, and familiarity with current treatment guidelines is essential for the proper management of asthma. All asthma management should begin with simple environmental control measures to prevent the patient from inhaling potentially allergenic or asthmagenic substances. After that, drug therapy should be instituted that attacks the eosinophilic inflammation underlying the disease. Although inhaled corticosteroids are the most effective in this regard, blockers of mast cell degranulation, such as cromolyn or nedocromil, or the new leukotriene modifying agents are good alternative choices, especially in children. Initial referral to a specialist may be helpful for all patients except those with the most mild asthma, to establish the diagnosis, identify and eliminate causative factors, and develop a therapeutic plan.

The most important thing to remember is that the vast majority of patients with asthma should be able to lead completely normal lives, with minimal symptoms, minimal adverse effects from drugs, and minimal interference with their daily activities. If this is not the case, it is incumbent on the physician to investigate the problem and to make appropriate changes in therapy until that ideal state of health is achieved.

Suggested Reading

Colasurdo GN, Larsen GL: Airway hyperresponsiveness. *In* Busse WW, Holgate ST (eds): Asthma and Rhinitis.

Boston, Blackwell Scientific Publications, 1995, pp 1044–1056

Gleich GJ: The eosinophil and bronchial asthma: Current understanding. J Allergy Clin Immunol 85:422, 1990

Guidelines for the Diagnosis and Management of Asthma. Second Expert Panel on the Management of Asthma. NIH Publication No 97-4051A, May 1997

Manian P: Genetics of asthma: A review. Chest 112:1397–1408, 1997

McFadden ER Jr, Gilbert IA: Asthma. N Engl J Med 327:1928–1937, 1992

McFadden ER, Gilbert IA: Exercise-induced asthma. N Engl J Med 330:1362–1367, 1994

National Asthma Education Program Guidelines for the Management of Asthma During Pregnancy. Bethesda, MD, National Heart, Lung and Blood Institute, Report No. NIH 93-3279A, 1993

Peat JK, Tovey CM, Mellis CM, et al: Importance of house dust mite and *Alternaria* allergens in childhood asthma: An epidemiological study in two climatic regions of Australia. Clin Exp Allergy 23:812–820, 1993

Rosenstreich DL, Eggleston P, Kattan M, et al: The role of cockroach allergy and exposure to cockroach allergen in causing morbidity among inner-city children with asthma. N Engl J Med 336:1356–1363, 1997

Weiss KB, Gergen PJ, Hodgson TA: An economic evaluation of asthma in the United States. N Engl J Med 326:862–866, 1992

Chapter 12

Asthma: Special Considerations— Pediatrics, Exercise- Induced Asthma, Pregnancy

Gail G. Shapiro

EPIDEMIOLOGIC CONSIDERATIONS

Childhood asthma remains a problem of growing incidence and prevalence in the United States today. Over 5 million children in the United States are affected. Asthma causes more days lost from school than any other chronic disease.

The consequences of chronic asthma impact the individual, family, and community in ways that cannot be taken lightly. A child with well-managed chronic asthma may lead a very close to normal life and may have normal pulmonary function as an adult, even though the airway hyper-responsiveness may well remain throughout his or her life. In contrast, a child with poorly managed disease may miss considerable school time and miss the educational and social opportunities that school provides. Not inconsequentially, such a child may cause parents to miss work and lose both the immediate financial rewards of work and also chances for advancement in the workplace, which may be tied to performance and attendance stability. The psychodynamics of family

life can be immeasurably upset by these school and work issues.

Another aspect of the dysfunctional spin that asthma can put on family life is fear of morbidity or even mortality. Just as emergency room visits and hospitalizations for asthma have been rising over the past two decades, so have deaths from asthma. The inner city African American population has been disproportionally represented in this adverse outcome group. The issues of lack of access to care, cultural mores that lead to crisis-oriented rather than preventive medicine, and negative environmental exposures all play a role.

Aside from inner city minority issues, there are also cross-cultural psychological profiles that are worrisome prognosticators for death from asthma. These include such features as depression, dysfunctional family dynamics, seizure disorder, and prior episode of assisted ventilation for acute asthma.

Asthma's cost to society is steep both in terms of the patient's and family's emotional and physical well-being and in terms of hard financial outcome figures. A large portion of this cost is related to emergent care in the hospital outpatient and inpatient sectors.

171

There is good reason to believe that physician and patient education regarding asthma management can cut these costs dramatically, simultaneously improving the patient's and family's quality of life.

PATHOGENESIS

Underlying efforts at asthma education and care today is the observation that asthma is essentially an inflammatory disease.

While years ago smooth muscle and bronchospasm were felt to be the prime targets of therapy, anti-inflammatory modalities now appear to be most important for asthma control. Bronchoalveolar lavage studies of patients with asthma before and after anti-inflammatory therapy, for example inhaled corticosteroids, show a significant decrease in inflammatory cells such as the eosinophil and in other cell markers that correlate with inflammatory activity. Treatment with bronchodilators alone fails to alleviate airway inflammation.

RECOGNIZING ASTHMA

History

Most children who develop asthma do so by 5 years of age. Many children begin by having episodes of wheeze and cough or both with viral infections during the first years of life. Although the majority of children in this situation will cease to show these signs with time, a substantial minority will develop worsening symptoms with infections, difficulty breathing after strenuous exercise, and perhaps wheezing with allergen exposure. Factors that weigh toward development of asthma include family history of asthma and allergy, an atopic predisposition, and exposure to tobacco smoke and allergens.

Although a child's most striking symptoms may be recurrent episodes of wheezing and shortness of breath, the findings may be more subtle. It is not uncommon to see chronic cough as the sole manifestation of asthma. When cough presents after every upper respiratory tract infection and when exercise tolerance markedly drops during these times, the

diagnosis of asthma should be entertained. When children present with night cough, it is important to consider asthma, but it is also important to consider upper airway causes such as allergic rhinitis and sinusitis.

The child who has a history of recurrent bronchitis or recurrent pneumonia may actually have asthma, as both of these terms are sometimes used as euphemisms, which can actually prevent families from dealing with the reality of a chronic disease. Although recurrent cough and wheezing in childhood are most likely to be caused by asthma, the clinician should be aware of other causes of airway obstruction that can produce wheeze (Table 12–1). When the history uncovers problems associated with the atopic state, including atopic dermatis, allergic rhinitis, or food allergy, the possibility of asthma is strengthened. Most children with asthma are atopic, and allergy becomes increasingly important as a trigger factor as the child ages.

Physical Examination

The physical examination of the child who may have chronic asthma should include an evaluation of the head, neck, chest, and skin. Since an atopic predisposition is common in children with asthma, the presence of atopic dermatitis and rhinoconjunctivitis strengthens

---

Table 12–1. **Differential Diagnosis of Recurrent Cough and Wheeze in Children**

Large Airway Involvement

Enlarged lymph nodes or tumor
Foreign body
Laryngeal webs
Laryngotracheomalacia
Tracheo- or bronchiostenosis
Vascular ring

Large and Small Airway Involvement

Asthma
Aspiration for swallowing mechanism disturbance
Bronchopulmonary dysplasia
Chlamydia infection
Cystic fibrosis
Gastroesophageal reflux
Obliterative bronchiolitis
Pulmonary edema
Viral bronchiolitis

From Shapiro GG: Childhood asthma: Update. Pediatrics in Review, Vol. 13 No. 11 November 1992; used with permission.

any impression of asthma that the history suggests.

Head and Neck

The results of the head and neck examination is often abnormal in children with asthma. There may be evidence of middle ear disease (which may be a complication of allergic rhinitis): middle ear fluid, otitis, or ventilating tubes. In both children and adults, the eyes may show conjunctival edema and injection compatible with allergic disease. There may be periorbital edema and discoloration because of the venous and lymphatic stasis that may accompany allergic rhinitis (so-called allergic shiners). The nose may show the pallor, edema, and clear secretions of allergic rhinitis or erythema and purulent secretions from infectious rhinitis or sinusitis. The presence of nasal polyps in children suggests cystic fibrosis, whereas in the adolescent and adult it suggests nonallergic eosinophilic respiratory disease (possibly with aspirin sensitivity), which may involve the upper and lower airway. Since sinusitis and viral upper respiratory infections both exacerbate asthma, it is important to diagnose and treat infections that are likely to be bacterial.

Chest

The examination of the chest may be totally normal between acute exacerbations. In children with long-standing chronic obstruction one may see bowing of the ribs and an increased anterior–posterior diameter of the chest, since growth and bony remodeling will accommodate chronic pulmonary hyperinflation. On auscultation one may notice an increased expiration phase of respiration. There may be wheezing on expiration or on both inspiration and expiration; coarse wheezes may take on the quality of rhonchi. Wheezing on forced expiration alone generally indicates less obstruction than wheezing throughout expiration; wheezing during both inspiration and expiration indicates more severe disease. Nevertheless, these correlations are only generalizations. It is not uncommon to hear normal breath sounds and inspiratory–expiratory

ratios in a child who has marked chronic airway obstruction. This complicates the task of assessing disease severity, particularly in younger children. In older children, the use of peak flow determination and spirometry add an important objective dimension to the understanding of the patient's status. Even with the additional information provided by these tools, however, asthma fluctuates in severity and is truly a dynamic problem. The traditional physical examination provides a view of only one moment in time.

Pulmonary Function Tests

Pulmonary function monitoring is essential in the diagnosis and ongoing care of children with asthma because both symptom scores and physical examination correlate poorly with the degree of airway obstruction. Unfortunately, currently available methods of monitoring are not applicable to young children, because peak flow determinations are of limited value before 4 years of age and spirometry is difficult before 5 years of age. PEFR measures air flow through large airways. Tables for predicting PEFR based on patient sex and height are available. Healthy children generally will have a PEFR greater than 90% of the predicted value. Any measurements below 80% of the predicted value suggest obstruction that requires follow-up and treatment; a decrease to 50% or lower heralds a severe attack.

This type of monitoring is helpful in the office and the home. Patients who have moderate or severe asthma should monitor their PEFR daily, measuring it at least each morning before taking medication. Even more information is obtained from monitoring before and after taking bronchodilator medication in the morning and at bedtime. The regimen chosen will depend on asthma severity and patient compliance. Both patient and physician awareness of fluctuations around the patient's personal best yields more information than judging performance based on predicted tables. A level that is more than 90% of the personal best PEFR indicates a comfortable position (in the safety zone), and one that is less than 80% signals the need for caution. As a patient's condition becomes stable on a chronic medication regimen for asthma, it is common to see both an increase in peak flow measures and a decrease in diurnal variation from morning (generally the lowest peak flow of the day) to night. Displaying this improvement visually on graph paper is gratifying to the patient, family, and physician (Figs. 12–1 and 12–2).

Spirometry provides more sensitivity than does peak flow monitoring. Also, it visually documents the quality of the expiratory maneuver. The patient's results are compared with predicted normal values for sex and size available in standardized tables, but as with peak flow monitoring, fluctuations around a personal best level are most revealing. In general, the forced expiratory volume in 1 second (FEV_1) measures larger airway flow and should be 80% or more of that predicted. Forced expiratory flow at 25% to 75% of vital capacity is mainly useful for following a patient's changes over time. Children who require chronic therapy for asthma and are old enough to perform the maneuver (usually ages 5 to 6 years) should have spirometry performed at least yearly in order to follow progress and determine how to modulate therapy. Spirometry is advisable more often than this

in patients with labile symptoms and whose medications are being changed.

Other Laboratory Tests in Diagnosing Asthma

Sometimes the diagnosis of asthma remains unconfirmed after weighing the information provided by the history, physical examination, and lung function tests. Additional testing is warranted in these situations.

Response to Bronchodilators

The simplest method to assess the degree of airway obstruction is to look for improvement in lung function after administration of bronchodilators. This procedure is useful to ascertain if patients with low pulmonary function test results have easily reversible disease and to decide what is a patient's optimal pulmonary function. In children too young for spirometry, listening for clearing of rales or cough after bronchodilator administration may give diagnostic information about reversible dis-

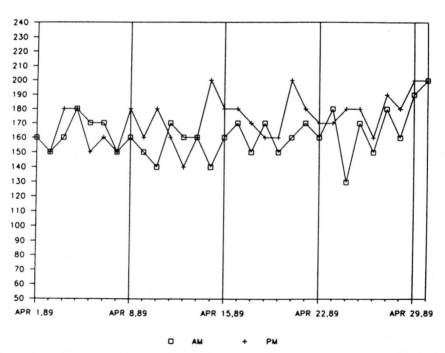

Figure 12–1. Example of a twice-daily peak flow chart depicting the type of fluctuation that can be expected from a child who has moderate, fairly well-controlled asthma. The child who generated this tracing is 5 years of age. (From Shapiro GG: Childhood asthma: Update. Pediatrics in Review 13 (11): November 1992, with permission.)

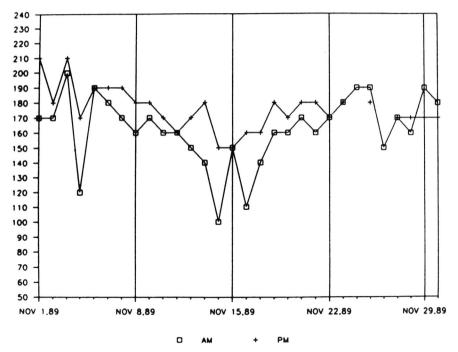

Figure 12–2. This peak flow chart was generated by the same child as in Fig. 12–1 and shows fluctuation during an acute asthma exacerbation. The dips during early and mid-November alerted the family to the need for increased attention to the condition and the pediatrician to the need for beta agonist bronchodilators. (From Shapiro GG: Childhood asthma: Update. Pediatrics in Review 13 (11) November 1992; with permission.)

ease. Beta-agonists can be delivered by a metered dose inhaler (MDI) (2 actuations) or compressor driven nebulizer (0.1 to 0.15 mg/kg albuterol solution or equivalent, maximum 5 mg). A greater than 12% improvement is consistent with asthma. In patients with long-standing obstruction, a one- to two-week course of oral corticosteroids may be necessary to demonstrate a reversible component to airflow obstruction and to reach the patient's personal best pulmonary function.

Provocation Challenges

Chemical Challenge Tests

Chemical challenges are valuable for the patient with presumptive asthma or chronic cough in whom baseline pulmonary function is normal and therapeutic trials with anti-asthma medications are inconclusive. Patients with asthma have airways that are overly sensitive to bronchoconstrictors. This feature can be used to distinguish people who are likely to have asthma from those with normal airway

reactivity. Methacholine and histamine challenges can be performed with standardized protocols that have high specificity and sensitivity for airway hyper-responsiveness and asthma. Patients inhale increasing concentrations of methacholine or histamine according to a standardized protocol and perform spirometry after inhaling each concentration of the drug. The challenge is complete when FEV_1 has dropped 20% or more from baseline or when one completes the dilutions of the protocol. A decline in FEV_1 of greater than 20% indicates bronchial hyper-responsiveness. When this information is melded with a supporting clinical history, the diagnosis of asthma becomes likely. On the other hand, a negative challenge test usually excludes asthma.

Distilled water inhalation, eucapneic hyperventilation of cold air and hypertonic water inhalation are alternative challenge procedures. These are less well standardized than chemical and exercise challenges. Inhalation challenge of specific antigens would seem to offer valuable diagnostic information regarding asthma triggers; however, in practice, antigen challenge has severe limitations. Antigen inhalation may produce bronchospasm in the laboratory, whereas only rhinitis occurs after natural inhalation. Also, late phase reactions that may occur after the patient leaves the laboratory are common. All bronchial challenge tests are potentially dangerous. They should only be performed by specialists who have had special training in their use and experience in this technique.

Exercise Tolerance Tests

Exercise-induced asthma is a common feature of childhood asthma, affecting the majority of children with chronic asthma. In certain situations, the extent of change in pulmonary function with activity may deserve evaluation. This evaluation can be done informally with free running or in a more standardized way in the laboratory using a treadmill or stationary bicycle. Typically the exercise period lasts 6 to 8 minutes, and pulmonary function is monitored for 20 minutes or more thereafter. The peak drop in pulmonary function will occur 5 to 15 minutes after exercise. A fall of greater than 12% in FEV_1 or in peak expiratory flow or, alternatively, 25% $FEF_{25-75\%}$ is diagnostic of exercise-induced asthma.

Nasal and Sputum Cytology

Nasal and sputum cytology may be helpful in sorting eosinophilic inflammatory disease from neutrophilic, infectious disease, since both of these may be concomitants of asthma and provide information regarding asthma etiology, e.g., allergic versus infectious exacerbations. For nasal cytology the patient blows his or her nose into plastic wrap, the secretions are applied to a glass slide, heat fixed, and stained with Hansel's stain, an eosin–methylene blue combination that stains eosinophils distinctively. Alternatively, a tiny nasal brush or rhinoprobe device can be used to obtain a specimen from the wall of the nasal vault. The presence of greater than 5% to 10% eosinophils suggests allergic or eosinophilic nonallergic rhinitis. The presence of large numbers of neutrophils and bacteria suggests infection. If the problem has been long-stand-

ing, the possibility of subacute or chronic sinusitis, which serves to aggravate bronchial hyper-responsiveness, should be considered. When dealing with sputum, which is only obtainable in older children, freshly expelled material is placed in a thin layer on a slide and then examined in the same fashion as nasal secretions. In sputum, one may see Curschmann's spirals, which are threads of glycoprotein, creola bodies, which are clusters of epithelial cells, or Charcot-Leyden crystals, which are derived from eosinophils.

Total Serum IgE

Total serum IgE determination may be helpful at times, although it is nonspecific and there are overlaps in the serum levels of normal and allergic individuals. Approximately 80% of children with allergen-induced asthma and 50% of adults will have a total serum IgE concentration greater than two standard deviations from the nonallergic population mean. The presence of an elevated IgE concentration suggests allergic bronchopulmonary aspergillosis (ABPA) or that environmental allergy may be an important trigger factor for asthma. More helpful, however, is evaluation of antigen-specific IgE.

Allergy Testing

Allergy skin testing is important in evaluating childhood asthma, because allergy has been shown to play an important role. Testing is done with extracts of selected allergens based on history and known or potential allergen exposure. Asthma in children is frequently exacerbated by exposure to environmental allergens. In a given patient, the same antigen-specific IgE that can trigger inflammatory events in the airway can be detected in the skin. Antigen applied to the skin reacts with specific mast cell-bound antibody, which induces mediator release. Histamine will create local vasodilation with a wheal-and-flare within 15 minutes, and a variety of chemotactic factors may create a delayed inflammatory response hours later. Although true positive skin test results indicate that a patient has antigen-specific IgE, it does not prove that exposure will create clinically significant disease. The predictive value of a positive skin test result is enhanced if the reactivity is intense and occurs in conjunction with a positive provocative history.

As an alternative to allergen-specific skin tests, serum IgE against a specific antigen can be measured with serologic tests such as the radioallergosorbent test (RAST). In this procedure, antigens are coupled to an inert carrier such as latex or cellulose and mixed with the patient's serum, after which binding of antigen and patient's antibody is measured.

Chest Radiograph

It is not unusual to see patchy atelectasis or peribronchiolar infiltrates during an acute asthma episode. Since these findings are not likely to alter therapy, the need for a chest radiograph is limited. Nevertheless, it is wise to obtain a chest radiograph at some time during the course of childhood asthma that is persistent and moderate to severe in intensity in order to rule out a structural abnormality.

MANAGEMENT OF CHRONIC ASTHMA

Education of the patient and family regarding the chronicity of asthma, the management of exacerbations, and the importance of ongoing therapy to minimize acute exacerbations and to maximize lung health and growth is an essential part of treatment. Allergens and irritants that may be driving the disease should be investigated thoroughly in children with asthma. It is important to consider environmental issues as being potentially as important as medication for treating this disease.

Environmental Control

Exposure to allergen and irritants at vulnerable times may significantly increase bronchial reactivity and adversely influence asthma control. The antigens most commonly implicated in chronic asthma are house dust mite, cockroach, pet-derived antigenic proteins (with cat being the most common), and airborne molds and pollens. Murray reported on the beneficial influence of bedroom dust control measures in 1983, and subsequent studies add to the information implicating dust mite antigen as a major factor in asthma.

Encasing mattresses in airtight covers, washing pillows and bedding weekly in hot water (over 130°F), and removing carpeting, particularly if laid on concrete slab floors, will reduce house dust mite levels in the home. Other valuable measures include reducing the humidity to less than 50% and using acaricides to kill the mites. When carpets cannot be removed, acaricides such as benzyl benzoate and products that denature mite antigen such as 3% tannic acid spray to the carpet and stuffed furniture may be helpful. Most physicians concentrate efforts on education that relates to keeping the bedroom and family area as free as possible of house dust mite antigens.

It is unfortunate that although pet removal may be necessary to effect major improvement in asthma symptoms for some highly atopic patients, carrying out this removal is so difficult. If a pet to which a patient is sensitive cannot be removed from the home, certain temporizing measures are worthwhile: keeping the pet out of the bedroom and considering an electrostatic or HEPA filter. Many pet antigens are tenacious molecules that travel easily and are difficult to eliminate from the home. The part-time indoor pet may produce the same antigen load as the full-time indoor pet, and it may take months after the pet is removed from the environment for residual allergen to decrease to nonproblematic levels.

Cockroach antigen is a problem primarily in the eastern and southern United States. Antigen concentration appears to be related in part to lower socioeconomic populations. Cockroach antigen may be more important than dust mite among this population. Attempts at environmental control include removing uncovered food sources and exterminating these insects.

Irritant exposure should be limited to achieve best asthma control. Tobacco smoke exposure has been linked to asthma exacerbations, decreased lung growth, and age of onset of asthma; therefore, smoking in the home should be forbidden. Wood stove heat has been linked to increased emergency room visits for asthma and should be avoided in favor of cleaner heating fuels. Atmospheric levels of ozone and sulfur dioxide may be related to asthma exacerbations, although correlations are modest.

The amount of counseling that one offers concerning the environment depends largely on historical issues, level of allergy skin test reactivity, and the ability of a family to make changes in their surroundings.

Pharmacologic Management Commonly Used Asthma Medications

The pharmacologic therapy of asthma involves using drugs that relax smooth muscle and dilate the airways and others that decrease inflammation and thereby prevent exacerbations.

Beta-Agonist Bronchodilators

Beta-agonist bronchodilators are valuable as intermittent therapy for children who have infrequent episodes of obstruction, as adjunctive therapy used intermittently or routinely in conjunction with anti-inflammatory agents for patients who have frequent exacerbations or chronic obstruction, before exercise for blocking exercise-induced asthma, and in the emergency setting for acute attacks. These drugs are available in formulations for oral administration and inhalation and are most effective when inhaled from a metered dose inhaler, dry powder inhaler, or nebulizer. Inhalation delivers a greater ratio of a dose to the pulmonary tree and minimizes the systematically delivered portion, which may cause such side-effects as tremor and irritability.

Beta agonists lack anti-inflammatory effects. Although symptoms are relieved, inflammatory changes, which aggravate bronchial hyper-responsiveness and underlie the clinical disease, are not prevented.

The most commonly used beta agonist bronchodilators used today are β_2-selective, relaxing bronchial smooth muscle without having appreciable beta$_1$ activity (i.e., cardiac-related effects such as producing tachycardia).

Metaproterenol does retain some β_1 activity, whereas the more β_2-selective drugs include albuterol, pirbuterol, terbutaline, and tornalate. Levalbuterol, the R-isomer of albuterol, is now available for nebulizer use and appears more potent than racemic albuterol with less β_1 activity. These drugs are relatively short acting, having rapid onset of action within minutes and having activity for 4 to 6 hours at most. Salmeterol is a long-acting β-agonist whose activity begins 20 to 30 minutes after administration, peaks by 1 hour and lasts for approximately 12 hours. Salmeterol offers prolonged bronchodilatation and relief from the need to use shorter acting agents repeatedly. Several reports support the ability of salmeterol to decrease the amount of inhaled steroid required by patients with moderate to severe asthma.

Nonsteroidal Anti-inflammatory Drugs

Cromolyn-like nonsteroidal anti-inflammatory agents appear to prevent release of mediators from mast cells, which induce acute bronchoconstriction and chronic inflammatory airway changes. In addition, these drugs may modulate the activity of proinflammatory molecules that upregulate airway hyper-responsiveness. Although these drugs have been shown to decrease asthma symptoms and improve disease control, the potency of their anti-inflammatory activity is much less well documented than that of inhaled corticosteroids. Cromolyn is useful as a maintenance, prophylactic agent for mild-to-moderate chronic asthma. In addition, cromolyn can be used intermittently to decrease exercise-induced asthma and to prevent antigen-induced episodes. Cromolyn is administered by inhalation from an MDI or nebulizer. The usual recommended dosage by MDI is 2 actuations (1 mg per actuation) four times per day, although it is often prescribed as 2 to 3 actuations three times per day, and then may be tapered to twice per day, if good asthma control has been achieved. The ampule for nebulization contains 20 mg/ml and probably provides more therapeutic efficacy per dose than the MDI, but no comparative studies have been published. Cromolyn does not have steroid-spacing capacity and need not be continued with inhaled corticosteroid in patients who are stepping up to more intensive therapy.

Nedocromil is a pyranoquinoline that has proven benefit for asthma symptom control and has probable anti-inflammatory effects on the airway. It has been shown to be effective in clinical trials of children and adults with chronic asthma. It appears to have prophylactic properties when used prior to antigen challenge as well as a variety of other challenges including sulfur dioxide, cold air, and exercise; nedocromil is similar to cromolyn in anti-asthma potency. It may have a faster onset of action and more therapeutic activity. It appears to have steroid-sparing capability, which cromolyn does not have. Approximately 13% of patients strenuously object to its taste and refuse to use it, whereas another subset find it unpleasant but tolerable. Nedocromil for asthma is currently available in the United States in MDI form only. A preparation for nebulization is currently under Food and Drug Administration review.

Inhaled Corticosteroids

Inhaled corticosteroids are very valuable anti-inflammatory agents for chronic asthma. They are appropriate for management of mild, moderate, and severe disease. Their use is increasing as more is known about their long-term safety and their potential for positively influencing long-term asthma outcome; benefits which have not been evaluated for cromolyn or nedocromil. Inhaled corticosteroid preparations currently available in the United States include beclomethasone, budesonide, triamcinolone, fluticasone, and flunisolide. Although each of these compounds is different and generalizations are imprecise, when these drugs are used in doses of less than 400 μg per day (beclomethasone equivalent), there is little likelihood of discernible systemic action. Doses greater than 800 to 1000 μg per day present risks of systemic corticosteroid activity to some extent and raise issues regarding endocrine function, growth, and bone density, as well as other less worrisome side-effects related to steroid usage. The goal with these medications is to use the least effective dose that maintains normal life-style and pulmonary function. In the most severe situations, one must compromise and choose the dose that gives the best risk-benefit ratio for the patient.

Tapering dosage is an important aspect of inhaled corticosteroid use. After a patient achieves good benefit from inhaled corticosteroid therapy, it is worthwhile to taper the dose by 25% every 3 to 6 months to establish the lowest effective dose.

Oral Corticosteroids

Oral corticosteroids are a mainstay of care during asthma exacerbations. In this setting, the patient usually receives a loading dose of 1–2 mg/kg of prednisone. This dose is then tapered over several days to a week or more, depending on the patient's particular situation (see Management of Acute Asthma). Oral corticosteroid use in chronic asthma is limited to patients with very severe disease in whom the use of inhaled agents is not adequate. Patients who require oral steroid therapy on a regular basis usually use this in conjunction with high dose inhaled corticosteroids and all other forms of adjunctive therapy. The oral dose is tapered to the lowest alternate-morning regimen that provides adequate control. This regimen minimizes the risk of pituitary–adrenal axis suppression.

Antileukotriene Agents

Antileukotriene agents are anti-inflammatory agents that work by either blocking the lipoxygenase enzyme responsible for converting arachidonic acid to the leukotrienes, which are proinflammatory molecules, or by blocking leukotriene receptors in the airway. Zileuton, of the former group, is approved for children 12 and older. It must be dosed four times per day. Liver enzyme abnormalities have been noted in some patients, so liver function must be monitored for several months after initiating therapy. Zafirlukast is a receptor antagonist approved for children 7 years and older. It is dosed twice per day on an empty stomach. Montelukast, also a receptor antagonist, is dosed at 5 to 10 mg at night. Pediatric studies show effectiveness for mild asthma and exercise-induced asthma. These drugs may have steroid-sparing potential and be a valuable adjunct in moderate and severe disease. At this point clinical anecdotes and optimism regarding the value of montelukast as a single daily dose anti-inflammatory for maintenance therapy outpace published documentation. It will be important to learn how this family of drugs compares to inhaled corticosteroids in terms of effects on long-term prevention of airway remodeling and the natural history of asthma.

Anticholinergic Agents

Anticholinergics are bronchodilators that counteract bronchoconstriction related to cholinergic innervation to the airways via the vagus nerve. These drugs also decrease mucus hypersecretion in some patients and counteract cough-receptor irritability. Ipratropium bromide is the anticholinergic agent that is approved for use in the United States. It is available in a MDI and in a nebulizer preparation. Despite data showing additive bronchodilatation of ipratropium with β-agonist for acute asthma, there is no information to support the chronic use of ipratropium by nebulizer or MDI for chronic disease. The drug has been useful, however, in treating adults who have chronic obstructive disease with a reversible component.

Theophylline

Theophylline is a bronchodilator that has been popular in the United States for a long time, perhaps more so than in any other part of the world. It is useful as a maintenance bronchodilator for mild chronic asthma and as an adjunct for more severe chronic asthma. Theophylline has lost some of its attractiveness, with the current focus on anti-inflammatory therapy for asthma. It does not appear to provide significant anti-inflammatory effect, although this point remains controversial. Theophylline is available in a wide variety of oral formulations, varying from rapidly released preparations with short durations of action to sustained release products that can be used twice per day. Although once-daily dosing is possible with certain preparations in people who clear theophylline relatively slowly, most children are fast metabolizers and require at least twice-daily dosing to maintain therapeutic serum concentrations.

Much has been written about theophylline pharmacokinetics and issues of dosing. Several points are essential to know: (1) Although there are age-related guidelines for dosing, only by following serum concentrations can one be certain of proper dosing. In general, children younger than 9 years of age require more theophylline per kg than do older children. (2) The ideal therapeutic range for maximizing effectiveness and decreasing adverse effects is 5 to 20 μg/mL, but many physicians prefer to narrow this 5 to 15 μg/mL to lessen the risk of adverse effects. (3) Disease and drugs that affect the P450 cytochrome system of the liver can alter theophylline clearance and change levels, sometimes drastically. Examples are certain febrile illnesses such as influenza and such drugs as erythromycin, cimetidine, and ciprofloxacin. (4) A variety of symptoms of intolerance can occur with theophylline, including headache, gastrointestinal upset, and irritability. To avoid these effects, begin therapy at a dosage level that is one third of the anticipated optimal dosage, then increase to full dosage. Determine the serum level after the patient's condition stabilizes at this dosage (e.g., after 2 to 3 days). If symptoms of intolerance develop during the increases, check the serum level sooner. The use of theophylline commits the physician to monitoring the patient closely and assessing serum levels accordingly. The appropriate period between assessments may be yearly for the stable patient but much more frequently for the patient who may experience adverse effects.

Allergen Immunotherapy

Allergen immunotherapy has been shown to decrease asthma symptoms and bronchial hyper-reactivity in a number of trials that have recently been summarized. Immunotherapy should be considered when environmental avoidance measures and appropriate pharmacologic interventions are not sufficiently helpful or cannot be maintained by the patient and family and where the history indicates a large environmental allergen influence on the disease. Immunotherapy has been shown to be effective for dust mites, certain molds, and pollens. It has been useful for cat allergy, although avoidance is a preferable solution. Allergen immunotherapy is typically given for 3 to 5 years. Although a positive effect should be seen within a year to justify continuation of this intervention, several years more of therapy appears to be needed to increase the likelihood of more persistent protection. Life-threatening reactions to immunotherapy are uncommon when the process is supervised by a specialist, but the risk of anaphylaxis still remains. Considering this, allergen immunotherapy must be administered in a clinic where facilities and personnel are available to treat a life-threatening reaction. Patients should wait for 30 minutes after each shot since this is the interval of highest risk.

APPROACH TO THERAPY

Very Young Children
(Fig. 12–3)

Therapy for children under 5 years of age is guided by concerns about delivery systems that are appropriate for the very young as well as by the need for medication. The most common stimulus for wheezing in this age group is a viral syndrome. The typical pattern of disease is onset of wheezing with a viral infection in the first year of life followed by the return of wheezing and cough with subsequent infections over the next 2 to 3 years. The majority of children who follow this pattern will eventually outgrow their airway hyper-responsiveness either totally or to a large degree. Approximately one-third will develop more frequent wheezing with more varied stimuli. Both those children who go on to a life-long problem and those who develop frequent wheezing and coughing for only a few years of life should be considered to have chronic asthma and should be given the benefit of anti-inflammatory therapy. At this time there is no way to screen for those patients who will certainly outgrow their problem. Therapeutic trials suggest that early intervention with chronic therapy yields the best outcome in terms of symptom control and long-term development.

Children with mild intermittent disease wheeze less than 3 times a week and can be treated with rescue medication alone, i.e., a β-agonist as needed. Medication can be given by mouth or by inhalation using a nebulizer or face mask and spacer. During viral syndromes, the frequency of dosing can be increased to up to every 4 hours. If this frequent medication use is needed more than every 6–8 weeks, the use of chronic anti-inflammatory medication should be considered. If a specific episode becomes severe or if the patient has a history of severe acute exacerbations, the use of systemic corticosteroids is an important addition. In using a β-agonist, the oral route of administration provides less active drug to the pulmonary tree and more systemic drug that can contribute to tremor and irritability.

When symptoms occur more than twice a week, there is enough evidence of airway inflammation to argue for chronic anti-inflammatory therapy. The choices of long-term preventive therapy include a montelukast chewable tablet (5 mg), cromolyn by MDI or nebulizer, or either nedocromil or a low-dose inhaled corticosteroid by MDI. In the near future, inhaled corticosteroid preparations for nebulizing will be available as an alternative for chronic therapy in the very young. Young children require the use of a face mask with a spacer attached to the MDI; the mask is held in place for 20 to 30 seconds after each actuation. The dose of inhaled medication that reaches the pulmonary tree is considerably lower with this method of administration in young children than in adults. In the United States there has been a preference to attempt nonsteroidal anti-inflammatory therapy prior to initiating corticosteroid therapy. The use of compressor–nebulizer devices has simplified delivery of cromolyn on a chronic basis, adding a β-agonist for acute exacerbations and sometimes regularly along with cromolyn. In a case in which the nonsteroidal agents and low-dose inhaled corticosteroid therapy is not adequate to control disease, the patient should be treated with higher doses of inhaled corticosteroid by face mask and spacer. The β-agonist should be delivered by face mask and spacer or nebulizer on an as needed basis. However, some patients may do better if the β-agonist is used regularly up to every 4 hours. There is no benefit to continuing cromolyn therapy in the patient who is taking chronic inhaled corticosteroid. In adults there appears to be steroid-sparing potential of nedocromil, but this has not been shown in young children, and

Step 1 Mild Intermittent	Step 2 Mild Persistent	Step 3 Moderate	Step 4 Severe	S T E P D O W N ⇩
■ Bronchodilator as needed for symptoms. Either: -- Inhaled short-acting beta₂ nebulizer or face mask and spacer or -- Oral beta₂-agonist prn for symptoms <3 times a week ■ With viral respiratory infection: -- Bronchodilator q 4-6 hours up to 24 -- Consider systemic corticosteroid or - If patient has history of previous severe attacks.	■ Daily long-term preventive medication. Either: -- Cromolyn (MDI or nebulizer) or nedocromil (MDI only) TID-QID (infants usually begin a trial of cromolyn or nedocromil) or -- Inhaled corticosteroid (beclomethasone) spacer and face mask 100-400 mcg/ day rescue ⇩ ■ beta₂-agonist as needed for symptoms up to every 4 hours (see Step 1).	■ Daily long-term preventive medication. Either: -- 400-800mcg/ day inhaled corticosteroid spacer and face mask -- beta₂-agonist tid-qid routinely or prn. -- Consider use of theophylline to minimize dose of inhaled steroid. -- Consider nedocromil to minimize dose of inhaled steroid. Consultation with an asthma specialist is recommended. rescue ⇩ ■ beta₂-agonist as needed for symptoms (see Step 1) up to every 4 hours.	■ Daily long term preventive medicine -- >800mcg/ day inhaled corticosteroid spacer and face mask. -- beta₂-agonist tid-qid routinely or prn. Theophylline to minimize steroid dose. Consider nedocromil to minimize dose of inhaled steroid. -- If needed, add oral corticosteroids at lowest alternate morning dose that stabilizes symptoms rescue ⇩ ■ beta₂-agonist needed for symptoms (see Step 1) up to every 4 hours.	

Note:
■ Patients should start treatment at the step most appropriate to the initial severity of their condition. Establish control as soon as possible; then decrease treatment to the least medication necessary to maintain control.
■ A rescue course of prednisolone may be needed at any time and step.
■ It is important to remember that there are very few studies on asthma therapy for infants.

⇩ **Step down**
Review treatment every 3 to 6 months. If control is sustained for at least 3 months, a gradual stepwise reduction in treatment may be possible.

⇧ **Step up**
If control is not achieved, consider step up. But first: review patient medication technique, compliance, and environmental control (avoidance of allergens or other trigger factors).

Figure 12-3. Stepwise approach to management of asthma in infants and young children.

the possible benefit must be weighed against the cost and compliance issues related to using an additional medication. The steroid-sparing potential of antileukotrienes has been reported in clinical trials that have not yet been published.

The patient with severe asthma will require high doses of inhaled corticosteroid through a face mask and spacer as well as a regular β-agonist. Theophylline may be used as a supplementary bronchodilator. Nedocromil may be considered as a means of decreasing the steroid requirement. In the most difficult disease situations, an oral corticosteroid may be used in addition to an inhaled corticosteroid. If an oral agent is required, it should be a short-acting agent such as prednisone or methylprednisolone. It should be given on an alternate-morning schedule to minimize the chance of pituitary–adrenal axis suppression.

Young children with moderate and severe disease should be evaluated by an asthma specialist. It is essential to rule out structural disease of the lung and other pathologic processes that may masquerade as asthma. It is very important to search for underlying causal factors in the environment such as irritants and allergens that may contribute to the disease. Also, it is valuable to obtain therapeutic advice from an expert in such difficult situations.

Older Children (Fig. 12–4)

The management of children over 5 years of age is very similar to the management of adults. Short-acting β-agonists effectively treat intermittent mild asthma. When these episodes occur less than twice weekly, the patient may receive a β-agonist from an MDI. Therapy can be repeated every 4 to 6 hours during viral syndromes or with asthma-inducing environmental exposures. Systemic corticosteroids may be needed during severe attacks of asthma. It is quite important to assess the frequency of β-agonist and corticosteroid use to determine if the patient actually has persistent mild to moderate disease, requiring chronic anti-inflammatory therapy.

Patients who are symptomatic more than twice a week should receive chronic nonsteroidal anti-inflammatory therapy or an inhaled corticosteroid. In some cases in which the use of inhaled medications is impossible, oral antileukotrienes and sustained release theophylline are alternatives. As with younger children, the nonsteroidal anti-inflammatory agents and low-dose inhaled corticosteroids are options for those with mild to moderate disease. A short-acting β-agonist should be available on an as needed basis. If this agent is being used regularly, particularly during the night, a longer acting bronchodilator is appropriate. In this situation, the short-acting beta$_2$-agonist would still be available as a rescue drug. One would need to be certain that the addition of the long-acting agent actually diminished the use of the short-acting drug. If not, its use would be superfluous and possibly negative, as excessive use of β-agonists may increase bronchial hyper-responsiveness.

For the patient with moderately severe disease, the dose of inhaled corticosteroid needs to be increased until symptoms abate and ideally, until pulmonary function returns to normal. To minimize the necessary dose of inhaled steroid, a β-agonist should be used regularly. Salmeterol has been shown to preclude the need for increased inhaled steroid in adults. It may also be advisable to consider sustained-release theophylline or nedocromil.

The patient with severe disease requires high-dose inhaled corticosteroid along with a regularly used bronchodilator. This may be a long-acting β-agonist, sustained-release theophylline, or both. A short-acting β-agonist will still be necessary for rescue. Some patients will require an alternate-morning oral corticosteroid in addition to these medications. Considering the relative risk these drugs pose, it is best to maximize inhaled corticosteroid and bronchodilators use in order to minimize the systemic corticosteroid. If an oral corticosteroid can be discontinued, the next target for tapering of medication should be the inhaled corticosteroid.

While the antileukotriene drugs are documented to be effective for mild, persistent asthma, their effectiveness as additional therapy to inhaled corticosteroids for moderate and persistent disease is currently being evaluated. Although anecdotal evidence appears to be positive there are no scientific data currently available.

Preferred treatments are in bold print

Step 1 Mild Intermittent	Step 2 Mild Persistent (milder end of spectrum)	Step 3 Moderate	Step 4 Severe
Long-Term Preventive - None needed	**Long-Term Preventive**	**Long-Term Preventive**	**Long-Term Preventive**
Short-acting bronchodilator: **inhaled beta₂-agonist** as needed for symptoms, but no more than twice a week. Intensity of treatment will depend on severity of exacerbation. Inhaled beta₂-agonist, cromolyn, or nedocromil before exercise or exposure to allergen. With viral infection: -- Inhaled beta₂-agonist q 4-6 hours up to 24 hours (longer with physician consult) but no more than every 6-8 weeks -- Consider systemic corticosteroid if current attack is severe or if patient has history of severe attacks with infection.	Daily medications ■ Either **inhaled cromolyn sodium or nedocromil or inhaled corticosteroid** 400-800mcg or anti leukotriene	Daily medications ■ **Inhaled corticosteroid** ■ Long-acting bronchodilator; especially for nighttime symptoms; either long-acting inhaled beta₂-agonist, sustained-release theophylline, or long-acting beta₂-agonist tablets. ■ Consider nedocromil to minimize inhaled steroid. * role of anti-leukotrienes not clear	Daily medications: ■ **Inhaled corticosteroid, 800-2000** mcg or more and ■ Long-acting bronchodilator: either long-acting inhaled beta₂-agonist, sustained-release theophylline, and/or long acting beta₂-agonist tablets and ■ Consider nedocromil to minimize dose of inhaled steroid. ■ Corticosteroid tablets or syrup long term (2mg/kg/day max. 60mg per day) - alternate morning doses. * role of anti-leukotrienes not clear
rescue ⇩	rescue ⇩ Short-acting bronchodilator: **inhaled beta₂-agonist** as needed for symptoms not to exceed 3-4 times in 24 hours.	rescue ⇩ ■ Short-acting bronchodilator: **inhaled beta₂-agonist** as needed for symptoms, not to exceed 3-4 times in 1 day.	rescue ⇩ ■ Short-acting bronchodilator: **inhaled beta₂-agonist** as needed for symptoms.

S T E P D O W N ⇩

⇩ **Step down**
Review treatment every 3 to 6 month; a gradual stepwise reduction in treatment may be possible.

⇧ **Step up**
If control is not achieved, consider step up. First, review patient medication technique, compliance, and environmental control (avoidance of allergens or other trigger factors).

Note:
■ Patients should start treatment at the step most appropriate to the initial severity of their condition. Establish control as quickly as possible; then decrease treatment to the least medication necessary to maintain control.
■ A rescue course of prednisone may be needed at any time and at any step.
■ Patients should avoid or control triggers at each step.

Figure 12–4. Stepwise approach for management of chronic asthma in children over 5 years old.

THE ACTION PLAN

At each level of severity, the patient and family must have a guide for both daily and crisis intervention. Daily therapy must be formulated in a spirit of communication and with adequate teaching of essential aspects of therapy, including proper use of nebulizers, spacers, and MDIs. These tasks require continual reinforcement to assure optimal technique and to motivate the patient and family for better compliance.

A peak flow meter is a valuable addition to all but the patient with the mildest asthma. Although not all patients will use the peak flow meter all the time, it may provide useful information in a variety of circumstances. For a mildly affected patient, normal peak flow rates will reinforce that there is no reason for anxiety about asthma. For a severely affected patient, the peak flow rate will clarify whether there is stability when the patient may not be able to perceive this on his or her own, since loss of sensitivity to obstruction is common with asthma.

It is valuable for the patient to have a written action plan that delineates the steps to take when peak flow rates or symptoms indicate deterioration. Usually, the patient will initiate use of a short-acting bronchodilator and repeat this until there is adequate improvement, usually restricting this to every 4 hours unless there is a frank acute episode. For this situation, the β-agonist can be used every 20 minutes for 3 times by MDI (2 actuations) or by nebulizer. The oral corticosteroid needs to be started if symptoms do not readily abate. Usually, the patient or family will need to contact the physician for guidance at this juncture, though educated families may have enough experience to start a burst of prednisone on their own and follow up with the doctor soon after.

Many communities have resources for families with asthmatic children. The Asthma and Allergy Foundation of America has local chapters and support groups. The American Lung Association provides educational sessions. AAN/Mothers of Asthmatics has an active membership and a valuable newsletter. Education and support from the community help the family that is dealing with asthma to overcome feelings of isolation as well as fears about serious consequences. Although it is true that asthma morbidity and mortality are increasing in the United States, it is also true that proper disease management leads to a normal lifestyle for most children with asthma.

EXERCISE-INDUCED ASTHMA

Although exercise is a well-known trigger of asthma in all patients, exercise-induced asthma (EIA) may be more readily apparent in children because of their typically active play. In one study, EIA was shown to occur in 63% of children with asthma and in about 40% of nonasthmatic, atopic children. A more recent assessment of the scope of this problem, however, suggests that all asthmatic patients can experience EIA given a sufficiently strenuous level of exertion. Nonetheless, most children and other patients with asthma can safely participate in athletic activities and other forms of exercise as long as their underlying condition is adequately diagnosed and treated.

Definition

Exercise-induced asthma, also known as exercise-induced bronchospasm, is defined as a temporary increase in airway resistance, which usually occurs after a period of sustained strenuous exercise. Typically, this response develops soon after the person has *stopped* exercising, although (as described later) some people experience a delayed response.

The strict definition of EIA, according to laboratory criteria, is a 15% reduction in PEFR or FEV_1 after exercise as compared with the pre-exercise values. A standard challenge involves measurements taken before and after 6 to 8 minutes of strenuous treadmill exercise. Pulmonary function is measured at 5-minute intervals after exercise for 20 to 30 minutes. The peak drop in lung function usually occurs 10 to 15 minutes after exercise, with recovery shortly after.

Signs and Symptoms

The main signs and symptoms of EIA are coughing; wheezing; and chest pain, discomfort, or tightness. There may be dyspnea, fatigue, and prolonged recovery time after exercising and (in some children) stomachache or chest pain. As previously noted, these responses are usually most pronounced immediately after the person has exercised, and they generally abate within 15 to 30 minutes after exercising.

Pathophysiology

Exercise-induced asthma, which follows a typical clinical pattern in predisposed patients, is characterized by transient bronchodilation (i.e., the initial response to exercise), followed by progressive bronchoconstruction that resolves within 30 to 60 minutes (i.e., recovery). Pulmonary function generally declines about 5 to 10 minutes after an asthmatic stops exercising, a reaction known as early phase response. Following this initial response, approximately half the patients with EIA experience a 2- to 4-hour refractory period, during which time they will not experience a significant drop in pulmonary function if they exercise again. Some patients experience a second, delayed episode of EIA 3 to 10 hours after exercising, a reaction known as late phase response.

Several factors appear to play an important role in the severity of exercise-induced airway bronchoconstriction. These include (1) environmental factors (e.g., temperature and humidity of inspired air, air quality, or allergen exposure), (2) type, duration, and intensity of exercise (e.g., high levels of minute ventilation), (3) the person's baseline level of airway reactivity, and (4) amount of time elapsed since prior exercise (Fig. 12–5).

Although the cause of EIA is probably multifactorial, several hypotheses have been proposed to explain the pathophysiology of this response. One theory, the water loss hypothesis, is based on the premise that evaporative water loss from respiratory mucosa during exercise briefly increases the osmolarity of the vasculature and release of inflammatory mediators from mast cells (Fig. 12–6). The latter event promotes further vasodilation and causes contraction of bronchial smooth muscle, thereby causing airway obstruction. Another theory, the postexertional airway re-

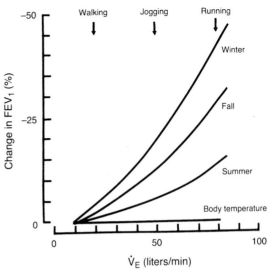

Figure 12–5. Effect of the interaction between the intensity of exercise and the thermal environment on the pulmonary mechanical response. FEV_1 denotes forced expiratory volume in one second, and V_E shows minute ventilation. Arrows indicate the levels of ventilation associated with increasingly strenuous exertion, such as walking, jogging, and running. As V_E rises, the severity of obstruction increases, except when respiratory thermal fluxes are prevented, as when one inhales fully humidified air at body temperature (37°C). The maximal obstruction occurs when air at a low temperature (e.g., in the winter) is inhaled, and the minimal obstruction occurs when hot, humid air (e.g., at body temperature in the laboratory) is inspired. (From McFadden ER, Gilbert IA: Exercise-induced asthma. N Engl J Med 330:1362–1367, 1994; with permission. Copyright © 1994 Massachusetts Medical Society. All rights reserved.)

warming hypothesis, is based on the observation that loss of heat from respiratory mucosa during exercise results in a decrease in bronchial blood flow. Following exercise, reactive hyperemia causes vascular engorgement and edema, which results in narrowing of the bronchial airway and leads to obstruction of airflow (Fig. 12–7).

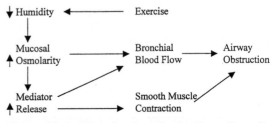

Figure 12–6. Water loss hypothesis. (From Cypar D, Lemanske RF Jr: Asthma and exercise. Clin Chest Med 15:351–368, 1994; with permission.)

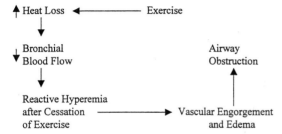

Figure 12–7. Postexertional airway rewarming hypothesis of EIA. (From Cypar D, Lemanske RF Jr: Asthma and exercise. Clin Chest Med 15:351–368, 1994; with permission.)

Treatment of Exercise-Induced Asthma in Children

The main goal of therapy in patients with EIA is to prevent episodes so that patients can participate in various activities without experiencing bronchospasm. Patients can benefit from a regimen that includes both pharmacologic and nonpharmacologic therapy.

Nonpharmacologic Therapy

Certain nonpharmacologic recommendations for treating EIA apply to *all* patients, including young children and adolescents. As previously mentioned, about half the asthmatic patients experience a refractory period following exercise, during which time the same activity does not induce EIA. Patients can use this nonresponsive period to their advantage by doing a series of warm-up exercises within an hour before resuming exercise or participating in athletic activities. Although this approach is helpful for scheduled activities, it is not practical for routine daily activities.

Another nonpharmacologic step to prevent EIA is to increase exposure to warm, humid air and to avoid breathing cold, dry air. This can be accomplished by wearing a facemask or scarf when exposed to cold, ambient temperatures or participating in indoor sports or other forms of exercise whenever possible.

Pharmacologic Therapy

In many patients, some form of pharmacologic therapy is needed to prevent the onset of EIA or to treat breakthrough episodes that occur after exercise. Asthma medications that are most effective in preventing EIA when used 10 to 15 minutes before exercise are listed in Table 12–2. Beta$_2$-adrenergic agonists are the therapy of choice for relief of acute symptoms and prevention of EIA. These agents prevent exercise-induced bronchospasm in more than 80% of patients. When used shortly before exercise, the short-acting inhaled beta$_2$-agonists (e.g., albuterol, terbutaline) provide protection for 2 to 3 hours, and the long-acting β_2-agonist salmeterol has been shown to prevent EIA for 10 to 12 hours. A recent study in children with EIA showed that inhaled salmeterol, 25 and 50 μg taken in the evening, improved baseline lung function the following morning and protected against exercise-induced bronchospasm. Another long-acting β_2-agonist, formoterol, which has not yet been approved in the United States, also provides protection against exercise-induced asthma for up to 12 hours. The duration of protection against EIA by salmeterol is often shorter than its bronchodilating effect so that patients taking salmeterol on a chronic basis may still need short-acting bronchodilators before exercise.

According to guidelines issued by the Expert Panel Report 2 in May 1997, both cromolyn and nedocromil also effectively prevent EIA when taken shortly before exercise. Two recent studies also compared the effectiveness of these agents and placebo, all delivered by a MDI, in preventing EIA in children. At clinically recommended doses, both cromolyn (10 mg) and nedocromil (4 mg) provided significant, comparable protection from EIA. Complete protection (defined as a drop in FEV$_1$ of <10% after exercise) was achieved in 53% of patients treated with either cromolyn or nedocromil in one study, and in 54% of patients treated with either drug in the other study. Duration of the protective effect with either drug was less than 2 hours. A primary advantage of both cromolyn and nedocromil is their excellent safety profile. Cromolyn and nedocromil may act additively when combined with β-agonists. Cromolyn combined with β_2-agonist terbutaline, for example, provided prolonged effective protection from moderate to severe EIA for up to 4 hours without any unwanted side-effects.

Table 12–2. **Effective Asthma Medications for the Treatment of Exercise-Induced Asthma**

Agent	Dose (puffs)	Time Before Exercise (min)	Effectiveness*	Duration of Protection (hr)†
β₂ aerosols				
Salmeterol‡	2	10–15	+ + +	10–12
Albuterol	2	10–15	+ + +	2.0–2.5
Terbutaline	2	10–15	+ + +	2.0–2.5
Cromolyn sodium	2	10–15	+ +	1.5–2.0
Nedocromil sodium	2	10–15	+ +	1.5–2.0
Methylxanthines	variable	30–60	±	?
Anticholinergics	2	30–60	±	?

*Effectiveness is rated as follows: + + +, ablation or substantial reduction in the obstructive response at the midpoint of the stimulus-response curve; + +, marked reduction in the obstructive response; ±, questionable efficacy.

†A question mark indicates that the duration of the effect is difficult to ascertain because of the variability of protection.

‡Salmeterol is a long-acting β₂-agonist drug available in many European countries but not in the United States or Canada.

From McFadden ER, Gilbert IA: Exercise-induced asthma. N Engl J Med 330:1362–1367, 1994; used with permission. Copyright © 1994 Massachusetts Medical Society. All rights reserved.

Other common medications used for long-term control of asthma, including theophylline and inhaled corticosteroids, will have some modifying effect on airway reactivity, but are not recommended for acute therapy before exercise. Likewise, the anticholinergic medications such as ipratropium bromide, which relieve acute bronchospasm, do not block exercise-induced bronchospasm.

A new class of agents, the leukotriene modifiers, have been shown to be effective in the prevention of EIA. Leukotriene receptors on the airways mediate bronchoconstriction, and participate in many of the pathologic changes of asthma. Although zafirlukast has been evaluated 2 hours before exercise, zileuton has been shown to be effective after chronic dosing for 2 days and montelukast after dosing the night before exercise.

Exercise Selection

Given the pathophysiology of EIA, it is evident that certain sports and other activities are less likely to elicit this response. Low asthmogenic activities, such as those listed in Table 12–3, are associated with a low level of minute ventilation and warm and humid climatic conditions, and are less likely to provoke EIA. In contrast, high asthmogenic activities, such as those listed in Table 12–4, are associated with a high level of minute ventilation and with cold, dry climatic conditions. Patients engaging in high asthmogenic activities, therefore, need to receive more aggressive medical pretreatment.

Summary

Exercise-induced asthma is a common problem in children, as well as adults, and may

Table 12–3. **Low Asthmogenic Activities**

Low-Minute Ventilation Activities

Tennis*	Karate	Football
Handball*	Wrestling	Baseball
Racquetball*	Boxing	Downhill skiing
Gymnastics	Sprinting	Isometrics
	Golf	

Activities Associated with Warm and Humid Climatic Conditions

Swimming	Water polo	Diving

*In the elite athlete, racquet sports may be associated with higher minute ventilation and an increased propensity for the development of exercise-induced asthma.

From Cypar D, Lemanske RF Jr: Asthma and exercise. Clin Chest Med 15:351–368, 1994; used with permission.

Table 12–4. **High Asthmogenic Activities**

High-Minute Ventilation Activities

Long-distance running
Cycling
Basketball
Soccer
Rugby

Activities Associated with Cool and Dry Climatic Conditions

Ice hockey
Ice skating
Cross-country snow skiing

From Cypar D, Lemanske RF Jr: Asthma and exercise. Clin Chest Med 15:351–368, 1994; used with permission.

have a serious impact on participation in physical and social activities. Many patients feel stigmatized by their condition, which may lead to ostracism or low self-esteem and withdrawal from their peers. It is imperative that every effort be made to allow these children and adults to engage in a wide variety of games and other sports shared by their peers.

The key to preventing the physical and psychological toll imposed by EIA is to diagnose and treat this disorder as early in life as possible. In young children, certain clinical signs and symptoms are highly prognostic, although exercise challenge testing may be warranted in older children. Beta$_2$-adrenergic agonists are a treatment of choice for preventing EIA; second choice agents are cromolyn and nedocromil and antileukotriene drugs. Regardless of which form of treatment is ultimately selected, judicious prescribing allows most of these children to live active and engaged lives, replete with all the physical endeavors that promote growth and development during these formative years.

ASTHMA AND PREGNANCY

The clinician who cares for teens and young adults must keep in mind that pregnancy is a serious concern of female patients. Many patients with chronic asthma will avoid optimal therapy before and during pregnancy because of the fear that medications will hurt their fetus. In truth, optimal care promotes the best outcome for mother and child.

Most studies show no significant changes in airway mechanics during pregnancy, FEV_1 and peak flow are unaffected. Pregnant women do experience an increase in minute ventilation, oxygen consumption, and CO_2 production. These changes result in a compensated physiologic respiratory alkalosis. This hyperventilation may cause some degree of dyspnea, which is unrelated to airway obstruction. Also, one should expect to find a mildly decreased CO_2 and elevated pH. Values that are more normal may actually indicate worsening asthma and relative acidosis. Although the fetus experiences oxygen tension that is only one fourth that of an adult, its oxygen needs are met because of a high rate of tissue perfusion and the high affinity of fetal hemoglobin

for oxygen. The dissociation characteristics of fetal hemoglobin allow for a small change in fetal O_2 partial pressure to produce significantly increased fetal O_2 saturation.

Nonpharmacologic Management

As with asthma in general, avoidance of irritants and allergens is a paramount feature of best care for the pregnant patient. This may be a time when the patient will be open to smoking cessation intervention to benefit her baby and herself. Dust, pet, and mold avoidance should be reviewed if these are pertinent, because this may be a window of opportunity for promoting these respiratory health measures.

Allergen immunotherapy may be continued at doses that have been well tolerated. To be cautious, it is reasonable to consider lowering the maintenance dose once it is achieved, and to halt any progression until after delivery. It is generally not wise to advance dosages or to initiate immunotherapy during this pregnancy when the risk of anaphylaxis has consequences for both mother and child. Although the risk of systemic reactions from skin testing are very small, it often is prudent to defer testing until after completion of the pregnancy or to perform *in vitro* testing.

Pharmacologic Management

Although most of the drugs that are used to treat asthma appear to be safe for mother and fetus, there are limited data regarding risk, particularly of newer agents. There is comforting information regarding medications that have been used for a substantial period of time. Also, there is evidence that the likelihood of fetal or maternal harm from undertreatment of asthma is much greater than the risks posed by appropriate pharmacotherapy. Several large projects have looked for an association between drug use in pregnancy and fetal risk, including congenital malformations. These data have been thoughtfully compiled

Table 12–5. **Working Group on Asthma and Pregnancy Recommendations**

Drugs "Preferred" for Use During Pregnancy	Drugs "That Generally Should Be Avoided During Pregnancy"
Anti-inflammatory: cromolyn, beclomethasone, prednisone Bronchodilator: inhaled β_2-adrenergic agonist, theophylline Antihistamine: chlorpheniramine, tripelennamine Decongestant: pseudoephedrine, oxymetazoline Cough: guaifenesin, dextromethorphan Antibiotic: amoxicillin	α-Adrenergic compounds (other than pseudoephedrine) Epinephrine (other than for anaphylaxis) Iodides Sulfonamides (in late pregnancy) Tetracyclines Quinalones

From Report of the Working Group on Asthma and Pregnancy: Management of Asthma During Pregnancy. Bethesda, MD, National Institutes of Health, 1993. Publication 93-3279.

and considered by the National Asthma Education Program (NAEP) Working Group on Asthma and Pregnancy (Table 12–5). The FDA has approved the antihistamines loratadine and cetirizine as having reasonable benefit to risk profiles (category B classification). The drugs listed in Table 12–5 also may be considered safe during lactation. A recent review of asthma and pregnancy summarizes the current status of relevant drugs and their classification status (Table 12–6).

Interrelation of Asthma and Pregnancy

Maternal asthma, particularly uncontrolled asthma, may increase the risk of such complications as pre-eclampsia, prenatal mortality, prematernity and small-for-gestational-date infants. Several studies of asthma and pregnancy in which asthma specialists managed the respiratory disease for optimal control showed no increase in adverse outcomes. Use of glucocorticoids in pregnancy also may increase adverse outcomes, although it is unclear whether they are secondary to severe asthma or to medication use. Failure to use oral corticosteroids in patients with severe asthma poses a great risk from uncontrolled disease with even mortality as a possible result.

A literature review and meta-analysis have concluded that one third of women have improvement in their asthma, one third deterioration, and one third stay the same during pregnancy. The effect of pregnancy on an individual's asthma will be similar in subsequent pregnancies. The peak time for asthma exacerbations is from 24 to 36 weeks of gestation with few problems in the last weeks and during labor and delivery.

Table 12–6. **Medications Introduced for Asthma and Allergy Since 1993**

Drug Type	Drug	Year Introduced	Route of Administration	FDA Class
Long-acting β_2-agonist	Salmeterol	1994	Inhaled	C*
NSAID	Nedocromil	1993	Inhaled	B†
Antileukotriene (lipoxygenase inhibitor)	Zileuton	1996	Oral	C
Antileukotriene (receptor antagonist)	Zafirlukast	1996	Oral	B
	Montelukast	1998	Oral	B
Corticosteroid	Fluticasone	1996	Inhaled or intranasal	C
	Mometasone	1997	Intranasal	C
	Budesonide	1997	Inhaled or intranasal	C
Anticholinergic	Nebulized ipratropium	1993	Inhaled	B
	Nasal ipratropium	1995	Intranasal	B
Antihistamine	Azelastine	1996	Intranasal	C
Nonsedating antihistamine	Loratadine	1993	Oral	B
	Fexofenadine	1996	Oral	C
Low-sedating antihistamine	Cetirizine	1995	Oral	B

*Animal studies demonstrate adverse effects.
†Animal studies do not suggest adverse effects.
From Schatz M, Zeiger RS: Managing asthma during pregnancy. J Resp Dis 19:731–738, 1998; used with permission.

The recommendations of the NAEP working group are summarized in Table 12–5. Although newer drugs have been released since this report, they lack a long track record. Inhaled glucocorticoids and β-agonists, which are not mentioned by the working group, may be considered if the risk-benefit ratio weighs toward the advantages of continuing them. Nedocromil and salmeterol may be benign, and their continued use in a patient who is benefiting from them should be considered. The leukotriene modifiers are a newer class of medication without a history of human use in pregnancy. Patients who require systemic glucocorticoids warrant special monitoring for gestational diabetes, pre-eclampsia, and intrauterine growth retardation.

Management of Asthma During Labor and Delivery

Patients should continue their chronic asthma therapy during labor. Inhaled beta agonists are appropriate for increased wheezing. Intravenous methylprednisone should be added if the patient fails to respond adequately. Patients who have had potentially suppressive doses of inhaled or oral corticosteroids should have supplemental intravenous hydrocortisone.

Medications used at delivery that are contraindicated in women with asthma include β-blockers, prostaglandin $F_2\alpha$, transcervical or intra-amniotic prostaglandin E_2, methylergonovine or ergonovine, and nonsteroidal anti-inflammatories in aspirin-sensitive patients. Intracervical prostaglandin E_2 has not been shown to cause difficulty at delivery. Magnesium sulfate and calcium channel blockers are well tolerated. Regional anesthesia is preferred to general anesthesia; if the latter is necessary it may be acceptably performed with atropine or glycopyrrolate pre-anesthesia, induction with ketamine and maintenance with low concentrations of halogenated agents.

Suggested Reading

Abramson MJ, Puy RM, Weiner JM: Is allergen immunotherapy effective in asthma? A meta-analysis of randomized controlled trials. Am J Respir Crit Care Med 151:969–974, 1995

Agertoft L and Pedersen S. Effects of long-term treatment with an inhaled corticosteroid on growth and pulmonary function in asthmatic children. Respir Med 88:373–381, 1994

Barnes PJ, Holgate ST, Laitinen LA, Pauwels R. Asthma mechanisms determinants of severity and treatment: The role of nedocromil sodium. Clin Exper Allerg 25:771–787, 1995

Barnes RT: Inhaled glucocorticosteroids for asthma. N Engl J Med 332:868–875, 1995

Chilmonczyk BA, Salmun LM, Megathlin KN, et al: Association between exposure to environmental tobacco smoke and exacerbations of asthma in children. N Engl J Med 328:1665–1669, 1993

Expert Panel Report 2: Guidelines for the Diagnosis and Management of Asthma. National Asthma Education and Prevention Program, February 1997

Haahtela T, Jarvinen M, Kava T, et al: Comparison of β_2-agonist terbutaline, with an inhaled corticosteroid budesonide in newly detected asthma. N Engl J Med 325:388–392, 1991

Kattan M, Keens TG, Mellis CM, Levison H: The response to exercise in normal and asthmatic children. J Pediatrics 72:718–721, 1974

Martinez FD, Wright AL, Taussig ML, et al: Asthma and wheezing in the first six years of life. N Engl J Med 332:133–138, 1995

Murray A, and Ferguson AC: Dust-free bedrooms in the treatment of asthmatic children with house dust or house mite allergy: A controlled trial. Pediatrics 71:418–422, 1983

Nelson HS: Beta adrenergic bronchodilators. N Engl J Med 333:499–506, 1995

Randolph C: Exercise-induced asthma: Update on pathophysiology, clinical diagnosis, and treatment. Curr Probl Pediatr 27:53–77, 1997

Report of the Working Group on Asthma and Pregnancy: Management of asthma during pregnancy. Bethesda, Maryland, National Institutes of Health, 1993. Publication 93–3279

Schatz M, Hoffman CP, Zeiger RS, et al: The course and management of asthma and allergic diseases during pregnancy. In Middleton (eds): Reed, Ellis, Adkinson, Yuninger, Busse (eds): Allergy: Principles and Practice, 5th ed, St. Louis, Mosby, 1998; pp. 938–952

Schuh S, Johnson DW, Callahan S, et al: Efficacy of frequent nebulized ipratropium bromide added to frequent high-dose albuterol therapy in severe childhood asthma. J Pediatr 126:639–645, 1995

Shapiro GG, Konig P: Cromolyn sodium: A review. Pharmacotherapy 5:156–170, 1985

Sporik R, Holgate ST, Platts-Mills TAE, Cogswell JJ: Exposure to house-dust mite allergen (Der p 1) and the development of asthma in childhood. N Engl J Med 323:502–507, 1990

Tal A, Golan H, Grauer N, Aviram M, et al: Deposition pattern of radiolabeled salbutamol inhaled from a metered-dose inhaler by means of a spacer with mask in young children with airway obstruction. J Pediatr 128:479–484, 1996

Weiss KB, Gergen PJ, Hodgson TA: An economic evaluation of asthma in the United States. N Engl J Med 326:862–866, 1992

Weiss KB, Wagener DK: Changing patterns of asthma mortality. Identifying target populations at high risk. JAMA 264:1683–1687, 1990

Woolcock A, Vo L, Ringal M, Jacques LA: Comparison of addition of salmeterol to inhaled steroids with doubling of the dose of inhaled steroids. Am J Respir Crit Care Med 153:1481–1488, 1996

Yoshihiro K, Okabe S, Tamura G, et al: Chemosensitivity and perception of dyspnea in patients with a history of near-fatal asthma. N Engl J Med 330:1329–1334, 1994

Chapter 13

Occupational Asthma

Nicholas Orfan, Anthony Montanaro, Stephen A. Tilles, and Jonathan A. Bernstein

Occupational asthma (OA) is characterized by variable airflow limitation and airway hyper-responsiveness due to particular occupational environment exposures and not to stimuli encountered outside the workplace. Occupational asthma can present by itself or in conjunction with other occupationally related disorders including rhinitis, contact dermatitis, or in the most severe circumstances anaphylaxis. An excellent example of the coexistence of these disorders is found in the case of a healthcare worker who develops sensitization to latex in the workplace. A latex-sensitized worker may initially present with symptoms of allergic rhinitis, hives, or cutaneous contact sensitization, which may later progress to asthma symptoms and in the most severe of circumstances anaphylaxis. In this scenario the onset of OA is preceded by a latency period of exposure during which time sensitization to latex occurs. Occupational asthma with a latency period is usually characterized by an underlying IgE-mediated mechanism. However, OA may present without a latency period of exposure, which has classically been referred to as Reactive Airways Dysfunction Syndrome (RADS) or irritant-induced asthma.

Occupational asthma must be distinguished from building-related illness and sick building syndrome. Building-related illness is induced by an agent not integrally related to the work process. An example of this disorder would be in a mold-sensitive allergic patient who develops allergic asthma after there has been water damage to his or her office at work. Sick building syndrome is a term used to describe a myriad of unhealthy factors in a building such as poor ventilation and humidity control leading to overgrowth of mold spores and bacteria, which can produce mycotoxins and endotoxins, respectively. Sick building syndrome has remained a poorly defined clinical entity that manifests as a constellation of non-specific symptoms but is not related to any particular work activity. It has a variable presentation without definable physical, laboratory, or pathogenic abnormalities.

PREVALENCE

According to the most recent prevalence statistics, OA is the most common occupational lung disease in Europe and the United States. Occupational asthma accounts for 5% to 15% of all new cases of asthma diagnosed each year in the United States. Given the rising prevalence of OA and the potential for severe chronic airway obstruction if the worker is not readily diagnosed and removed from further exposure, it is not surprising that the associated healthcare costs to manage this disease are substantial. These costs include lost productivity in the workplace, increased utilization of healthcare resources, and the adjudication of Worker's Compensation and disability cases.

Over 250 agents in the workplace have now been associated with OA. The prevalence of OA is generally determined by cross-sectional studies and varies among occupations. For example, studies have found the prevalence of OA among laboratory animal workers is approximately 20%, whereas western red cedar asthma occurs in approximately 5% of workers. The prevalence of OA has been estimated to occur in 7%–9% of bakers, 5%–10% of isocyanate-exposed workers, 20%–50% of platinum-exposed workers, and in up to 60% of enzyme-exposed workers.

The prevalence for OA within a specific occupation depends on many factors, including environmental conditions within the plant, exposure levels, and the number of exposed workers. For example, at first glance, it might appear that isocyanate-exposed workers have a lower prevalence of OA compared with platinum-exposed workers. The absolute number of workers exposed to isocyanates (>100,000) each year results in a greater absolute number of workers who develop isocyanate-induced OA compared with platinum-exposed workers who develop OA.

Unfortunately, cross-sectional studies can underestimate the prevalence of OA owing to the healthy worker effect. This effect occurs because symptomatic workers leave the workplace, resulting in a misleadingly low prevalence rate. To obtain more accurate prevalence statistics and information about the causes, risk factors, and natural course of OA, surveillance programs have been established in developed countries including the United Kingdom, United States, and Finland. The SWORD (Surveillance of Work-Related and Occupational Respiratory Disease) program established in the United Kingdom involves voluntary reporting of occupational illnesses from a variety of industries by pulmonologists and occupational medicine physicians. This program has already yielded useful prevalence data owing to the excellent response rate from participating physicians. Thus far, SWORD has identified OA as the most frequently reported occupational respiratory illness and isocyanates as the most common specific cause of OA. The SEHNSOR (Sentinel Health Notification System for Occupational Risks) program established in the United States has not been as successful in obtaining useful epidemiological data because of a poor response rate from participating physicians. This is in contrast to Finland's program, which has already compiled enough data to estimate the country's yearly incidence of OA and hypersensitivity pneumonitis.

PHYSIOLOGIC PRESENTATION OF OCCUPATIONAL ASTHMA

The diagnosis of OA can often prove elusive because workers may experience various physiologic patterns of airway responsiveness depending on their exposure to an offending antigen. An immediate response or early asthmatic reaction (EAR) is characterized by a maximal decline in forced expiratory volume in 1 second (FEV_1) 30 to 60 minutes after exposure. This decline usually subsides within 2 hours but can occasionally persist for several hours. The late asthmatic reaction (LAR) begins 2 to 8 hours after exposure and generally resolves over a 24-hour period. A dual asthmatic response (DAR) refers to an EAR followed by an LAR.

The difficulty of establishing a diagnosis of OA can best be demonstrated in the worker who remains asymptomatic during his or her workshift but later develops symptoms at home during the night. This particular scenario is characteristic of an isolated LAR, which is a common presentation for certain forms of OA such as those that are isocyanate-induced. However, there are other clinical scenarios that a clinician might encounter while evaluating a worker suspected of having OA. The worker might manifest a classic EAR with symptoms that begin within 1 to 2 hours after entering the workplace and then subside or may experience an EAR in conjunction with an LAR, resulting in a DAR. Figure 13–1 illustrates a DAR exhibited by a worker undergoing specific bronchoprovocation to toluene diisocyanate. IgE-mediated causes of OA usually present as either an EAR or a DAR, whereas non–IgE-mediated OA usually manifests as a LAR or a DAR.

Occupational asthma should not be confused with aggravation of pre-existing asthma in a worker from exposure to one or more nonspecific workplace irritants. However, pre-existing asthma does not preclude a diagnosis of OA as it is also possible that a worker with stable pre-existing asthma could experience deterioration directly as a result of a specific occupational exposure. It is also possible that a worker could develop newly diagnosed asthma entirely unrelated to the workplace or suffer

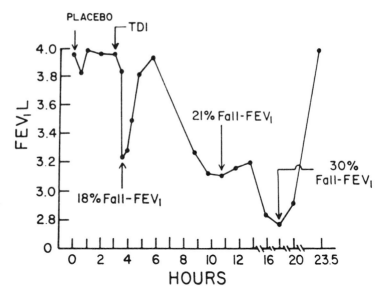

Figure 13–1. A dual-asthmatic response in a polyurethane foam worker after bronchoprovocation to toluene diisocyanate (TDI). The early asthmatic response is followed by spontaneous recovery and then a late asthmatic response.

from a pulmonary condition other than asthma that is either work-related (e.g., hypersensitivity pneumonitis) or nonwork-related (e.g., sarcoidosis or chronic bronchitis).

MECHANISMS

Occupational asthma has been demonstrated to occur through immunologic and nonimmunologic mechanisms. Examples of nonimmunologically mediated mechanisms include vagally mediated reflex bronchospasm, which can be induced by exposure to inert dusts, sulfur dioxide, or cold air or pharmacologically induced bronchoconstriction described in workers exposed to organophosphates as a result of the potent cholinergic agonist effect of these compounds.

Direct injury to the bronchial epithelium leading to chronic airway inflammation and bronchial hyper-responsiveness has been well documented to occur after a single excessive exposure to a noxious gas or chemical exposure which is referred to as reactive airways disease syndrome (RADS) or irritant-induced asthma. Inciting agents include ozone, nitrogen dioxide, anhydrous ammonium gas, and isocyanates. Reactive airways dysfunction syndrome may be distinguished from other forms of OA and non-OA by a significantly greater degree of basement membrane thickening caused by collagen deposition. A common feature of nonimmunologic OA is the absence

of an asymptomatic latency period following initiation of exposure.

A significant proportion of OA cases have been explained by an underlying immunologic mechanism. Typically, workers suffering from immunologically induced OA experience an asymptomatic latency period of variable duration during which time they become sensitized to a specific agent. Immunologically induced OA can occur through either an IgE-mediated or a non–IgE-mediated mechanism. IgE-mediated OA involves the binding of one or more relevant antigenic determinants to antigen binding sites located on specific IgE antibodies that have been fixed to tissue mast cells located in the bronchial airways. The resultant activation of mast cells leads to the release of bioactive mediators, including histamine, prostaglandin D2, and sulfidopeptide cysteinyl leukotrienes, which can cause bronchoconstriction, airway mucosal edema, vascular permeability, and mucous hypersecretion. Chemotactic factors and interleukins function to attract proinflammatory cells such as eosinophils and lymphocytes into the lung parenchyma, which become activated. With repeated exposure to the offending agent, an inflammatory cascade of events occurs that leads to chronic airway inflammation that is histologically indistinguishable from non-OA.

IgE-mediated OA often is induced by high molecular weight (HMW) antigens such as proteins or glycoproteins, but also may involve low molecular weight (LMW) highly reactive chemicals that have haptenic side chains capable of reacting with endogenous tissue proteins to form complete antigens, which can then elicit an immunogenic response.

Non–IgE-mediated OA always involves LMW chemical agents. The mechanism for non–IgE-mediated immunologic OA is not as clearly defined but has been postulated to occur through T cell-mediated mechanisms. For instance, increased CD8+ lymphocytes and eosinophils in the bronchoalveolar lavage fluid have been demonstrated in workers with isocyanate-induced OA. The confirmation of this observation by other investigators provides further support for the role of a cell-mediated mechanism for isocyanate-induced OA. Another postulated non-IgE immunologic mechanism may involve the release of neuropeptides from afferent nerve endings. Neuropeptides such as substance P, calcitonin gene-related peptide (CGRP), and neurokinin A are capable of activating mast cells, resulting in bronchoconstriction and neurogenic inflammation. Table 13–1 compares characteristic features of HMW- and LMW-induced OA.

CLINICAL EVALUATION FOR OCCUPATIONAL ASTHMA

In order to accurately make a diagnosis of OA, the clinician must first establish that the worker has asthma. Once the diagnosis of asthma has been demonstrated, it is then necessary to prove that the patient's asthma has been caused or aggravated by one or more workplace exposures. Therefore, a stepwise, systematic approach is recommended for making a diagnosis of OA as outlined in Figure 13–2. Although this algorithm serves as a useful guide for establishing a diagnosis of OA, it is important to emphasize that each worker's evaluation should be tailored to the history and the suspected causative agent. The extent of the OA evaluation should always be guided by good clinical judgment.

History and Physical Examination

The first step in evaluating a worker for OA requires a thorough and accurate history. Standard occupational questionnaires have proved useful for elucidating relevant clinical and exposure information. These questionnaires elicit information regarding the worker's symptoms such as cough, wheeze, chest tightness, or dyspnea in addition to any ocular, nasal, dermal, or constitutional complaints. They also include questions about duration of symptoms and their temporal relationship to workplace exposure. The clinician should inquire whether the worker's symptoms improve when the worker is away from work for extended periods of time such as on weekends or holidays. A detailed past medical history should elicit information about asthma, atopy, and smoking. Information regarding the patient's current work process and work environ-

Table 13–1. Features of HMW and LMW Antigen-Induced OA

HMW Antigen-Induced OA	LMW Antigen-Induced OA
Antigen >1000 kds	Antigen <1000 kds
IgE-mediated mechanism	IgE- or non–IgE-mediated mechanism
Antigen is a protein or glycoprotein	Antigen is a hapten which combines with tissue proteins to form immunogen
Atopy is often a risk factor	Atopy not often a risk factor
Symptoms of allergic rhinitis frequently precede symptoms of asthma	Asthma without preceding rhinitis
The antigen is adequate for immunologic testing by either in vivo or in vitro methods	Must combine with carrier protein for in vitro or in vivo immunologic testing
Causes EAR or DAR	Airway response may be EAR, DAR, or isolated LAR
Examples	Examples
Foods, egg, shellfish, flour, coffee	Pharmaceuticals, antibiotics
Enzymes, papain, trypsin, lactase	Inorganic compounds, nickel, platinum
Animal proteins, rodent urine	Organic compounds, colophony, plicatic acid,
Insect proteins, meal worm, fruit fly	acid anhydrides, isocyanates

EAR, early airway response; DAR, dual airway response; LAR, late airway response.

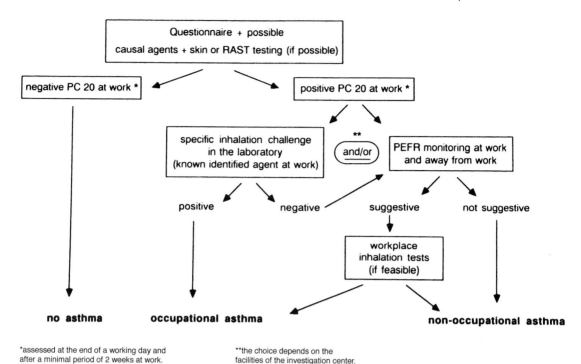

Figure 13–2. An algorithmic approach for the assessment and diagnosis of occupational asthma.

ment, previous employment history, and prior occupational exposures including any chemical spills should be obtained. It is also important to identify whether protective equipment or clothing such as respirators or gloves has been routinely worn by the worker. Table 13–2 summarizes the key elements of the occupational history in the evaluation of OA.

If available, results of environmental monitoring routinely conducted in the workplace should be obtained. Material safety data sheets (MSDSs) are often helpful for identifying agents known to cause OA that are routinely used in the workplace. Material safety data sheets must be made accessible to the employee by the employer. The employer also is required to train their employees on proper handling techniques of all hazardous materials. Although MSDSs should provide specific information about toxic and sensitizing properties of a given agent or its constituents, they are often incomplete. Consulting with an industrial hygienist or safety officer familiar with the workplace, therefore, may provide valuable added information about specific agents used by the worker and the worker's inherent exposure risk.

The physical examination of a worker sus-

pected of having OA should focus on identifying clinical findings indicative of asthma and other potential pulmonary conditions. The clinician should be alert to signs of atopic disease such as ocular, nasal, and dermal findings, which often precede or occur concomitantly with OA. It should be emphasized, however, that the physical examination is often entirely normal, similar to what is found for patients with non-OA.

Imaging Studies

The chest radiograph is usually normal in workers with OA. Abnormal findings may include hyperinflation and peribronchial cuffing, which are characteristic of advanced non-OA. A chest radiograph is most useful for excluding other pulmonary conditions such as pneumoconiosis, bronchiolitis obliterans, or pulmonary sarcoidosis.

Pulmonary Function Testing

The purpose of pulmonary function testing is to document the presence of reversible airway

Table 13–2. **Key Elements of the Occupational History in the Evaluation of Occupational Asthma**

Demographic Information
  Identification and address
  Personal data including sex, race, and age
  Educational background with quantitation of the number of school years completed
Employment History
  Current department and job description including dates begun, interrupted, and ended
  List all work processes and substances used in the employee's work environment. A schematic diagram of the
    workplace is helpful to identify indirect exposure to substances emanating from adjacent work stations
  List prior jobs at current workplace with description of job, duration, and identification of material used
  Work history describing employment preceding current workplace. Job descriptions and exposure history must
    be included
Symptoms
  Categories
    Chest tightness, wheezing, cough, shortness of breath
    Rhinorrhea, sneezing, lacrimation, ocular itching
    Systemic symtoms such as fever, arthralgias and myalgias
  Duration should be quantitated
  Duration of employment at current job prior to onset of symptoms
  Identify temporal pattern of symtoms in relationship to work
    Immediate onset beginning at work with resolution soon after coming home
    Delayed onset beginning 4–12 hours after starting work or after coming home
    Immediate onset followed by recovery with symptoms recurring 4–12 hours after initial exposure to suspect agent
      at work
  Improvement away from work
Identify Potential Risk Factors
  Obtain a smoking history along with current smoking status and quantitate number of pack years
  Asthmatic symptoms preceding current work exposure
  Atopic status
    Identify history of nasal or ocular symptoms
    Family history of atopic disease
    Confirmation by epicutaneous testing to a panel of common aeroallergens
  History of accidental exposures to substances such as heated fumes or chemical spills

disease and to differentiate between other forms of obstructive and restrictive pulmonary diseases. Spirometry, which includes evaluation of forced vital capacity (FVC), forced expiratory volume in the first second of exhalation (FEV_1), FEV_1/FVC ratio, and forced expiratory flow rate (FEF_{25-75}), usually provides adequate information for this purpose. Spirometry should be performed before and after administration of a bronchodilator medication to document the necessary 12% to 15% improvement in FEV_1 required to make a definitive diagnosis of asthma. It may be useful to obtain lung volumes and diffusion capacity (DLCO) in order to exclude the presence of other pulmonary disorders such as interstitial fibrosis. These tests are usually normal in patients with OA.

Measurement of Bronchial Hyper-responsiveness

Frequently, workers with a history suggestive of OA have a normal physical examination, a normal chest radiograph, and normal spirometry results without improvement in their FEV_1 after administration of bronchodilators. However, a negative, initial, cursory evaluation does not exclude the diagnosis of OA. Establishing the presence of bronchial hyper-responsiveness is the essential next step for confirming or excluding a diagnosis of OA. Methacholine, a synthetic analogue of acetylcholine, is the agent most commonly used when testing for bronchial hyper-responsiveness because of its general lack of side-effects and short half-life. A methacholine challenge test is a useful screening test for detecting OA early in its course, because bronchial hyper-responsiveness often precedes obstructive lung changes detected by simple spirometry. All workers with OA should demonstrate some degree of bronchial hyper-responsiveness by methacholine challenge test if they are symptomatic with ongoing workplace exposure. Similarly, the absence of bronchial hyper-responsiveness confirmed by a negative methacholine challenge test in a worker with ongoing workplace exposure is a strong negative predictor for OA. After removal of the worker from the workplace, bronchial hyper-responsiveness can continue to persist for varying lengths of time, but also may diminish or completely disappear after an extended period of time.

The interpretation of a methacholine challenge test result requires a certain degree of expertise, because of the potential for overlapping results between asthmatic and normal individuals. It should be emphasized that a positive methacholine challenge test, although indicative of asthma, is not diagnostic of OA; a normal methacholine test does not exclude the possibility of a worker developing OA in the future. However, a positive response to a methacholine challenge performed while the worker is regularly exposed to a known agent in the workplace that reverts to a negative challenge result after the worker has been removed from the work environment, is strong evidence supporting a diagnosis of OA.

Cross-Shift Spirometry

Once the diagnosis of asthma has been established for the worker, additional investigative techniques are necessary for determining the presence or absence of an occupational cause. Cross-shift spirometry involving pre- and postworkshift measurements of FEV_1 during the workweek has been commonly used to determine a relationship between asthma and the workplace. This approach has been found to lack sensitivity in confirming a diagnosis of OA, largely because it overlooks workers who predominantly manifest a LAR. Furthermore, workers with OA who have had prolonged occupational exposure may have persistent airway obstruction that obscures the FEV_1 variability between workdays and nonworkdays.

Serial Peak Expiratory Flow Rate Monitoring

Serial peak expiratory flow rate (PEFR) monitoring is the most frequently used objective method for measuring lung function at and away from work, because it is easy and inexpensive to perform. PEFR measurements should be recorded for at least 2 to 3 weeks while at work and at home. The worker should be instructed to measure and record the PEFR every 1–2 hours while at work and every 2–3 hours while awake at home. Special attention should be placed on documenting workplace exposure and medication usage with each recorded PEFR measurement. Peak expiratory flow rate variability greater than 15%–20% over a 24-hour period, which corresponds to work exposure is considered an abnormal response compatible with OA. Serial PEFR measurements have been shown to correlate well with specific bronchoprovocation testing in establishing a diagnosis of OA provided they are performed properly. Proper testing requires that the worker be instructed in the proper PEFR technique and understands the importance of accurately recording the results. A major limitation of serial PEFR measurements is that patients can falsify their readings. Therefore, workers must be closely supervised and monitored for compliance. Another limitation of PEFR monitoring is that it does not identify the specific causative agent.

Immunologic Evaluation

Immunologic studies can serve as useful adjunctive tests for establishing a diagnosis of OA; therefore, it is important to be knowledgeable about specific in vivo and in vitro tests that are available for confirming exposure or sensitization to known causative agents of OA. Table 13–3 summarizes specific HMW and LMW causes of OA and the in vivo and in vitro immunologic tests that are used for confirming a diagnosis. The most commonly performed immunologic studies are in vivo skin tests, predominantly used for evaluating OA induced by HMW proteins, and in vitro immunoassays, which are usually the preferred methods for detecting the presence of specific IgG and IgE antibodies to LMW agents.

Detection of specific IgE antibodies by in vivo skin testing requires proper characterization of the allergen source, extraction procedure and, if possible, its biochemical composition. All reagents require prior testing to establish their sensitivity and specificity using known sensitized and nonsensitized volunteers

Table 13–3. **Etiologic Agents of Occupational Asthma and Reported Immunologic Tests**

	In Vivo	In Vitro
HMW Agents		
Baby's breath *(Gypsophila paniculata)*	Intradermal titration testing	RAST/histamine release
Bacillus subtilis enzymes	Prick tests with 0.05, 0.5, 5 and 10 mg/ml	RAST/radial immunodiffusion
Buckwheat flour	Prick test with 10 mg/ml	Reverse enzyme immunoassay/histamine release
Castor bean	Prick test with 1:100 extract	Not done
Coffee bean	Intradermal titration to coffee bean extract	RAST to coffee bean extract
Douglas fir tussock moth	Cutaneous tests with 1:25 extract	Histamine release
Egg proteins	Prick tests with 1:10 w/v egg white, egg yolk, whole egg; prick tests to 10 mg/ml egg white fractions	RAST to egg proteins
Garlic	Prick test titrations beginning at 10^{-5} garlic extract	RIA* for IgE against garlic extract
Grain dust, grain dust mite	Prick and intracutaneous tests with grain dust and grain mite	Not done
Grain weevil	Skin test to weevil extract	Not done
Gum acacia	Skin tests with gum arabic	Not done
Guar gum	Prick tests with 1 mg/ml guar gum	RAST with guar gum
Hog trypsin	Skin test to trypsin	Histamine release
Laboratory animals	Skin tests with serum and urine extracts from animals	ELISA
Latex	Prick test using low ammonia latex solution	Not done
Locusts	Prick tests with locust extract at 0.1, 1 and 10 mg/ml	ELISA
Mealworm	Prick test titration beginning at 1:20 w/v Tenibrio molitor (TM) extract	RAST to TM extract
Mushroom	Prick test with mushroom extract	Not done
Papain	Skin test with papain at 1.25 to 20 mg/ml	RAST to papain
Pancreatic extract	Prick tests with 1:100 and 1:1000 extracts	Not done
Poultry mites	Skin test with 1:10 w/v Northern fowl mite (NFM)	RAST to NFM
Protease bromelain	Prick test with bromelain at 10 mg/ml	RAST to bromelain
Redwood	Prick test to redwood sawdust extract	Not done
Tobacco	Skin tests with green tobacco extract 10 mg/ml	RAST with green tobacco extract
Wheat flour	Prick tests with 10% w/v extract	RAST to wheat flour and wheat flour components
LMW Agents		
Azodicarbonamide	Prick tests with 0.1, 1 and 5% azodicarbonamide	Not done
Carmine dye	Skin test with *Coccus cactus*	RAST to dyes
Chloramine-T, halazone	Scratch test at 10^{-5} dilution	Not done
Chromate	Prick test at 10, 5, 1 and 0.1 mg/ml $Cr_2(SO_4)_3$	RAST to HSA-chromium sulfate
Cobalt	Patch tests	RAST to HSA-cobalt sulfate
Diazonium tetrafluoroborate (DTFB)	Not done	RAST to HSA-DTFB
Dimethylethanolamine	Prick tests to dimethylethanolamine undiluted at 1:10, 1:100 and 1:1000	Not done
Dyes, textiles	Prick or scratch tests to dyes at 10 mg/ml in 50% glycerine	HSA-dye
Ethylenediamine	Intracutaneous test to 1:100 ethylenediamine	Not done
Furan binder	Not done	RAST to catalyst, sand, and furfuryl alcohol
Hexamethylene-diisocyanate (HDI)	Prick tests to HSA-HDI	ELISA to HSA-HDI
Hexahydrophthalic anhydride (HHPA)	Not done	RAST to HSA-HHPA
Nickel	Prick tests with $NiSO_4$ at 100, 10, 5, 1 and 0.1 mg/ml	RAST to HSA-$NiSO_4$
Penicillin	Prick tests to ampicillin at 10^{-3} to 10^{-2} mol/l, benzyl penicilloyl polylysine at 10^{-6} mol/l and minor determinants at 10^{-2} mol/l	Not done
Penicillamine	Prick tests with penicillamine, major and minor penicillin determinants at 0.01, 0.1 and 1 mg/ml	Not done
Phthalic anhydride (PA) and tetrachlorophthalic anhydride (TCPA)	Prick and intradermal tests to HSA-PA and HSA-TCPA	ELISA; RIA to HSA-PA only
Platinum	Prick tests with complex platinum salts from 10^{-3} to 10^{-11} g/ml	RAST to $(NH_4)_2PtCl_2$, RAST to HSA-platinum and histamine release
Spiramycin	Prick tests with 10 and 100 mg/ml spiramycin	Not done
Toluene diisocyanate (TDI)	Prick test to 5 mg/ml HSA-TDI	RAST and ELISA to HSA-TDI, histamine release
Trimellitic anhydride (TMA)	Prick tests to 3.4 mg/ml HSA-TMA and TMA in acetone	RIA with HSA-TMA
Western Red Cedar (WRC)	Prick tests with 25 mg/ml WRC extract; intracutaneous testing with 2.5 mg/ml WRC	Not done

*Radio Immuno Assay; RIA Kit.

as controls. Reagents should be sterile filtered to ensure that they are free of biological contaminants. High molecular weight antigens (molecular weight > 1,000 kd) should be suspended in phosphate-buffered saline to achieve a final concentration range of 0.1–10 mg/ml. This concentration range has been demonstrated to be nonskin irritating for prick skin testing. Skin testing to confirm IgE sensitization has also proved useful for select LMW antigens (molecular weight < 1,000 kd), including platinum salts and acid anhydrides (see Table 13–3). Most LMW agents, such as acid anhydrides, require prior conjugation to an endogenous protein carrier, such as human serum albumin, to form a conjugate before it can be used as a reliable skin test reagent. An exception to this rule are platinum salts, which can be used in their native form to elicit an accurate skin test response.

In vitro testing requires use of either the radioallergosorbent test (RAST) or the enzyme-linked immunosorbent assay (ELISA) to determine the presence of a specific serum IgG or IgE antibodies to a particular occupational agent. Both techniques involve the binding of a known protein or hapten–protein conjugate to a solid medium with subsequent demonstration of specific binding to the bound antigen by specific antibodies present in the worker's serum. RAST testing, because it involves the use of radioisotopes, has been largely replaced by ELISA testing, which relies on nonradioactive colorimetric changes. In vitro tests require stringent standardization methods to ensure their validity. Characterization of the specific test reagent to determine the degree of chemical linkage to protein and the ratio of chemical ligand to protein carrier must be established because antigenicity and allergenicity of the final conjugate varies with ligand density. The same guidelines for establishing the sensitivity and specificity of a skin test should be applied to in vitro tests. Appropriate negative and positive control sera should be included with each run to establish reproducibility and validity of the test results. It is essential that the clinician thoroughly investigate the clinical laboratory where specimens are sent for in vitro assays to ensure that the laboratory adheres to proper quality control guidelines. In general, in vitro immunoassays for specific IgE to HMW OA agents

are less sensitive and specific than skin testing and are seldom necessary to perform.

Fewer tests are available for the evaluation of non–IgE-mediated immunologic causes of OA. Measurement of IgG precipitating antibodies has been found in workers exposed to trimellitic anhydride (TMA) that develop hemolytic anemia and pulmonary hemorrhage. These antibodies also have been found in TMA-exposed workers who develop late systemic symptoms, suggesting a mechanistic role of these antibodies in cytotoxic or immune complex mediated reactions. The use of additional in vitro tests, such as lymphocyte proliferation assays, to evaluate the role of cell-mediated responses in OA, has been used primarily in the laboratory by researchers and these tests have not been established as reliable methods for routine use by clinicians.

Workplace Evaluation

Visiting the workplace is an effective method for assessing the worker's direct and indirect exposure to potential occupational allergens. An on-site walk through can provide a clearer perspective of the work process and environmental conditions such as ventilation and relative humidity that can enhance the worker's exposure and risk for developing OA. If available, the physician should be accompanied by a trained industrial hygienist experienced in air sampling. Methods for air sampling are available for detecting levels of airborne gases and vapors in parts per billion. Personal air sampling devices can be worn by the worker in order to obtain more accurate measurements of his or her exposure to a particular agent. Permissible exposure levels (PEL) or threshold limit values (TLV) are enforced by the Occupational Safety and Health Administration for all potentially dangerous chemicals in the workplace. This information, which can be obtained from MSDSs, typically focuses on the known toxic effects of chemicals but often omits their potential sensitizing properties. It is important to recognize that although a worker's total exposure to a specific agent is measured as a time-weighted average (TWA) over an 8-hour workshift, this measurement does not always reflect brief episodes in which a worker may be exposed to high concentrations of an offending agent that can occur in relationship to a specific work activity.

Specific Bronchial Provocation Test

The specific bronchial provocation test (SBPT) is the gold standard test for establishing a clear causal relationship between a suspected agent in the workplace and the development of asthma. The SBPT is especially useful for identifying index cases in which a suspected agent has not yet been proved as a cause of OA. It is also frequently relied on as an important determinant for deciding whether a worker is eligible for Worker's Compensation or disability. Although the SBPT is a very specific diagnostic test, it is not 100% sensitive for making a diagnosis of OA. The diagnosis of OA can be missed if the worker has been absent from workplace exposure for a prolonged period of time and bronchial hyper-responsiveness to a specific agent has diminished. Therefore, it is important to perform an SBPT while the worker is actively exposed or within a short time after removal from the workplace.

The SBPT has significant risks and should be conducted only in specialized centers by experienced personnel. One must select the correct offending agent and expose the patient to a concentration that resembles the workplace environment. An SBPT is contraindicated if the worker's baseline FEV_1 is <60% of predicted or if the worker has significant cardiac disease. An SBPT also should not be performed if the worker has had a recent respiratory infection. Bronchodilators, cromolyn and nedocromil sodium, leukotriene modifying agents, and inhaled corticosteroids should be withheld for at least 24 hours before the challenge. Currently, there are no well-standardized methods available for performing an SBPT. However, a sensible protocol that is widely used by many experienced centers begins obtaining serial FEV_1 measurements on day 1 every hour for 8 hours to establish lung function stability (<10% variation). On day 2, a 15–30 minute exposure to a control agent should be performed followed by monitoring of FEV_1 similar to that on day 1. On day 3, specific challenge to the sus-

pected agent should be performed with subsequent monitoring of FEV_1 as on days 1 and 2. Because of concerns about an isolated LAR, exposure to LMW agents should be limited to a single concentration per day with progressive increases over consecutive days. This is in contrast to HMW agents in which exposure can be progressively increased on the same day with appropriate monitoring and dosing intervals. Aqueous solutions may be nebulized at different concentrations, and special chambers are available to maintain constant airborne particle concentrations to help avoid irritant responses or severe bronchospasm from overexposure. A greater than 20% decrement in FEV_1 from baseline to challenge with the suspected agent strongly supports a diagnosis of OA. A positive SBPT result to one agent does not exclude the possibility that the worker also has been sensitized to other agents in the workplace.

TREATMENT

Treatment of OA requires complete avoidance of exposure to the offending agent, as even minimal concentrations may exacerbate the asthma and perpetuate airway inflammation. Workers with OA induced by isocyanates, acid anhydrides, western red cedar, or colophony have been demonstrated to be more susceptible to persistent progressive asthma if there is a delay in their diagnosis and a prolongation of their workplace exposure. Pharmacologic therapy is not considered a substitute for avoidance of the causative agent, but is effective at reducing symptoms and airway hyper-responsiveness. The treatment of OA uses the same medications used to treat non-OA, with emphasis on controlling airway inflammation. Immunotherapy has been shown to be effective in controlled studies for animal laboratory workers with OA and may be effective for workers with OA induced by other HMW antigens such as shellfish.

PREVENTION

Prevention of OA will be best achieved by implementation of engineering and industrial hygiene control measures to ensure minimal exposure to sensitizing agents or chemicals in the workplace. Such strategies have been successfully implemented in the detergent and isocyanate industries with dramatic reductions in occupational allergic disease. Effective prevention techniques have included: (1) enclosure of previously open work processes; (2) providing full protective suits with separate air supplies to heavily exposed workers; (3) providing gloves, masks, and uniforms to workers who have lower exposure potential; (4) performing frequent, random samplings to monitor levels of airborne irritants and allergens and; (5) initiating immunosurveillance programs designed to identify sensitized workers early in the course of the disease. Effective prevention programs have also used prescreening procedures of workers for known risk factors such as atopy prior to assigning job tasks within the workplace where they may be at increased risk for developing OA. Atopy is a well established risk factor in industries in which workers are exposed to enzymes, animal proteins, and latex proteins, whereas smoking has been demonstrated to be a risk factor for OA in platinum workers.

MEDICAL AND LEGAL CONSIDERATIONS

Frequently, physicians are asked to provide expert testimony for Worker's Compensation evaluations or personal injury lawsuits. The legal standard of medical probability is greater than 50% likelihood that occupational exposure was a significant contributing factor. Ultimately, the clinician must determine whether asthma is work-related based on the worker's history and supportive objective testing. Although worker's impairment can often be defined in medical terms, a physician asked to render a judgment about disability also must consider the effect that the worker's impairment from asthma has on his job activity and general life-style. For many cases of OA, impairment can be difficult to assess because airway obstruction may be variable, depending on exposure to other nonspecific triggers or improvement by the use of medication. Once the diagnosis of OA has been established, attention should be focused on the practical tasks of determining what restrictions, accom-

modations, or changes in job activity will allow the individual to continue to work. Often a worker will be required to leave the job, as this is the only satisfactory option that will guarantee total avoidance of future exposure to the offending OA agent.

CONCLUSION

The diagnosis of OA represents a formidable challenge for both the primary care physician and specialist. It is important that primary care physicians be able to recognize a potential diagnosis of OA and have a firm understanding of the algorithmic approach advocated for establishing a diagnosis of OA since they often have the first medical contact with the worker (see Fig. 13–2). The success of future immunosurveillance programs established in the United States to identify the prevalence of OA and specific worker risk factors will rely heavily on primary care physicians' diligent reporting of OA cases they encounter. Earlier recognition of OA by the primary care physician will inevitably reduce the morbidity and legal and health care costs associated with this disease.

Suggested Reading

Bernstein DI: Clinical assessment and management of occupational asthma. *In* Bernstein IL, Chan-Yeung M, Malo J-L, Bernstein DI (eds): Asthma in the Workplace. New York, Marcel Dekker, 1999, pp. 145–158

Bernstein DI, Korbee L, Stauder T, Bernstein JA, et al: The low prevalence of occupational asthma and antibody-dependent sensitizers to diphenylmethane diisocyanate in a plant engineered for minimal exposure to diisocyanates. J Allergy Clin Immunol 92:387–396, 1993

Bernstein IL, Chan-Yeung M, Malo J-L, Bernstein DI: Definition and classification of asthma. *In* Bernstein IL, Chan-Yeung M, Malo J-L, Bernstein DI (eds): Asthma in the Workplace. New York, Marcell Dekker, 1999, p. 1–4

Bernstein JA, Bernstein IL: Clinical aspects of respiratory hypersensitivity to chemicals. *In* Dean JH, Luster MI, Munson AE, Kimber J (eds): Immunotoxicology and Immunopharmacology. New York, Raven Press, 1994, pp. 617–642

Bernstein JA, Bernstein DI, Bernstein IL: Occupational asthma. *In* Bierman CW, Pearlman DS, Shapiro GG, Busse WW (eds): Allergy, Asthma, and Immunology from Infancy to Adulthood. Philadelphia, WB Saunders, 1996, pp. 529–548

Bernstein IL, Kes H, Malo J-L: Medicolegal and compensation aspects. *In* Bernstein IL, Chan-Yeung M, Malo

J-L, Bernstein DI (eds): Asthma in the Workplace. New York, Marcel Dekker, 1999, pp 279–298

Gautrin D, Boulet L-P, Boutet M, Dugas M, et al: Is reactive airways dysfunction syndrome a variant of occupational asthma? J Allergy Clin Immunol 93:12–22, 1994

Grammar LC, Patterson R, Zeiss CR: Guidelines for the immunologic evaluation of occupational lung disease. J Allergy Clin Immunol 84:805–813, 1989

Menzies D, Bourbeau J: Building-related illnesses. New Engl J Med 21:1524–1531, 1997

Montanaro A: Chemically-induced nonspecific bronchial hyperresponsiveness. Clin Rev Allergy Immunol 15:187–203, 1997

Chapter 14

Hypersensitivity Pneumonitis

Michael C. Zacharisen and Jordan N. Fink

Hypersensitivity pneumonitis or extrinsic allergic alveolitis describes an immunologically mediated, inflammatory alveolar lung disease. A wide variety of inhaled organic dusts, low molecular weight chemicals, and medications may induce this disease of the pulmonary interstitium, terminal airways, and alveoli. Depending on the duration and degree of exposure to the offending agent, the nature of the agent, and the immunologic response of the patient, one of three forms—acute, subacute, or chronic—may result. Hypersensitivity pneumonitis is distinct from asthma or other immunologic pulmonary diseases in immunopathogenesis and clinical presentation.

PRESENTATION AND PROGRESSION

Causative Antigens

Numerous antigens derived from microorganisms, animal and plant products, low molecular weight chemicals, and medications are capable of inducing hypersensitivity pneumonitis (Table 14–1). Sensitization occurs after repeated inhalation of respirable antigens into the alveoli of susceptible persons. Medications administered orally or parenterally may induce acute lung disease, resembling hypersensitivity pneumonitis. Risk factors for sensitization are not clear, and a history of atopy is not seen. Of interest is the observation of lower prevalence in patients who smoke.

The most frequently implicated antigens are the thermophilic actinomycetes that cause farmer's lung. These organisms are found in moist soil, manure, grain, compost, hay, straw, cornstalks, sawdust, and forced-air heating systems. Any organic material that has molded and then warmed up to 50°C to 60°C is an abundant source. In farming, the antigen load may be heavy and, for example, shoveling moldy hay in silos provokes an acute episode of farmer's lung. Other organisms implicated include fungi such as *Alternaria, Penicillium,* and *Aspergillus.* Residential compost piles have been documented as a cause of hypersensitivity pneumonitis. Children have developed hypersensitivity pneumonitis from exposure to a moldy basement shower contaminated with *Epicoccum nigrum.*[1] Suberosis has been described in the cork industry, and sequoiosis occurs in the redwood lumber industry. Cheese worker's lung is related to inhaling *Penicillium* spores. Metal working fluids contaminated with *Pseudomonas* or *Acinetobacter lwoffii* are responsible for outbreaks in machine shops,[2] and therefore this manifestation is called machine operator's lung. Spray air-conditioning systems contaminated with amebae or fungi are responsible for outbreaks in building-related illness. Stagnant water and debris continuously exposed to temperatures of greater than 60°C provide an environment suitable for the proliferation of thermophilic actinomycetes. Room humidifiers and home ultrasonic humidifiers that generate microaerosolized water droplets also have been implicated, although the organisms in these cases may not necessarily be thermophilic actinomycetes.

Table 14–1. **Representative Antigens in Hypersensitivity Pneumonitis (HP)**

Disease	Environmental Antigen	Source Material
Bacteria		
Farmer's lung	Thermophilic actinomycetes	Moldy hay, compost, grain
Bagassosis	*T. sacchari*	Moldy sugarcane
Residential composter's lung	*T. vulgaris*	Compost
Ventilation pneumonitis	*T. candidus, Klebsiella*	Humidifier/air conditioner
Fungi		
Farmer's lung	*Penicillium brevicompactum*	Moldy hay
Malt worker's lung	*Aspergillus* species	Moldy malt dust
Woodworker's lung	*Alternaria* species	Moldy wood dust
Cheese worker's lung	*Penicillium caseii*	Cheese mold
Maple bark stripper's disease	*Cryptostroma corticale*	Moldy maple bark
Machine operator's lung	*Pseudomonas fluorescens*	Used metalworking fluid
	Acinetobacter lwoffii	
Basement shower HP	*Epicoccum nigrum*	Moldy basement shower
Animal Proteins		
Bird breeder's disease	Avian serum proteins (pigeon, duck, turkey, lovebird)	Avian dust
Laboratory worker's lung	Rat urine protein	Rat urine–contaminated dust
Oyster shell lung	Oyster shell protein	Oyster shell dust
Insect Proteins		
Wheat weevil disease	*Sitophilus granarius*	Infested wheat flour
Sericulturist's lung	Silkworm larvae	Cocoon fluff
Amebae		
Ventilation pneumonitis	*Naegleria gruberi, Acanthamoeba castellani*	Contaminated humidifier
Medication-Induced	Amiodarone, gold, beta-blockers, sulfasalazine, BCG,* nitrofurantoin, minocycline, procarbazine, methotrexate, chlorambucil, mesalamine, fluoxetine	Drug
Chemicals		
Paint refinisher's disease	Toluene diisocyanate (TDI)	Paint catalyst
Epoxy resin worker's lung	Phthalic anhydride	Epoxy resin
Plastic worker's lung	Trimellitic anhydride	Plastics industry
Grass		
Stipatosis	Esparto grass	Wet plaster/stucco
Other	Soybean hull	Veterinary feed

*BCG, bacillus Calmette-Guérin: intravesical administration.

Animal proteins are an important group of antigens. Avian proteins of serum or intestinal origin may be inhaled from dried excreta of pigeons, doves, ducks, chickens, parakeets, or lovebirds. Up to 15% of bird breeders become ill after repeated exposure. Children are susceptible when the coop is in or connected to the home.

Volatile low molecular weight reactive chemicals, such as isocyanates or phthalic anhydride, that are used in the plastics industry may act as haptens, combining with proteins in respiratory tissue when inhaled or may alter respiratory protein structure and form new antigens, causing sensitization and subsequent disease. These chemical antigens also can induce an IgE-mediated occupational asthma. Occupational exposure may occur in such in-dustries as polyurethane foam production, paint spraying, and molding in foundries. Diverse medications including amiodarone, gold salts, beta-blockers, sulfonamides, nitrofurantoin, chlorambucil, minocycline, and procarbazine have been associated with pulmonary diseases resembling hypersensitivity pneumonitis.

With the increased recognition of sources of antigens, the number of inhaled organic dusts, chemicals, or medications known to be able to sensitize susceptible individuals will undoubtedly increase.

PRESENTATION

The signs and symptoms are similar regardless of the inhaled organic dust. They will, however, vary with the stage of disease, designated as acute, subacute, or chronic (Table 14–2). Patient sensitization and ensuing clinical features also depend on several factors including (1) the nature (particle size, solubility, antigenicity) of the inhaled dust, (2) the frequency and intensity of exposure, (3) the intensity of the patient's immunologic response, and (4) a concomitant exposure such as a respiratory infection.

Acute Form

The clinical features of the acute form are explosive in nature, mimicking acute viral pneumonia. The period of sensitization to the offending antigen is variable and may take months or even years, but after sensitization has developed each subsequent exposure reproducibly triggers a nonproductive cough, dyspnea, fever, chills, myalgia, and malaise. The symptoms may persist for 18 to 24 hours then resolve spontaneously. The severity of the episode depends on the degree of exposure and the sensitivity of the individual. Anorexia, weight loss, and progressive dyspnea may be prominent when frequent and severe attacks occur. A common scenario is the patient who dramatically improves within 48 hours into the hospital admission while on antibiotics for an atypical pneumonia only to experience symptoms after rechallenge at home or the workplace. During an acute attack the patient appears ill and dyspneic. Bibasilar end-inspiratory rales are prominent and may persist for several hours, days, or weeks after an episode. Between attacks the examination and laboratory study results may be completely normal. During the acute episode, leukocytosis as high as 20,000 to 30,000 per mm^3 with a marked left shift is common. Eosinophilia is typically absent. Serum immunoglobulins are usually elevated except IgE. Erythrocyte sedimentation rate (ESR) and C-reactive protein (CRP) may be elevated. Arterial blood gases often demonstrate a respiratory alkalosis with hypoxemia. Although chest films may be normal if acute exacerbations are widely separated, they more commonly reveal sharp nodulations, reticulation, and general coarsening of the bronchovascular markings. During an acute attack, patchy, ill-defined parenchymal infiltrates appear to coalesce, giving rise to a ground glass appearance (Fig. 14–1). The most common pulmonary function abnormalities in acute disease occur 4 to 6 hours after exposure, when a decrease in both forced vital capacity (FVC) and 1-second forced expiratory volume (FEV$_1$) occur consistent with a restrictive pattern. Expiratory flow rates are not changed. A dual response has been observed in patients

Table 14–2. **Characteristics of Hypersensitivity Pneumonitis**

	Acute	**Subacute**	**Chronic**
Time	Episodic, 4–6 hours after exposure	Days to weeks	Months
Symptoms	Chills, fever, dyspnea, cough, myalgia, nausea, sweating, headache	Cough, dyspnea, mild systemic symptoms	Progressive dyspnea, dry cough, malaise, weight loss, anorexia, weakness
Examination	Ill, end inspiratory rales	Ill, inspiratory rales	Dry crackles
Chest x-ray	Normal to interstitial infiltrates	Interstitial infiltrates	Diffuse interstitial fibrosis to honey-combing
Spirometry	Restriction	Restriction	Restriction and/or obstruction
DLCO*	Decreased	Decreased	Decreased
BAL†	CD8 + Lymphocytic alveolitis	CD8 + Lymphocytic alveolitis	CD8 + Lymphocytic infiltrate
Lung biopsy	Interstitial pneumonitis; lymphocytic/foamy macrophages	Interstitial pneumonitis, noncaseating granulomas	Diffuse interstitial fibrosis and noncaseating granulomas
Laboratory	Leukocytosis, elevated ESR,‡ serum precipitins present	Serum precipitins present	Normal WBC Serum precipitins present
Reversibility	Good	Good to fair	Poor

*DLCO, diffusion capacity to carbon monoxide.
†BAL, bronchoalveolar lavage.
‡ESR, erythrocyte sedimentation rate.

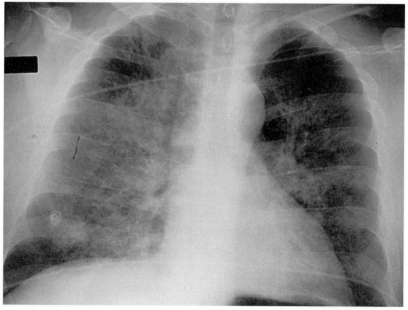

Figure 14–1. Chest radiograph of a patient with acute hypersensitivity pneumonitis. Bilateral interstitial infiltrates are evident, more on the right side than the left. Note the absence of pleural effusion, hilar adenopathy, and hyperinflation.

with pigeon breeders' disease and rarely with actinomycetes sensitivity, in which an immediate asthmatic-like response with a decrease in FEV_1 and expiratory flow rates is observed. This response is then followed by the late reaction as described previously. A decreased diffusion capacity is characteristic compared with an increase as seen in asthma. The abnormalities resolve as the attack subsides.

Subacute Form

The subacute form is intermediate between the acute and chronic forms. Symptoms appear gradually over several days to weeks and are marked by cough and dyspnea. Disease may progress to severe symptoms and cyanosis, prompting urgent hospitalization. Physical examination and laboratory evaluation results are similar to those found in acute hypersensitivity pneumonitis although less impressive.

Chronic Form

Prolonged low-level antigen exposure characterizes the chronic form, which presents as insidious, progressive respiratory disease with-out acute explosive episodes. The chronic form can result in irreversible pulmonary damage with fibrosis. Chronic disease is common in bird breeders in situations in which the birds are kept in the home or in cases of ventilation pneumonitis in which there is continuous exposure to a contaminated system. Symptoms include progressive dyspnea on exertion, cough, malaise, weakness, anorexia, and weight loss. Fever is often absent. On examination, features of interstitial fibrosis are seen, such as crackling bibasilar rales, dyspnea, cyanosis, and occasionally nail clubbing. Chest films typically show diffuse fibrosis or even honey-combing in end-stage disease. With sufficient parenchymal damage, spirometric abnormalities may be found during asymptomatic phases. A predominately restrictive ventilatory impairment with a decrease in diffusing capacity (DLCO) accentuated with exercise is found. With severe restrictive impairment, the expiratory flow rates and diffusing capacity decrease, and hypoxemia and hypercapnia may be observed especially with exercise.

PATHOLOGY

Despite quite different antigens, hypersensitivity pneumonitis is characterized by similar histologic changes. These changes largely depend on the intensity of antigen exposure and the stage of the disease when the biopsy is performed. In acute hypersensitivity pneumonitis the alveolar and interstitial inflammation is comprised of lymphocytes, activated foamy macrophages, plasma cells, and neutrophils.

In the subacute and chronic stages, a CD8+ lymphocytic alveolitis predominates. Also observed are intra-alveolar foamy macrophages, increased mast and plasma cells, interstitial inflammation, noncaseating granulomas, and interstitial fibrosis (Fig. 14–2). The granulomas differ from those found in sarcoidosis by appearing smaller and more loosely arranged; they have a higher predominance of lymphocytes and are more frequently located in alveolar tissue than in the vicinity of bronchioles and blood vessels. The severity of fibrosis varies and is associated with minimal epithelial cell necrosis or connective tissue destruction, suggesting a reparative process. Even in the late stages of hypersensitivity pneumonitis, characteristic features seen in the early stages may persist, helping to distinguish hypersensitivity pneumonitis from idiopathic pulmonary fibrosis.

The exact immunologic mechanisms involved in the pathogenesis of hypersensitivity pneumonitis have not been clarified. There may be multiple immunologic and even non-immunologic factors, depending on the stage of the disease. The inhaled organic dusts stimulate alveolar macrophages, directly activate the alternative pathway of complement, function as immunologic adjuvants, and induce enzymatic activity in lymphocytes through endotoxin or other toxic substances. The sequence of inflammatory events is likely multifaceted. The initial presentation follows repeated antigen exposure at the level of terminal bronchioles and alveoli. Presumably antigen processing cells, including alveolar macrophages, engulf and process the antigen releasing cytokines and chemoattractants. These cytokines, including interleukin 1 and interleukin 2 are likely responsible for the ensuing cellular infiltration. In the acute phase, there is a marked increase in neutrophils within the alveoli. This is replaced with CD8+ lymphocytes and other activated T cells as the disease process continues.

As the initial inflammatory response resolves with a decrease in neutrophils, the total number of cells recovered in lavage fluid continues to be elevated, with a predominance of lymphocytes. The initiation and maintenance of the granulomatous response is likely because of the dynamic interaction between the inhaled agent, the release of inflammatory mediators, attraction of leukocytes, and the resident structural airway cells.

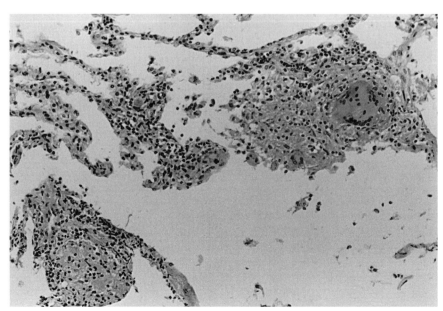

Figure 14–2. Lung biopsy specimen of a patient with acute hypersensitivity pneumonitis shows diffuse lymphocytic infiltration of the alveolar walls and noncaseating granulomas. (Hematoxylin and eosin stain, magnification ×120.)

Host factors play a role in the pathogenesis because the majority of individuals exposed to organic dusts remain asymptomatic.

DIAGNOSIS

Hypersensitivity pneumonitis should be considered in patients with recurrent pneumonia, intermittent pulmonary and systemic symptoms, or with progressive unexplained pulmonary symptoms and evidence for interstitial lung disease. Table 14–3 outlines a diagnostic algorithm. A complete history exploring temporal relationships between symptoms and an occupation, hobby, medication, or inhabitation of a building with forced-air equipment may provide clues. A site visit to the home or workplace may be necessary to discover the source of an offending agent and obtain material for culture. No single diagnostic laboratory test is available. A combination of clinical findings, radiographic abnormalities, pulmonary function changes, and immunologic testing supports the diagnosis. Inhalational challenge, bronchoalveolar lavage, and lung biopsy may be necessary in some cases to confirm the diagnosis. Laboratory findings that are helpful in the acute stages include elevated ESR, positive CRP, increased white blood cell count, and arterial hypoxemia.

The demonstration of serum precipitating antibodies against the specific offending antigen is the characteristic immunologic finding. This is done by traditional Ouchterlony double immunodiffusion gel system using the patient's sera and the specific antigen. A positive test result confirms exposure but not necessarily disease. False-negative precipitin studies may result from improper quality controls, insensitive techniques, use of the wrong antigen, or underconcentrated sera. More sensitive assays for IgG-specific antibodies include immunoelectrophoresis; yet these must be interpreted cautiously. A reliable laboratory may avoid the need for additional, expensive, or invasive procedures. Specific antigen preparations, made from dusts or fungi cultured from the furnace, humidifier, or the place of employment, may be needed when traditional antigens are negative or not suspected. Skin testing is not practical because both false-positive and -negative reactions may occur, and commercial antigen preparations for this purpose are not available. Allergy testing for an immediate reaction is not indicated because the disease is not IgE mediated.

Results of pulmonary function tests and findings on chest radiographs vary depending on the stage of the disease. They may be normal if obtained during an asymptomatic period related to avoidance or corticosteroid treatment. When a specific environment is suspected as the cause, it may be necessary to perform pulmonary function tests before and several hours after exposure. If significant changes occur in vital capacity, FEV_1, diffusing capacity, or even flow rates, the environment should be suspected and further investigated with cultures and immunologic studies. Peak flow measurements alone are not helpful.

A high resolution computed tomography (CT) scan of the chest may be useful when the chest film appears normal or nonspecific findings are identified. It is also useful as a guide for a lung biopsy or to detect suspected complications when clinical conditions or lung functions deteriorate.

Removal of the patient from the suspected environment or the agent from the patient's environment as a therapeutic trial may be extremely helpful. Improvement occurs in most acute cases within days. Using corticosteroids as a therapeutic trial is not recommended because this approach lacks specificity and may be hazardous in those patients with an underlying infectious etiology.

Fiberoptic bronchoscopy with alveolar lavage may help distinguish hypersensitivity

Table 14–3. **Diagnostic Algorithm for Hypersensitivity Pneumonitis**

History: occupation, hobbies, medications
Physical examination
Chest film, consider chest CT scan
Spirometry including lung volumes and diffusing capacity
Exercise pulmonary function testing with arterial blood gases
Laboratory: serum precipitins, ESR, WBC count, CRP
Bronchoalveolar lavage: T-cell markers (CD4, CD8)
Inhalational challenge (experimental, special situations)
Lung biopsy

CT, computed tomography; ESR, erythrocyte sedimentation rate, WBC, white blood cell; CRP, C-reactive protein.

pneumonitis from sarcoid lung or other lung diseases by evaluating T cell subsets CD4 and CD8. A predominance of CD8+ cells suggests hypersensitivity pneumonitis; a predominance of CD4+ lymphocytes suggests sarcoidosis. The presence of neutrophils in lavage fluid suggests hypersensitivity pneumonitis when the symptoms are acute and idiopathic pulmonary fibrosis when the symptoms are chronic and progressive.

Lung biopsy should be carried out only if the other diagnostic efforts fail to establish the diagnosis or to rule out other diseases that require different treatment. Since the histopathologic features of hypersensitivity pneumonitis are not entirely specific, they must be considered in light of the overall case.

Inhalation challenge using suspected antigenic materials should be done in selected hospital laboratories because of the potential for severe reactions and the need for experienced personnel.

To summarize, the main diagnostic test is restrictive ventilatory impairment and an abnormal chest film during times of symptoms both of which normalize relatively rapidly with avoidance of the antigen. The diagnosis of acute hypersensitivity pneumonitis is based on the clinical history of intermittent pulmonary symptoms with systemic features that correlate temporally with a particular environmental exposure. Therefore, a detailed history of occupational exposures is critical to quickly and accurately diagnose the condition.

Differential Diagnosis

Several other disorders should be considered when evaluating patients with recurrent pneumonias or interstitial lung diseases. The possibilities are many and depend on the individual's particular environment. Building-related illnesses may induce symptoms by immunologic, infectious, toxic, or irritant mechanisms.[3] For example, sick building syndrome is characterized by rather vague and subjective symptoms of eye irritation and respiratory complaints of chest tightness, coughing, and shortness of breath in many workers in the same building. Other predominately subjective complaints include memory loss, headache, depression, and dizziness. Physical findings

and radiographic and pulmonary function abnormalities are uncommon. The sick building syndrome appears to result from decreased fresh air intake in highly energy-efficient office buildings. There is a consequent increased concentration of a variety of multiple contaminants, usually volatile organic chemicals and microbes. Increased ventilation and modification of the extreme energy conservation measures usually resolve the situation.

Immune deficiency syndromes can present with recurrent pneumonias. In particular, common variable immune deficiency with hypogammaglobulinemia should be excluded by measuring quantitative immunoglobulins.

Organic dust toxic syndrome (ODTS) refers to a group of noninfectious febrile illnesses that occur in workers after exposure to agricultural dusts and toxins generated from organic materials contaminated with ammonia, hydrogen sulfide gases, and multiple bacterial and fungal species. Various descriptive terms have been coined including pulmonary mycotoxicosis, silo unloader's disease, grain fever, mill fever, humidifier fever, and animal house fever. ODTS is up to 50 times more common in farmers than hypersensitivity pneumonitis. It occurs more commonly in the summer months and in younger individuals than those affected with hypersensitivity pneumonitis. Although symptoms of delayed fever, malaise, cough, and chest tightness are similar in both diseases, chest radiographs are normal and pulmonary function tests are either normal or show mild airway obstruction without impairment in diffusing capacity in ODTS. Furthermore, in ODTS the symptoms generally clear within a few hours, and inhalation challenge with microbial antigens does not consistently reproduce symptoms. Inhalation of endotoxin will provoke effects in nearly half of previously unexposed persons. Lavage fluid from ODTS patients reveals increased numbers of total cells, polymorphonuclear cells, fungal elements, and a predominately CD8+ lymphocytic alveolitis can be seen after the first week. Cultures of lung biopsy specimens in patients with ODTS can grow large numbers of a variety of fungi, but the acute disease is quite different from farmer's lung. Lung biopsy specimens lack granulomas.

In the differential diagnosis of chronic hypersensitivity pneumonitis, one should consider conditions that produce interstitial lung disease with progressive pulmonary and systemic symptoms. These conditions include sarcoid, pulmonary histiocytosis, allergic bronchopulmonary aspergillosis (ABPA), and idiopathic pulmonary fibrosis.

Distinguishing characteristics for sarcoidosis include hilar adenopathy, elevated serum angiotensin-converting enzyme level, subtle differences in histopathology, CD4+ T-cell alveolitis and abnormal gallium scans with involvement of the parotid gland, lymph nodes, and extrathoracic tissues. Primary pulmonary histiocytosis, in contrast to hypersensitivity pneumonitis, is characterized by wheezing, hemoptysis, and Langerhans cells in bronchial lavage fluid and open lung biopsy specimens. These patients have a 10% spontaneous pneumothorax rate. Gallium scans are usually negative. Allergic bronchopulmonary aspergillosis is immunologic pulmonary inflammation resulting from sensitivity to *Aspergillus* in patients with asthma. Typical features distinguishing ABPA from hypersensitivity pneumonitis include a history of asthma, positive immediate skin test response to *Aspergillus,* elevated total serum IgE levels, and specific IgG to *Aspergillus,* peripheral blood eosinophilia, central bronchiectasis, and sputum revealing hyphae that is culture-positive for *Aspergillus.* Similarities with hypersensitivity pneumonitis that can cause confusion are precipitating antibodies to *Aspergillus* and recurrent infiltrates on chest radiographs. Granulomas are not found in ABPA, and ABPA can almost always be ruled out by a negative *Aspergillus* immediate skin test result. Idiopathic pulmonary fibrosis is differentiated from hypersensitivity pneumonitis by nail clubbing on physical examination, bronchoalveolar lavage fluid dominated by neutrophils and macrophages, and lung biopsy specimens with a significant increase in the total number of inflammatory cells. Gallium scans showing a diffuse pattern are positive in approximately 70% of patients. Frequently a fatal outcome occurs within 6 years after onset. Other chronic lung diseases should be ruled out. These include tuberculosis, berylliosis, silicosis, asbestosis, alveolar proteinosis, chronic eosinophilic pneumonia, alpha$_1$-proteinase inhibitor deficiency (alpha$_1$-antitrypsin deficiency), cystic fibrosis, and psittacosis. By means of radiologic examination, pulmonary function studies, and immunologic assays along with close observation of the patient during periods of exposure and avoidance, the appropriate diagnosis can be made.

NATURAL HISTORY

In general, in acute disease, the majority of individuals can expect complete resolution of symptoms and a return to normal pulmonary function after the exposure is stopped. A 14-year follow-up of patients with farmer's lung found that diffusion capacity in patients was significantly decreased compared with control farmers, especially if recurrent symptomatic episodes had occurred.[4] Similarly, subacute hypersensitivity pneumonitis is often completely reversible spontaneously with avoidance or with treatment. Poor prognostic factors include symptoms occurring for longer than 1 year before diagnosis, evidence of pulmonary fibrosis at diagnosis, and symptomatic recurrences. If the disease is left unrecognized or untreated and coupled with continued antigen exposure, there may be progression to irreversible lung damage and a fatal outcome.[5] Reversal of the disease process depends on how quickly the diagnosis is made so that avoidance, drug therapy, or both may be instituted.

TREATMENT

Avoidance of the offending antigen is the most important and effective treatment. A variety of precautions may be attempted once the inciting antigen is identified. If the antigen is an airborne dust, the use of air-cleaning systems, personal masks, or alterations in forced-air heating or cooling systems may be of benefit. A change in a hobby or occupation also may be necessary.

Specific environmental changes can be important and include improving ventilation in pigeon coops, wearing protective respirators, and changing farming techniques.

Pharmacologic treatment is indicated when the offending antigen cannot be avoided or if the disease is progressing despite avoidance measures. Oral corticosteroids are the mainstay of therapy in patients with acute flares of hypersensitivity pneumonitis. The clinical and laboratory responses to these drugs are dramatic. The duration of corticosteroid therapy is based on the clinical and laboratory improvement of each individual. Chronic use of corticosteroids should be reserved for situations in which the antigen cannot be avoided such as with a farmer or bird breeder who refuses to change his or her practices. Allergen injection immunotherapy with the offending antigen is not recommended because of the potential adverse effects from injected microbial or fungal toxins or the development of an immune-complex vasculitis. Early detection of clinical illness, and identification and subsequent avoidance of the offending antigen are most important.

WHEN TO REFER TO A SPECIALIST

An allergist, immunologist, or pulmonologist with experience in diagnosing interstitial lung disorders is invaluable in performing and interpreting specific laboratory tests. Early referral is encouraged when the diagnosis is entertained because prompt identification and avoidance of the offending antigen is key to preventing ongoing exposure and potential chronic lung disease.

Guidelines for the clinical evaluation of hypersensitivity pneumonitis were published in 1989; these guidelines are still relevant.[6]

KEY POINTS

▶ Hypersensitivity pneumonitis is a non-IgE-mediated inflammatory lung disease primarily affecting the alveoli and interstitium caused by the interaction of environmental organic dusts with a susceptible individual's immune system.

▶ Symptoms characteristic of the acute form are cough, dyspnea, fever, chills, and malaise, whereas the chronic form manifests as insidious onset of dyspnea exacerbated by exercise.

▶ Characteristic findings helpful in diagnosis include patchy infiltrates on the chest film, restrictive lung disease, and precipitating antibodies in gel diffusion studies.

▶ Acute, subacute, or chronic forms relate to the degree and frequency of exposure.

▶ Antigen avoidance results in complete recovery in nearly all cases. Treatment with oral corticosteroids results in dramatic improvement.

References

1. Hogan MB, Patterson R, Pore RS, et al: Basement shower hypersensitivity pneumonitis secondary to *Epicoccum nigrum*. Chest 110:855–856, 1996
2. Zacharisen MC, Kadambi AR, Schlueter DP, et al: The spectrum of respiratory disease associated with exposure to metal working fluids. J Occup Environ Med 40:640–647, 1998
3. Seltzer JM: Building-related illnesses. J Allergy Clin Immunol 94:351–362, 1994
4. Erkinjuntti-Pekkanen R, Kokkarinen JI, Tukiainen HO, et al: Long-term outcome of pulmonary function in farmer's lung: a 14-year follow-up with matched controls. Eur Respir J 10:2046–2050, 1997
5. Nakagawa-Yoshida K, Ando M, Etches RI, Dosman JA: Fatal cases of farmer's lung in a Canadian family. Chest 111:245–248, 1997
6. Richerson HB, Bernstein IL, Fink JN, et al: Guidelines for the clinical evaluation of hypersensitivity pneumonitis. J Allergy Clin Immunol 84:839–844, 1989

Suggested Reading

Fink JN, Zacharisen MC: Hypersensitivity pneumonitis. *In* Middleton E, Reed CE, Ellis EF, Adkinson NF, Yunginger JW, Busse WW (eds): Allergy: Principles & Practice. St. Louis, Mosby-Year Book 1998, pp 994–1004
Kreiss K, Cox-Ganser J: Metalworking fluid-associated hypersensitivity pneumonitis: A workshop summary. Am J Ind Med 32:423–432, 1997
Parker JE, Petsonk L, Weber SL: Hypersensitivity pneumonitis and organic dust toxic syndrome. Immunol Allergy Clin North Am 12:279–290, 1992

Chapter 15

Atopic Dermatitis

Vincent S. Beltrani

Atopic dermatitis (AD) is a common, chronic disease that is usually easy to recognize. Because of its characteristic exacerbations and remissions, the primary care physician should be familiar with its routine management, and also be aware of the many aggravating triggers and potential serious complications. Unfortunately, the treatment of patients with AD must be individualized. The primary care physician plays an important role in the routine care of patients with uncomplicated AD and ensures continuity of care in those patients whose disease requires more specialized management.

Some insight into the pathogenesis will help the reader to better understand the therapeutic modalities available in the management of AD. The importance of managing the entire family of patients with AD will be stressed; oftentimes an accessible support system can be as important as the medical management of the patient. Knowledge of the pathophysiology and management of AD also can be helpful in the care of patients with the other eczemas, which tend to occur more often in atopic individuals (Fig. 15–1). Given this information, a treatment plan that indicates when to refer to the appropriate specialist (i.e., dermatologist or allergist) can be derived.

PATHOGENESIS

Atopy is a genetic predisposition in which there is an exaggerated inflammatory response to many extrinsic (both immunologic [allergic] and nonimmunologic [pseudoallergic]) stimuli. The distinguishing immunologic (allergic) response results from an increased production of specific IgE antibodies by B-cells to a specific antigen, which then activate (hyperreleasable) mast cells, basophils, and Th$_2$ cells. Atopic individuals can be objectively identified by their elevated IgE levels, and by positive results of skin tests, radioallergosorbent tests (RASTs) to specific antigens, or both. These are reliable markers and can support a suspected family history of the atopic diathesis. It must be recognized that these positive skin or RAST results are not always clinically relevant; that is, they do not always cause allergic symptoms and are often considered false-positive results. Concomitantly, the mast cells and basophils of atopic individuals also can be activated by nonimmunologic stimuli, which produce a clinical picture indistinguishable from the immunologic IgE triggered symptoms; thus, these nonimmunologic triggers can be considered pseudoallergens.

Hours after a sensitized mast cell is activated by its specific allergen, it produces newly formed mediators, which cause the influx of inflammatory cells, including many eosinophils. This is known as the late-phase reaction, and it is believed to play an important role in AD, as measured by the large amounts of eosinophilic major basic protein in their upper dermis.

The genetic atopic predisposition to produce large amounts of IgE is the result of a T lymphocyte imbalance known as the Th1/Th2 ratio reversal. The dominance of helper T2 (Th2) cells, noted in the atopic patient, with its cytokine profile including interleukin 4 (IL-4) and interleukin 5 (IL-5), promotes the production of IgE antibodies and attracts eosinophils, respectively. In the nonatopic person,

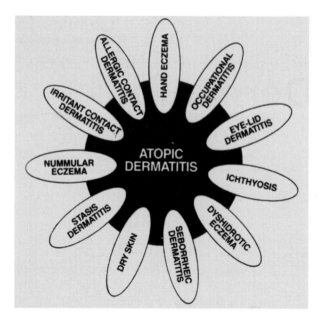

Figure 15–1. The occurrence of common eczematous eruption frequently associated with the atopic diathesis.

who has a predominance of Th1 cells, the cytokine profile includes IL-2 and interferon-gamma (INF-γ), which inhibit IgE production.

Clinically, atopy has been associated with seasonal perennial allergic rhinitis, "extrinsic" asthma, and AD. This group of diseases has been referred to as the atopic triad. Patients have been noted to have one, or two, or all three components of the atopic triad (Fig. 15–2). At present, there is no reliable way to predict which symptoms, or the severity of symptoms, an atopic individual will experience.

Atopy does not fit a simple autosomal dominant model, and complex interactions among multiple genes are involved in the expression of atopic symptoms. The incidence of AD in childhood has been reported to be 10% to 15%, and there seems to be a steady increase in recent decades. In a study of 270 adults with AD, 60% of their offspring also were affected. The prevalence of AD in children was 81% when both parents were affected, 59% when one parent had AD and the other had respiratory atopy, and 56% when one parent had AD and the other parent had no atopic history. In atopic individuals, it has been found that the incidence of allergic rhinitis is ten times, and asthma five times more common than AD. But, the risk of patients with AD developing respiratory symptoms in later years has been reported to be 40% to 60%. In one study, it was noted that when asthma worsened, the AD tended to improve, whereas allergic rhinitis appeared to be independent of the AD.

No benefit has been observed from eliminating major food allergens from the maternal diet during the third trimester of pregnancy for the prevention of AD in the developing fetus. However, placing both the lactating mother and her infant on a food allergen (e.g., cow's milk, egg, peanut) elimination diet results in significantly less AD at 1 year of age compared to high-risk infants who have no dietary restrictions, but the difference is no longer apparent after age 2 years.

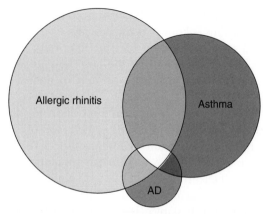

Figure 15–2. Venn circles. Relative prevalence of atopic diseases after puberty. During infancy, atopic dermatitis (AD) takes the place of allergic rhinitis.

Although the role of allergens as (immunologic) triggers for rhinitis and asthma is universally accepted, their role in AD remains a source of contention. It is well recognized that the same symptoms caused by mast cell, basophil, and Th2 cell activation, such as itching, sneezing, and wheezing, can be elicited by nonimmunologic triggers, and these can be considered pseudoallergic. Thus, the patient with hay fever sneezes when exposed to perfumes, soap, and so forth, and the asthmatic patient wheezes with a viral infection. The many non-IgE triggers for AD are described in subsequent paragraphs.

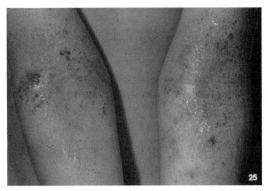

Figure 15–3. Atopic youngster with chronic eczema of the antecubital fossae since childhood. The long-standing scratching resulted in the thickened, exaggerated skin markings, known as lichenification, and the linear crateriform, dug-out excoriations reflect the aggressive scratching elicited by the itch.

CLINICAL PRESENTATION

Although AD can be seen at any age, it is predominantly a disease of the pediatric age group. The majority of cases (55%) occur in the first year of life, and another 30% develop before the age of 5 years. Interestingly, the prevalence of AD has risen dramatically over several decades, from 5.1% in the mid 1940s to 12.2% in 1970.

Signs and Symptoms

The most consistent symptom of AD is pruritus, that extremely unpleasant sensation that provokes the desire to scratch. The pruritus of AD is often noted as early as the newborn period, by the newborn's increased crying and restlessness in the nursery. The earlier onset often signals a more severe course. Pruritus in AD is variable, but can be extremely intense. Scratching is not observed before 2 months of age, but the pruritus may be the cause of the young infant's inability to get a good night's sleep. In older children the pruritus often interferes with socialization and school performance.

Most of the chronic lesions of AD are secondary to scratching, leading to excoriations and lichenification (Fig. 15–3), which increases the inflammation, and in turn provokes more itching. Thus itching is the central phenomenon in AD. Hanifin has graded the itch of AD as 4 + when compared with the itch of urticaria (graded a 2 +). This difference in severity also makes the author suspect that the

pruritogenic mediators of AD and urticaria may be different (see below). Itching may be elicited by all kinds of stimuli, and to complicate matters, the underlying neurophysiologic mechanisms of itch are not fully understood. Itch is considered a hyperalgesia, and the atopic individual is made to itch from stimuli that do not usually provoke itch in nonatopic individuals. Hagermark has proposed to label this kind of itch *alloknesis* (Gr. *allos* = other, and *knesis* = itch). Once AD patients have started to itch, itching increases the liability of the surrounding skin to (hyper)react to the lightest stimulus with more itching. This itch is not the same as a lowered itch threshold, which implies that pruritus is evoked by milder pruritogenic stimuli.

The most common provokers of itch in patients with AD are:

- Heat and perspiration   96%
- Wool   91%
- Emotional stress   81%
- Certain foods   49%
- Alcohol   44%
- Common cold   36%
- Dust mite   35 + %

The complete list of recognized triggers of itch in AD also includes:

- All "irritants," such as:
  Lipid solvents (especially soap)
  Disinfectants (e.g., chlorine in swimming pools)
  Occupational irritants
  Cigarette smoke (especially for eyelid dermatitis)

- Xerosis (dry skin)
- Aero- and contact allergens
  Dust mites—contact>aeroallergenic
  "Hairy" pets—cat>dog
  Pollens—"seasonal"
  Molds
  ??Human dander (dandruff)
- Microbial agents
  Viral infections
    especially URI's in children
  Staphylococcus aureus
    (both as a superantigen, and/or agent
    of impetiginization)
  Pityrosporon yeast—a "normal" resident of
    greasy skin
  Candida—(rarely)
  Dermatophytosis—(rarely)
- Others
  Foods (as a contact irritant>>vasodila-
    tor>allergen)
  Psyche
  Climate
  Hormones (e.g., menstrual cycle)

As is emphasized later in this chapter, the best results of any treatment regimen can only be attained by identifying, and then removing, each stimulus that initiates the scratch/itch cycle.

Since antihistamines have been so successful in relieving the itch of hives, they unfortunately, have earned the reputation of being the universal antipruritic agent. However, antihistamines are specifically effective in antagonizing the single mediator *histamine,* which is the cause of most urticarial eruptions. The beneficial effects of antihistamines in pruritic rashes other than urticaria are only marginal, and this raises the question of whether histamine is involved in the itch of AD.

In atopics there is more histamine in plasma and skin, and more mast cells in skin. This finding suggests that histamine ought to play an essential role in the pathogenesis of AD; however, intradermal injections of histamine in patients with AD produce the "triple response of Lewis," the same itch, wheal, and flare seen when histamine is injected into the skin of nonatopic individuals. Also, when histamine is repeatedly injected into the skin, the itch receptors become tachyphylactic; this condition is not compatible with the chronic itch that lasts for hours which occurs in AD. Lastly, controlled trials with antihistamines (H1- and H2-antagonists) indicate that they have a very

limited effect in itching diseases other than urticaria.

Proteases (tryptase, chymase), kinins (kallikrein), prostaglandins, neuropeptides, and opioids (β-endorphins) all induce itch or potentiate histamine release when injected into atopic skin. Both glucocorticoids and cyclosporin A inhibit the release and production of cytokines, so their strong therapeutic effect supports the idea that cytokines produced by the T-cell infiltrate may be the cause of the itch of AD.

Eczema is a symptom, not a specific disease. The terms *dermatitis* and *eczema* are often used synonymously; however dermatitis is really less specific, meaning any type of skin inflammation, whereas eczema is a nonspecific T-cell inflammatory response. Eczema is derived from the Greek *Ek zein* meaning "to boil over," and clinically, all eczemas may be identified by tiny (microscopic) bubbles or vesicles to large bullae in the skin. The clinical spectrum of eczema includes three frequently overlapping stages: acute, subacute, and chronic. Histopathologically, the three stages all show different degrees of epidermal intercellular edema, which is referred to as *spongiosis.* The dermis demonstrates a perivascular infiltrate, which is made up of T-cells. All the eczemas are histologically quite similar; thus, a biopsy specimen has its greatest value in ruling out noneczematous rashes (Table 15–1).

A common dermatologic dictum that atopic dermatitis is an itch that erupts, rather than an eruption that itches is not exactly true. AD is an itch that erupts when scratched. If

Table 15–1. **Histopathologic Differential Diagnosis of Spongiotic (Eczematous) Dermatoses**

Contact dermatitis (allergic or irritant)	Photoallergic dermatitis
	Photocontact dermatitis
Seborrheic dermatitis	Polymorphous light
Atopic dermatitis	eruption
Nummular eczema	Dilantin-induced eczema
Stasis dermatitis	Wiskott-Aldrich disease
Dyshidrotic eczema	Acrodermatitis
Asteatotic eczema	enteropathica
Lichen simplex chronicus	Vitamin deficiencies
Autosensitization or id reactions	Pellagra
	Riboflavin deficiency
Dermatophytosis	Hartnup's disease
Pityriasis rosea	Hyper IgE syndrome

the itch is not rubbed or scratched, the skin may get red (vasodilate), but no eczema appears until the site is traumatized. This reaction can be equated to the isomorphic response (Koebner phenomenon) seen in psoriasis and other skin conditions. The distribution of the eczema is determined by the accessibility to scratching the itch; thus, the typical, accessible antecubital and popliteal fossa involvement. The reactive eczema supports the description of AD being a "twitchy" skin syndrome similar to the asthmatic who is considered to have a "twitchy" lung syndrome. Regardless of the itch trigger, scratched or rubbed atopic skin reacts by producing an eczematous eruption. Listing specific sites of involvement, such as hand, eyelid, foot (Fig. 15–4), or nipple (Fig. 15–5), in an atopic individual may be confusing, because eczema is the characteristic response, irrespective of the site that itches and then is scratched or rubbed.

The characteristic clinical features of the eczema of AD are:

1. Distribution. Can be highly variable, but is generally age related, with facial (Fig. 15–6) and extensor involvement during infancy and childhood, and flexural and linear involvement in adolescence. Hot and sweaty fossae and folds almost always are involved, whereas the nose and surrounding skin are almost always spared. This distribu-

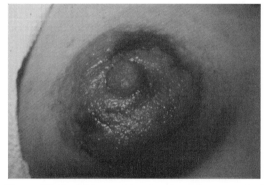

Figure 15–5. A 14-year-old asthmatic patient was scheduled for a biopsy because of this itchy, oozing nipple rash of 3 weeks' duration. Her atopic background should have made eczema the most likely diagnosis (rather than Paget's disease). Eczema disappeared after 5 days of 1% hydrocortisone cream twice a day.

tion is referred to as the headlight sign (Fig. 15–7). The diaper area is usually spared.

2. Excoriations. Indicate the intense scratching or rubbing (see Fig. 15–3).

3. Diverse stages of the eczema:

   Acute. Oozing or crusting little bubbles (spongiosis) in an area of papular erythema.

   Subacute. Thicker, less erythematous

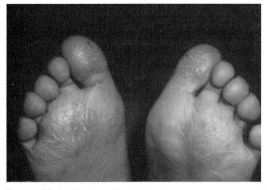

Figure 15–4. Despite the lack of response to repeated courses of topical and systemic antifungal agents, this (atopic) youngster was persistently treated for athlete's foot. The latter condition is rarely seen before puberty; the diagnosis should never be made without a fungal culture whenever the interdigital spaces are spared. This condition has been referred to as juvenile plantar dermatosis and responds best to topical steroids.

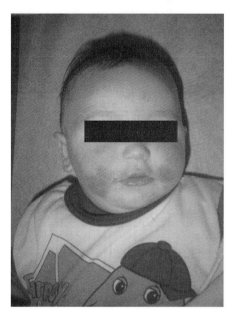

Figure 15–6. A 6-month-old atopic boy with scaly red patches on both cheeks of 2 months' duration. Atopic youngsters constantly rub their faces on the mattress to relieve the itch. It is not unusual for this presentation to be the only sign of atopic dermatitis.

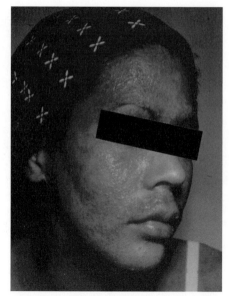

Figure 15–7. A 17-year-old girl with long-standing atopic dermatitis. She is experiencing an acute flare-up of her extensive facial eczema; notice the sparing of the nose and adjacent skin, the headlight sign.

plaques, with visible remnants of the tiny bubbles. More linear excoriations.

<u>Chronic.</u> Thickened (lichenified), dry, scaly, papular plaques, with old (scarred) and newer excoriations. Absent hairs if hairy areas were scratched or rubbed.

Dry skin *(xerosis)* is virtually universal and is most apparent when the humidity is low. Inflamed skin causes epidermal hyperproliferation, manifesting itself as scale. Keratosis pilaris, which feels like chicken skin, is most often noted on the upper arms and thighs, but can be generalized. This condition is caused by horny plugs that fill the skins' follicular openings. *Allergic shiners* have been noted in 60% of all atopic individuals (and 38% of people who are not atopic). *Dennie-Morgan lines* are symmetric, prominent folds of the lower eyelids (similar to those seen in Down syndrome) that occur in 60% to 80% of people with atopy. *Palmar or plantar hyperlinearity* is believed to occur independent of the xerosis.

These associated findings, (except for the xerosis) have greater cosmetic significance than being pathogenic or clinically significant.

DIAGNOSIS OF ATOPIC DERMATITIS

In order to have some diagnostic consistency, a standardized set of criteria have been agreed

on, with some variation for infants and adults. To make the diagnosis of AD, the patient must manifest *all* of the three major criteria.

1. Personal or family history of atopy
2. Pruritus (alloknesis)
3. Eczema that is chronic, relapsing, and is in the typical areas of distribution.

Non-essential for the diagnosis of AD are these findings—which while not exclusive to atopics—are noted to occur more often in atopic individuals:

1. Xerosis (dry skin)
2. Keratosis pilaris
3. Palmar or plantar hyperlinearity
4. Allergic shiners
5. Dennie-Morgan (infraorbital) lines
6. White dermatographism
7. Th1-cell defect—increased susceptibility to viral and fungal infections.
8. Anterior capsular cataracts
9. Keratoconus

Thus, it is evident that the diagnosis of AD is made from the history and physical examination, whereas the management of AD may require some testing to confirm a suspected trigger. Laboratory tests are rarely relied on to make the diagnosis, but an elevated IgE level, or positive response to a prick or RAST test can support the clinical impression. A mild eosinophilia can be seen in atopic diseases, but it is not pathognomonic of allergies; therefore, a routine complete blood count is rarely helpful. The differential diagnosis of eosinophilia includes: parasitic diseases (highest counts), cancer, drug reactions, the hypereosinophilic syndrome, and atopy (the most common cause). A skin biopsy, as noted previously, will not be diagnostic of AD but supportive. The biopsy specimen should be reviewed by a dermatopathologist, because a specialist is more apt to be able to differentiate the noneczematous (perivascular dermatitides, cutaneous T-cell lymphoma, and so forth) diseases.

Despite the enthusiasm of some who believe aeroallergens play an important role in the causation or perpetuation of AD, the routine use of either prick testing or patch testing with aeroallergens has been of limited value. There are some patients with AD whose eczema can be exacerbated by allergens. The suspicion of an allergen should be considered from a characteristic distribution of the ec-

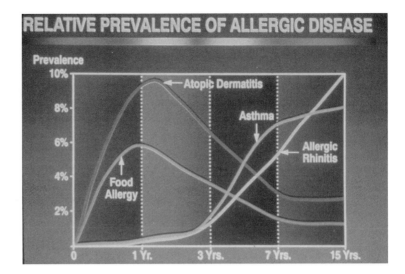

Figure 15–8. Relationship of food allergy, age, and atopic disease.

zema, for example, dust mite contact allergy when the eczema persists on the face, head, neck, and exposed parts of the extremities.

Food allergy is seen most often in infants before age 3 (Fig. 15–8) and should be considered when the eczema is generalized and is poorly responsive to routine management. Fifty percent of food-allergic infants have gastrointestinal symptoms: colicky, abdominal pain, vomiting, and diarrhea. Their eczema characteristically seems to flare *always* after the ingestion of a particular food. Five foods (egg, milk, peanut, soy, and wheat) account for 87% of positive food challenge responses; therefore, extensive food testing is unwarranted. Of note, half the children with proven (double-blind placebo-controlled food challenged [DBPCFC]) food allergy outgrow their food hypersensitivity (especially to soy, milk, eggs, and wheat) by age 2 years. Children who are allergic to peanut, nuts, and seafood are less likely to outgrow their allergies.

The colonization of skin by *Staphylococcus aureus* is a major feature in patients with AD. Routine cultures from atopic skin can cause confusion. The skin carriage rate of *S. aureus* in patients with AD is 75% on uninvolved skin, 90% on chronic lichenified lesions, and 100% on acute, exudative lesions. Thus, in AD patients, it is difficult to interpret between pure colonization by *S. aureus* and infection. Forty percent of healthy individuals are *S. aureus* nasal carriers, and chronic nasal carriers expose patients with AD to an increased risk of skin infections. Specimens from full-blown

infections should be cultured; these infections are easy to recognize by their classic symptoms, such as pustules and severe crusting (Fig. 15–9) but at times the *S. aureus* infection may just produce a weeping or oozing discharge on acute eczematous lesions (Fig. 15–10). Occasionally, patients may develop regional adenopathy. It should be noted that bright erythema, lateral spread of pustules, cellulitis, and fever rarely occur in skin infections caused by *S. aureus* (these signs are suggestive of strepto-

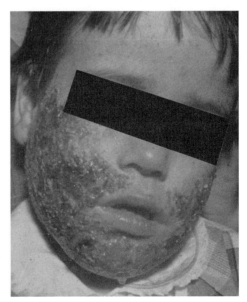

Figure 15–9. This 4-year-old presented with a history of 24 hours of increased itching and thick, crusted scabs overlying his facial eczema. Within 24 hours of starting penicillin G, the eruption had improved dramatically.

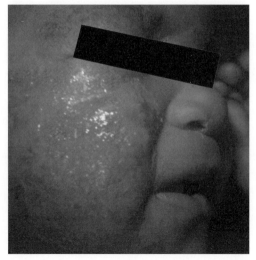

Figure 15–10. A 3-year-old youngster with a history of generalized pruritus for 48 hours prior to his visit. Objectively he had no fever, and the skin revealed no purulence, but only a shiny, "oozy" dermatitis. (Note sparing of the nose, the headlight sign.) This exacerbation of atopic dermatitis was due to the superantigenicity of *S. aureus* and required therapy with both penicillin and prednisone.

coccal impetiginization). Staphylococcal products that can produce inflammation have been identified recently. These products belong to a class of proteins collectively termed superantigens, which activate Th2 cells, releasing large amounts of IL-4 and IL-5, thus exacerbating the AD.

It has been speculated that *Pityrosporon,* a member of the normal skin flora, may act as an environmental allergen and trigger to aggravate AD, particularly on the head and neck. This organism is lipophilic and is found predominantly on greasy, oily skin of teenagers and seborrheic individuals. The possible etiologic role is supported by the therapeutic effectiveness of ketoconazole in some patients.

Candida albicans is another organism frequently cultured from atopic and nonatopic skin; some investigators suspect it plays a role in AD, but others doubt it. Dermatophytes, the cause of ringworm and athletes foot, have been found to be more common among all atopic patients. This finding is attributed to the lower Th1 cell population in atopic patients; it is the Th1 cell that protects against viral and fungal infections. There is no evidence that dermatophytes can act as a triggering factor for the aggravation of AD, but a fungal culture is certainly warranted in atopic

patients with recalcitrant hand and foot eczema (see Fig. 15–4).

In general, patients with AD do not have a major deficiency in defending against viral infections; however, some viral infections of the skin can have a dramatic, serious course, such as Kaposi's varicelliform (chicken pox) eruption and Kaposi's herpetiform (herpes simplex) eruption (Fig. 15–11). The question of whether patients with AD are infected more often with herpes simplex virus (HSV) than normal individuals is unanswered. Whenever a herpetic infection is suspected in an atopic individual, it should be confirmed by a Tzanck smear, and then treated aggressively with systemic antiviral medications.

Molluscum contagiosum and human papilloma virus (warts) are common skin infections that mainly infect children. Like the other viral skin infections, the incidence of these infections in patients with atopy, with or without AD, has been reported as greater, the same, and less than in normal individuals; thus, the incidence remains controversial.

NATURAL HISTORY OF ATOPIC DERMATITIS

Approximately 60% of patients develop AD before their first birthday, and another 30%

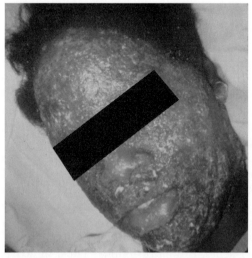

Figure 15–11. Kaposi's herpetiform eruption in a 28-year-old woman with a past history of atopic dermatitis and active eczema of her face and antecubital fossa. Within 48 hours after developing a "fever sore" on her lip, the patient's fever spiked to 104°F and she developed herpetic lesions in every eczematous lesion of her body. The patient died; this episode occurred before acyclovir was available.

have eruptions before age 5 years. There is a correlation between age of onset of AD and its severity. The earlier onset portends a more severe course. The natural course of AD is highly variable. Many cases resolve before age 2, and significant improvement at puberty is common; after the second decade there is a tendency for AD to resolve almost completely. It is unusual to see AD after age 50. Although the eczema may resolve with age, many of the minor features (i.e., xerosis, keratosis pilaris, and so forth) of AD can persist lifelong.

Predicting the course of AD is generally quite difficult. Exacerbations can occur in some patients after many years of remission. Patients with an atopic background have proved to be at a higher risk for developing occupationally induced skin diseases, particularly hand dermatitis. Individuals with atopic dermatitis have a reduced threshold for developing irritant contact dermatitis from soaps, detergents, solvents, and chemical irritants. Exacerbations and remissions can be seen with pregnancy, menses, and menopause.

MANAGEMENT OF ATOPIC DERMATITIS

Control of the pruritus should be the goal of all treatment plans. This control involves the characterization and elimination of as many endogenous and exogenous provocative factors (triggers) as possible. Eliminating the trigger should do away with the need to scratch. Without scratching, the eczema should resolve spontaneously. Some of the identifiable triggers are listed above; these usually can be identified by taking a careful history; occasionally some selective testing may be required. Modalities to help relieve the itch and reduce the inflammatory response are offered to make the patient comfortable until the trigger is no longer activating the inflammatory reaction.

Managing patients with any stage or severity of AD should include consideration of (1) Environmental factors; (2) Personal factors; and (3) Pharmacotherapy.

1. Environmental Factors
   a. Ambient temperature and humidity
   b. Irritant exposure (soaps, wool, cigarette smoke, Playdoh)
   c. Work and/or hobby exposures
   d. Allergen exposure (pets, dust mites, molds, pollens)
2. Personal Factors
   a. Bathing habits
   b. Emotional stress
   c. "Staph" carrier and/or exposure
   d. Viral infections (especially URIs)
   e. Seborrheic propensities (?*Pityrosporon*)
   f. Chronic dermatophytic or candidal infections
   g. Eating habits (?vasodilatory foods)
3. Pharmacotherapy
   a. Topical antipruritics
   b. Topical lubricants
   c. Topical anti-inflammatory drugs
   d. Systemic antipruritics
   e. Systemic immunomodulators

Environmental Considerations

Atopic patients are intolerant to heat, they have difficulty with thermal sweating, and are more apt to experience heat exhaustion. Sweat retention can be a complicating factor of most inflammatory diseases, and patients with atopy have difficulty acclimating to warmer temperatures. Eczema, therefore, is usually localized to the hot, sweaty folds in patients with AD, and exacerbations are noted with exertion and sweating.

Management

1. Modify activities and surroundings to minimize sweating.
2. Do not overdress. Wear loosely fitting, open-weave clothing.
3. Recommend an air-conditioned work and sleep environment (for summer).
4. Recommend use of a humidifier when indoor heat is used (for winter).

It has been well established that patients with AD have a lowered threshold of irritant responsiveness. Identifying and avoiding irritants is integral to successful management of AD. These irritants include soaps, detergents, chemicals, smoke, abrasives, and tight clothing. In the patient with atopy, xerotic, fissured skin results in an impaired barrier function, permitting access of many external agents, which can act as allergens, or irritants. Identifying all the irritants in a patient's environment often requires careful, time-consuming detective work but can be most rewarding.

Atopic patients who are apt to develop irritant contact dermatitis from job-related exposure should be advised to avoid such employment. Homemakers, food handlers, and bartenders are constantly in contact with water and juices from fresh fruits, meats, and vegetables (especially onions and garlic), each of which can perpetuate eczema on the hand. Wearing loosely fitting rubber gloves for less than 3 minutes at a time may be helpful, but the occlusion resulting from longer periods of use can be very harmful. Young people with atopy who are contemplating a career in any field (especially cosmetology) should be appropriately apprised of the occupational hazards.

Health care workers with atopy often develop intractable hand dermatitis; it is essential that they avoid contact with all the above-mentioned irritants. Their daily use of latex gloves predisposes them to the risk of developing IgE-mediated latex reactions. These reactions are triggered by aerosolized latex, not from contact, and they have been the cause of several anaphylactic fatalities. Unfortunately, barrier creams have been inconsistently effective.

Management

1. Identify all irritants in patients' home and work environments.
2. Offer substitutes for all irritants in patients' environment.
3. Counsel young atopic patients regarding potential occupational hazards.
4. Try barrier creams (e.g., Derma-Shield).
5. Discuss all latex precautions pertaining to atopy.
6. Update changes in work conditions.

Allergen avoidance is especially recommended for those patients with proven allergen-induced AD. More than 80% of youngsters with AD go on to develop respiratory allergies, so allergen avoidance should be instituted during infancy, not to prevent, but to postpone the allergen-triggered respiratory symptoms. Dust mites, which are found on all fomites, are reported to be the most common indoor allergen causing perennial respiratory allergy; the cockroach is the most common indoor allergen in inner-city homes. Dust mites can act both as a contact irritant and as a contact allergen, especially in patients whose eczema is most persistent on the face, head, neck, and extremities.

Fifty percent of homes have been reported to have a cat. Animal dander and saliva can be both an allergen and an irritant. There are no nonallergic breeds of cats or dogs. It takes approximately 3 months to rid the dander from an indoor environment after removal of the pet.

There is a small percentage of patients with AD who experience seasonal exacerbations to pollens (e.g., in the northeast USA during tree season in April and May; grasses in May and June; and ragweed in mid August until the first frost). Ragweed can act both as a contact and an inhalant allergen, whereas grasses and trees are inhalant allergens.

Management

1. Dust mite–free environments should be strongly encouraged. Provide patient with manufacturers (e.g., Allergy Control Products, Danbury, CT) who can provide them with a complete list of products available to significantly reduce the mite count.
2. Atopic patients should not have any "hairy" pet in the home. Since it is virtually impossible to get rid of pets once they are in a home, emphasize the importance of avoiding all exposure *before* a child becomes allergic.
3. Pollen-sensitive individuals should be instructed to sleep with closed windows and to drive in cars with closed "vents" during pollen seasons.

Personal Considerations

Bathing habits are mandated by one's family, and society. No other national population bathes as much as Americans. Bathing in the United States is more ritualistic than truly purposeful. Although this frequent bathing can be well tolerated by individuals with normal skin, it can be harmful to those with abnormal skin. Preventing dehydration of atopic skin remains a basic principle of management. Bathing, especially with soaps and cleansers, is a very effective way to remove moisture and protective skin oils that are present on the skin. The use of mild soaps or detergent bars and a reduction in the number of washings per day will minimize the drying effects of washing. Recent studies continue to show that Dove soap is the least irritating among 18 soaps and detergent bars tested. The author, however, strongly recommends that no soap or cleansers be used on eczematous skin; even the mildest soap will be irritating to irritated skin. Bath oils, bath salts, or any bath preparation (i.e., Burow's soaks) have little to no benefit. Bathing in a chlorinated pool can be beneficial, but the patient must rinse off the chlorine immediately and apply a lubricant while the skin is still moist. Rubbing the skin dry can initiate the itch–scratch cycle; affected patients must gently pat their skin dry.

Bathing does create a paradox, because soaking in tepid water for 20 to 30 minutes can hydrate the epidermis, especially if an effective moisturizer is applied to the skin surface within 3 minutes (to prevent evaporation). Petrolatum is the gold standard moisturizer and its use should always be encouraged. Alternatives include Crisco, Elta, Aquaphor, and Albolene. These moisturizers should be used frequently and they should be applied to the entire skin, especially in dry winter weather. Unfortunately, there is no miracle lubricant, and patient acceptance is most important for greatest compliance. Fashionable ingredients (such as aloe, vitamin E, and so forth) have not proved to be any better than their vehicle. The bath is important in providing a 10-fold better penetration of topically applied corticosteroids (see subsequent discussion).

Management

1. Recommend short, not hot, showers; or 20- to 30-minute soaking, tepid baths
2. No soap to eczematous skin; mild soaps may be used sparingly to intertriginous areas.
3. Pat dry; do not rub skin dry.
4. Apply an unscented lubricant, especially vaseline, to the entire skin, within 3 minutes of bathing.

Emotional stress has been identified as a common initiator of itch. (The itch is probably caused by the release of neuropeptides, which can induce vasodilatation, erythema, and an increase in skin temperature.) Patients with AD can have significant problems with anxiety, anger, and hostility. Although these emotional factors do not cause AD, they often trigger an exacerbation. Oftentimes, scratching is associated with significant secondary gain, or persists as a result of habit.

It was recently recognized that "because they wake up often, children with AD often sleep in their parents' bed. This and their constant scratching can lead to a no-sleep, no-sex syndrome for parents." This pattern can contribute to an unconscious rejection of the child with AD by an ambivalent and hostile parent, resulting in excessive and inappropriate indulgence by the parent, leading to the child's uncontrolled, demanding behavior, which further distorts the parent–child relationship. The impact of AD on a child can be quite significant and can manifest as problems with social interaction and low self-esteem. Patients who display self-serving, intentional noncompliance, or missing school or work that is not warranted by skin changes should prompt one to consider recommending more aggressive psychiatric assistance. Psychopharmacologic agents, such as doxepin, or fluoxetine have been useful.

It has been shown that when "any" psychological support is part of the management of patients with moderately severe to severe AD, greater improvement is noted in the skin condition when compared with comparable patients treated solely with dermatologic or standard medical care. This psychological support, for both the patient and family, may be provided by the primary care physician or the office nurse.

Psychological evaluation should be considered in patients who have difficulty with emotional triggers or psychological problems that contribute to difficulty in managing their AD. It may be especially useful in adolescents and young adults who may consider their skin disease disfiguring.

Management

1. Provide psychological support for patient and family.
2. Alleviate guilt with patient education.

Remind those involved of the pathogenesis and natural history of AD.

3. Refer for psychiatric support should inappropriate behavior be noted.

Being a carrier of *Staphylococcus* and/or being exposed, as noted previously, influences disease activity. A very effective and simple way to control the staph carrier condition is to apply mupirocin (Bactroban) cream to the external nares of the patient and all the household members, twice a day for 5 consecutive days a month. Antibacterial soaps and cleanser have been of little value prophylactically.

Infections with *Staphylococcus aureus* are frequent causes of exacerbations of AD. Oral antibiotics are often indicated at the initial visit for treatment of acute dermatitis or for flare-ups. The antibiotics of choice are the penicillinase-resistant penicillins such as dicloxacillin or the oral cephalosporins. For those patients with penicillin sensitivity, erythromycin is an alternative, although approximately 20% of *S. aureus* strains are resistant to this drug. Other drugs to consider are the newer quinolones, such as ciprofloxin.

Management

1. Recommend intranasal mupirocin b.i.d. to all household members of children with AD (especially if family member works in the health-related field).
2. Take a culture from the eczema, then use appropriate doses of dicloxacillin or other antibiotics for at least 10 days for any acutely flaring eczema.
3. Use appropriate alternative drugs if patient is allergic to penicillin.

It is well accepted that viral respiratory infections can precipitate asthma and allergic rhinitis. There is some disagreement as to the role of upper respiratory infections in causing exacerbations of AD. Several reports describe a definite increase of upper respiratory infections in children with a past or present history of AD, particularly in those with severe disease; however, another report did not confirm those results. The importance of the association is useful in identifying a cause for sporadic exacerbations. It is recommended that patients be questioned about symptoms of viral respiratory infections that occurred before each flare-up of their eczema.

Pharmacotherapy

Treatment regimens for AD have included the entire gamut of standard and alternative medical care, such as psychoanalysis, hypnosis, and behavior modification. Unfortunately, none of the modalities has proved to be a panacea. At best, proselytized cures, when evaluated scientifically, prove to be no better than a placebo.

Topical corticosteroids, because of their anti-inflammatory actions, are the mainstay of treatment of all eczematous lesions and should be used in conjunction with emollients that promote hydration of the skin. Their proper use must be emphasized to avoid potential side-effects. Potent fluorinated corticosteroids should be avoided, especially on the face, the genital skin, and all intertriginous areas. It may be medicolegally prudent for primary care physicians to restrict topical corticosteroid use to 1 to 2½% hydrocortisone preparations, or continue the preparation recommended by an AD specialist. Patients who do not respond to the above mentioned recommendations plus a low potency corticosteroid should be evaluated by an AD specialist. As a general rule, the lowest potency topical corticosteroid that is effective should be used; however, using a topical corticosteroid that is too low in potency may result in persistent or worsening AD.

There are seven classes of topical steroids, ranked according to their potency based on vasoconstrictor assays. Topical corticosteroids are safe when used judiciously. The more potent the corticosteroid, the greater the potential for side-effects, both localized and systemic, such as adrenal suppression. In general, topical ointments have a greater potential to penetrate the skin and, therefore, for systemic absorption when compared with topical creams. Creams and lotions are easier to spread and more cosmetically acceptable by patients, but they may be less effective and can contribute to xerosis. Solutions can be used on the scalp or intertriginous areas. Thinner skin, such as in the genital area, the eyelids, and intertriginous skin, especially in the acute phase of the dermatitis, has great potential for penetration, and for this reason corticosteroids should be applied sparingly to these areas. The maximal effect from topical steroids occurs when the skin is hydrated; whether the dermatitis is localized or generalized, the steroids are best applied immediately after bathing. Local side-effects include the development of striae and atrophy of the skin, perioral dermatitis, rosacea, and steroid acne. Systemic side-effects are related to the potency of the topical steroid, the site of application, the total area of skin treated, the occlusiveness of the preparation, and the length of use. Although it is uncommon, it is possible for prolonged use of topical steroids to cause adrenal suppression, and the risk of these side-effects is greater in small children and infants. It is useful, therefore, to see the patient within a week of clearance of the eczema with topical corticosteroid use to re-evaluate therapy and maintain control without corticosteroids.

Topical corticosteroids should be economical, and prescriptions should provide adequate amounts for treating the full course of inflammation. Most flares occur when supplies are exhausted. Application of topical corticosteroids more than twice a day increases the chance of side-effects, makes the therapy more costly, and usually does not increase efficacy. Patients often require use of several strengths at once—a higher potency corticosteroid for resistant areas and a lower potency one for well-controlled areas. As the dermatitis improves (e.g., after 3 to 7 days), the frequency of use may be decreased or a less potent topical preparation can be substituted. When the inflammatory process resolves, within 10 to 14 days of beginning therapy, the topical corticosteroid can be discontinued, but hydration and moisturizer therapy should continue. Applying an emollient immediately before or over a topical corticosteroid preparation may decrease the effectiveness of the topical corticosteroid.

Coal tar preparations may offer an antipruritic effect on the skin. Prior to the availability of topical steroids, crude coal tar extracts were used to reduce inflammation. Although the anti-inflammatory properties of tars are not as pronounced as those of topical corticosteroids, they are cytostatic (inhibit lichenification), their effects are longer lasting, and the side-effects are fewer. Tar preparations are still used to reduce topical corticosteroid use during maintenance therapy of AD.

Newer coal tar products (Estar gel, Tar Doak Lotion) are better tolerated with respect to odor and staining of clothing. It is recommended that a moisturizer be applied over the tar preparation to decrease the drying effect on the skin. Tar preparations are best used at bedtime and washed off in the morning, or used in the bath (Zetar Emulsion, 2 capfuls per 8 inches of bath water). Tar preparations should not be used on acutely inflamed skin, because this may result in further skin irritation. Tar shampoos (T/Gel, Pentrax Gold) are often beneficial for scalp involvement. Side-effects associated with tars include inflammation of hair follicles (folliculitis) and photosensitivity.

Topical antipruritic agents can offer some temporary symptom relief in some patients with AD. Cold compresses are most effective for acute episodes of pruritus. It is also helpful to suggest this treatment in place of scratching. Itching seems to be worst when the patient is not distracted, so patients should be strongly advised to place a cold compress next to them when they watch television, or do their homework, or as they fall asleep. Topical anesthetics, which are very commonly used as over-the-counter antipruritic agents should be avoided on inflamed skin because they are ineffective if applied to an intact epidermis and although they can be possibly useful on inflamed skin, the more effective drugs (e.g., benzocaine) are potential potent sensitizers. Topical antihistamine (Benadryl) has been used for its mild local anesthetic effect, but it too becomes a sensitizer when applied to a disrupted epidermis, and should be avoided.

Pramoxine is an active ether-like topical anesthetic that may be of value for relieving the itch of some cutaneous lesions. It is less sensitizing than the topical anesthetics and antihistamines, and its duration of action is 2 to 4 hours. It is available as a lotion or a cream with 1% or 2½% hydrocortisone (Pramosone).

Doxepin, a most effective systemic H1- and H2-antagonist, has been available as a topical preparation (Zonalon); it is promoted for its antihistaminic, antipruritic effect. Favorable clinical results have been inconsistent, and when applied to large areas of abnormal skin sedating amounts of the drug may be absorbed. More importantly, there have been several reports of up to 13% of patients who use this preparation becoming contact sensitized.

The role for anti-infective agents is discussed previously. Neomycin is such a potent contact sensitizer that its use should be discouraged on any abnormal skin. Most of the old combination Neo-corticosteroid preparations are no longer available, but patients can obtain over-the-counter antibiotic preparations and self-medicate, which can result in sensitization to the antimicrobial agent. It has been well documented that nondermatologists prescribe more of the expensive combination corticosteroid/anti-infective products for all skin conditions than dermatologists. It is known that for fungal skin infections a combination corticosteroid/antifungal preparation is less effective than monotherapy and may even exacerbate the disease.

Systemic antibiotics for *staphylococcus* should be considered whenever the patient with AD experiences an unexplainable exacerbation of their eczema. Staph can be more readily suspected when the patient presents with draining, purulent scabs, but when the same organism acts as a superantigen, it frequently presents only as generalized severe itching. Pus is not seen, and occasionally only a serous sticky exudate can be identified. The increasing incidence of resistance to erythromycin and oxacillin suggests that 10 days of oral dicloxacillin or cephalosporins (e.g., cephalexin) may be the most practical first-line therapy.

Oral antihistamines have been prescribed for patients with itch for years, yet there is little evidence that all itches are caused by histamine. Researchers who continue to study the itch of AD consistently conclude that the beneficial effects of systemic antihistamines in pruritic dermatoses other than urticaria are only marginal. Nonsedating antihistamines and anxiolytics may offer some symptomatic relief, probably through the placebo effect. The reputation of diphenhydramine (Benadryl) and hydroxyzine (Atarax) as relieving itch is believed to be related to their sedative effects.

The tricyclic antidepressant doxepin is both a very effective H1- and H2-receptor antagonist and can be quite sedating. Whenever nocturnal pruritus is severe, short-term use of doxepin (50 mg hs [weight-dependent]) to induce sleep may be warranted.

Systemic corticosteroids should be reserved as the effective rescue drug. The author recommends the exclusive use of prednisone (0.5–1.0 mg/kg/d) for that purpose. Improvement should be noted within 48 hours, and with the concomitant identification and removal of the trigger, and re-institution of routine topical care, it can be discontinued in 4 to 5 days without the need to wean. Systemic prednisone may be used for short periods, in selected severe cases, to bring patients with poorly controlled disease under better control. The primary care physician should contact the AD specialist before prescribing this effective immunomodulator. Should the patient seem to require prednisone more than once or twice a year, phototherapy (psoralen + UVA, or UVB light) should be considered. This therapy requires the expertise of a physician familiar with the administration of light therapy.

A short course of cyclosporin A (3–5 mg/kg/d) has proved to be as effective as prednisone, but should be reserved for patients who cannot tolerate prednisone, and then should be administered by a physician familiar with the use of this drug. A most exciting, related drug, tacrilimus—which is applied topically, is more effective than cyclosporine, and has virtually no side-effects—is in the final stages of clinical trials and may be available by mid-2000.

Unlike allergic rhinitis and extrinsic asthma, immunotherapy (allergy shots) with aeroallergens has not proved to be efficacious in the treatment of AD.

When to Refer a Patient to a Specialist

Cooperation between the patient and/or the patients' representatives, the primary care physician, and the AD specialist is important in the implementation of strategies for the care of patients with chronic AD. The primary care physician plays an important role in the routine care of patients with uncomplicated AD. Consultation with a specialist (dermatologist or allergist) is warranted for patients with mildly severe to severe AD who have significant dysfunction as a result of their skin disease. Not all dermatologists or allergists are comfortable managing complicated cases of AD; thus, finding a physician who can educate the patient regarding the many triggers of pruritus, and who can emphasize the importance and method of continuous skin care (bathing, hydration, and so forth), is an important consideration. Routine use of allergy testing will be most often disappointing, but can be rewarding for selected patients. Access to phototherapy may be another consideration for the management of the patient with severe AD. Biopsy specimens must be taken when the diagnosis is in doubt.

Patient Education

To achieve effective control of a patient's AD, it is essential to educate the patient and family members about the disease, exacerbating factors, and appropriate treatment options. The physician needs to provide written information that includes both detailed skin care recommendations as well as general disease information. Without written instructions, most patients or parents will forget or confuse the skin care recommendations given them. Patients should be educated on how to monitor their skin disease and know how to respond to changes in their status.

The treatment plan should be reviewed during follow-up visits, and the patient or parents should demonstrate an appropriate level of understanding to ensure a good outcome. Patient support organizations that provide updates on progress in AD research are important resources for these patients. Educational pamphlets and videos may be obtained from the Eczema Association for Science and Education (1221 SW Yamhill, Suite 303, Portland, OR 97205; [503] 228–4430), a national nonprofit, patient-oriented organization.

Suggested Reading

Hagermark O, Wahlgren CF: Itch in atopic dermatitis: The role of histamine and other mediators and failure of antihistamine therapy. Dermatol Therapy 1:75–82, 1996

Hanifin JM: Atopic dermatitis in infants and children. Pediatr Clin North Am 38:763–789, 1991

Leung DYM: Atopic Dermatitis: From Pathogenesis to Treatment. Austin, RG Landes Company, 1996

Morren MA, Przybilla B, Bamelis M, et al: Atopic dermatitis: Triggering factors. J Am Acad Dermatol 31:467–473, 1994

Ring J, Darsow U, Abeck D: The atopy patch test as a method of studying aeroallergens as triggering factors of atopic eczema. Dermatol Therapy 1:51–60, 1996

Romagnani S, DelPrete GF, Maggi E, Ricci M: Th1 and Th2 cells and their role in diseases. Allergy Clin Immunol 5:19–22, 1993

Rothe MJ, Grant-Kels JM: Atopic dermatitis: An update. J Am Acad Dermatol 35:1–13, 1996

Wuthrich B: Epidemiology and natural history of atopic dermatitis. Allergy Clin Immunol Int 8:77–82, 1996

Chapter 16

Urticaria and Angioedema

Mary V. Lasley, Michael S. Kennedy, and Leonard C. Altman

Urticaria and angioedema are very common conditions affecting up to 20% of the general population at some point during their lifetime. Urticaria, commonly called hives or welts, is characterized by pruritic, raised, erythematous lesions with pale centers. The lesions vary in size and can occur at any location on the body. Typically, urticaria arises suddenly and may leave quickly in 1 to 2 hours, or can last for as long as 24 hours. A similar process in the deeper dermis or subcutaneous tissue that has swelling as the predominant manifestation is called angioedema. Generally, angioedema is not pruritic, may be mildly painful, and lasts longer than 24 hours. In rare cases, it may become life threatening when swelling affects the upper airway. In half of the patients, urticaria and angioedema occur together, whereas urticaria occurs alone in 40% and angioedema alone in 10%. Urticaria and angioedema are best considered as symptoms because they may have a variety of causes.

Urticaria and angioedema are usually divided into two categories: acute and chronic. By definition, acute urticaria and angioedema are present for less than 6 weeks, whereas chronic urticaria and angioedema are episodes that have lasted for a longer period. Acute urticaria and angioedema are more common in children and young adults; chronic urticaria and angioedema are more common in adults, especially women. Contrary to common opinion, atopic patients, namely those with a family or personal history of asthma, allergic rhinitis, or atopic dermatitis, do not have an increased incidence of urticaria.

PATHOPHYSIOLOGY

Urticaria occurs in response to the release of inflammatory mediators from cutaneous mast cells. These inflammatory substances include histamine, leukotrienes, prostaglandins, platelet activating factor, and chemotactic factors for eosinophils and neutrophils. Release of these mediators results in vasodilatation, increased vascular leakage, and pruritus. Basophils from the circulatory system also can localize in tissue and release mediators analogous to those in mast cells. Patients with urticaria have elevated histamine content in their skin that is more releasable.

A variety of stimuli can trigger mast cells and basophils to release their chemical mediators. Typically, mast cell degranulation results when cross-linking of the membrane-bound IgE occurs. It is important to recognize, however, that not all histamine release is IgE mediated. Immunologic, nonimmunologic, physical, and chemical stimuli can produce degranulation of mast cells and basophils. For example, it is well known that C3a and C5a are anaphylatoxins that can cause histamine release in a nonIgE-mediated reaction. Anaphylatoxins are generated in serum sickness, which occurs in reactions to blood transfusions and in infectious, neoplastic, and rheumatic diseases. In addition, mast cell degranulation can occur from a direct pharmacologic effect or through physical or mechanical activation. Urticaria after exposure to opiate medications and dermatographism are examples.

ACUTE URTICARIA

By definition, acute urticaria and angioedema are hives and diffuse swelling that last less than 6 weeks. Often, the patient's history will be quite helpful in eliciting the cause of this acute reaction (Table 16–1). Allergy is a common cause of acute urticarial reactions but rarely a cause of chronic urticaria.

Foods and Food Additives

It is well recognized by both physicians and patients that foods are a common cause of urticaria. In children, the most common offenders include milk, egg, soy, wheat, peanut, and tree nuts, whereas in adults the most common foods include peanut, tree nuts, shellfish, and fish. Case reports are found in the literature describing a variety of foods as the offending agent. In situations of food-induced urticaria or angioedema, the onset of symptoms begins within minutes to a few hours after the food ingestion, and only small quantities of the food will induce the reaction. Food additives such as sulfites, vegetable gums, and food colors also have been implicated as a cause of urticaria; however, double-blind placebo-controlled challenges with food additives rarely substantiate these as a cause.

Urticaria and angioedema also can result from nonIgE-mediated food reactions. Strawberries contain a histamine-releasing substance that can result in urticaria. Other foods that are thought to induce a nonIgE-mediated urticarial reaction include tomatoes, shellfish, oranges, and alcohol. In contrast to IgE-mediated food reactions, these occur after ingestion of large quantities of food, sometimes called gluttony urticaria.

Medication

Numerous medications can cause urticaria and angioedema by various mechanisms (see Chapter 20). Penicillins, cephalosporins, and sulfa-based medications are most often implicated in type I, or IgE-mediated urticarial reactions.

Type II reactions, which are the result of cytotoxic antibodies and complement activation, also can induce urticaria. Captopril, rifampin, D-penicillamine, and blood transfusions have been involved. Often, the cause is obvious and symptoms are self-limited.

Type III or immune complex reactions also can be a cause of acute urticaria and angioedema. Classic serum sickness can occur and cause urticaria and angioedema approximately 7 to 10 days into a course of antibiotic therapy. In addition to urticaria and angioedema, serum sickness is associated with fever, lymph node enlargement, and proteinuria. Urticaria presenting in this setting may persist for several weeks. The drug cefaclor is noteworthy for producing serum sickness-like adverse reactions in up to 0.5% of patients.

Mast cell degranulation can occur when certain drugs directly cause mediator release without IgE or any immunologic involvement. The medications most commonly involved include codeine and other opiates, dextran, radiocontrast media, and nonsteroidal anti-inflammatory agents (i.e., aspirin, ibuprofen). In patients with chronic urticaria and angioedema, aspirin may cause exacerbations in 20% to 40% of those affected. Nonsteroidal anti-inflammatory agents may produce urticaria and angioedema by shunting arachidonic acid from the prostaglandin pathway to the lipoxygenase pathway. This shift results in the generation of leukotrienes, which can stimulate mast cells to degranulate.

Medications may be blamed for causing

Table 16–1. **Causes of Acute Urticaria**

Cause	Examples
Foods	Egg milk, wheat, peanut, tree nuts, soy, shellfish, fish
Medications	Suspect all medications, even over-the-counter or homeopathic ones
Insect stings	*Hymenoptera*
	Papular urticaria
Infections	Bacterial—Streptococcal pharyngitis, *Mycoplasma*
	Viral—Hepatitis B, mononucleosis, Coxsackie A & B
	Parasitic—*Ascaris, Ancylostoma, Echinococcus, Fasciola, Filaria, Schistosoma, Strongyloides, Toxocara, Trichinella*
	Fungal?—Dermatophytes, *Candida*
Contact allergy	Latex, pollen
Idiopathic	About 50% of cases

urticaria and angioedema when, in fact, it is the underlying illness rather than the medication that is responsible. This is particularly true in the case of infectious illnesses being treated with antibiotics.

Insect Stings

The most common manifestation of a stinging insect anaphylactic reaction is urticaria and angioedema. The hymenoptera stinging insects include yellow jackets, wasps, hornets, honeybees, and fire ants. The urticaria can be localized or systemic, and the mechanism can be IgE-mediated or immune complex-induced. This subject is discussed in detail in Chapter 21. Papular urticaria is a pruritic eruption that occurs as a delayed hypersensitivity reaction to insect bites. This reaction is commonly seen in children on their extremities and is caused by the bites of fleas, lice, mites, or mosquitoes. Typically, papular urticaria is more persistent than ordinary hives.

Inhalants

Occasionally, urticaria and angioedema may be caused by inhalant allergens. These reactions are nearly always accompanied by upper or lower respiratory tract symptoms, for example, a patient who develops wheezing and urticaria after exposure to a cat. Infrequently, some patients with seasonal hay fever will develop seasonal urticaria. Some patients who are highly allergic to grass pollen develop urticaria from contact with grass.

Infection

Infections also can be a cause of urticaria. In children, viral infections are a frequent cause of acute urticaria. Any infectious agent (viral, bacterial, fungal, or parasitic) can serve as an antigen that forms immune complexes, leading to complement activation. It is well known that urticaria may develop in the preicteric phase of hepatitis B and in the early stages of mononucleosis. There have been reports associating urticaria with herpes infection, coxsackie A and B viral illnesses, mycoplasma in-

fections, and streptococcal pharyngitis. Treatment or resolution of the infectious disease process often results in clearing of the urticaria.

Contact Urticaria

Contact urticaria is elicited after an antigen comes in contact with the skin. A person who is extremely allergic to pets may develop hives where they were licked by the animal. Recently, there have been reports identifying contact with latex as a cause of urticaria and angioedema. In latex sensitization of health care workers, many patients demonstrate contact urticaria before manifesting other systemic reactions to latex. A more thorough discussion of latex allergy is found in Chapter 22. As for nonimmunologic reactions that cause contact urticaria, many substances in the workplace and home have been identified as causative agents. This specialized area is covered in detail in the text *Contact Dermatitis* by Alexander Fisher.

CHRONIC URTICARIA AND ANGIOEDEMA

Chronic urticaria and angioedema are characterized by persistence of symptoms beyond 6 weeks. Some patients may have daily symptoms of hives and swelling, whereas others will have recurrent episodes (Table 16–2).

Chronic Idiopathic Urticaria

Chronic idiopathic urticaria accounts for 75% to 90% of all chronic urticaria cases and should be considered a diagnosis of exclusion (Fig. 16–1). Although both the patient and physician want to demonstrate a cause, these are patients in whom a careful history, physical examination, and laboratory evaluation fail to determine an etiology. Nonetheless, it is necessary to perform these procedures to determine if other medical conditions are a potential cause for this chronic symptom. For many patients, their symptoms will abate within 6 months. Nearly 50% will have persistence of

Table 16–2. **Causes of Chronic Urticaria**

Cause	Examples
Idiopathic	75–90% of cases
Physical	Dermatographism
	Cholinergic urticaria
	Cold urticaria
	Delayed pressure urticaria
	Solar urticaria
	Vibratory urticaria
	Aquagenic urticaria
Autoimmune	Rheumatologic
	Thyroid
	IgG antibody to IgE and IgE receptor
Malignancies	Lymphoproliferative disorders
	Neoplasms
Angioedema	Hereditary
	Acquired
	Angiotensin-converting enzyme inhibitors

urticaria beyond 6 months, and one-fifth of these patients will have symptoms lasting longer than 10 years.

Physical Urticaria and Angioedema

Physical urticaria and angioedema are characterized by environmental factors that trigger these reactions. The most common physical urticaria is dermatographism, which affects 2% to 5% of the general population. Dermatographism means "writing on the skin," and it is easy to diagnose if one firmly scratches the skin with a blunt point such as the wooden tip of a cotton swab or tongue depressor. It is characterized by an urticarial reaction local-

ized to the site of skin trauma. It has been suggested that trauma induces an IgE-mediated reaction causing histamine to be released from mast cells.

Cholinergic urticaria is characterized by the appearance of 1- to 3-mm wheals surrounded by large erythematous flares after an increase in core body temperature, commonly seen in young adults. Lesions may develop during strenuous exercise, after a hot bath, or following emotional stress (Fig. 16–2). Severe reactions that progress to exercise-induced anaphylaxis have been reported, although rarely.

Urticaria also occurs with exposure to cold. Urticaria may develop within minutes on areas directly exposed to cold or on rewarming of the affected parts (Fig. 16–3). Ingestion of cold drinks may result in lip swelling. Cold urticaria syndromes can be categorized into acquired and familial disorders. Severe reactions that result in death can occur with swimming or diving into cold water. It is imperative that patients avoid total body exposure to cold to prevent life-threatening reactions.

Delayed pressure urticaria is manifested by deep, painful swelling approximately 4 to 6 hours after pressure is applied to the skin. The palms, soles, and buttocks are most often involved. Other symptoms may develop during attacks including malaise, fever, chills, arthralgias, headache, and leukocytosis. Unlike most urticarias, this disease does not respond to antihistamines; instead, patients may require treatment with prednisone.

Less common types of physical urticaria include solar, vibratory, and aquagenic.

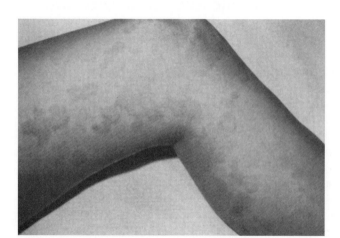

Figure 16–1. Typical rounded, slightly indurated lesions of chronic urticaria demonstrating variability in size and shape. (From Kaplan AP: Urticaria and angioedema. *In* Kaplan AP [ed]: Allergy, 2nd ed. Philadelphia, WB Saunders, 1997, p 585.)

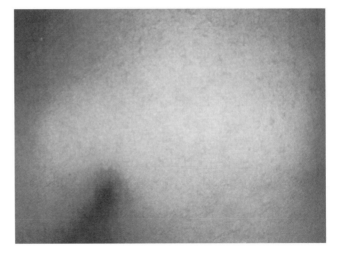

Figure 16–2. Urticarial lesions induced in a patient with cholinergic urticaria by running in place for 10 minutes. (From Kaplan AP: Urticaria and angioedema. *In* Kaplan AP [ed]: Allergy, 2nd ed. Philadelphia, WB Saunders, 1997, p 578.)

Autoimmune Disease

Autoimmune diseases have been associated with urticaria and angioedema. For some patients, the skin findings will precede other symptoms by months. The connective tissue diseases that have been associated with chronic urticaria and angioedema are systemic lupus erythematosus, Sjögren's syndrome, polymyositis, and various forms of leukocytoclastic vasculitis.

Approximately 15 years ago, researchers reported the association of chronic urticaria and angioedema with thyroid autoimmunity. In fact, patients may express an elevation of thyroid antibodies (antimicrosomal or antithyroglobulin antibodies or both) with or without an actual deficiency in thyroid hormone. It appears that the thyroid antibodies serve as an indicator of autoimmunity rather than being responsible for the urticarial lesions themselves.

Another autoimmune disorder that causes urticaria has been identified in patients who develop anti-IgG antibodies directed against IgE or the α subunit of the IgE receptor ($Fc_\epsilon R1\alpha$) (Fig. 16–4). These antibodies trigger mast cells and basophils to degranulate. Skin testing with autologous serum elicits a wheal-and-flare response and mast cell degranulation. It is not known why these autoantibodies develop in some patients.

Malignancies

Neoplastic disease also has been linked to urticaria and angioedema. For adult patients, urticaria and angioedema have been reported in association with lymphoma; leukemia; my-

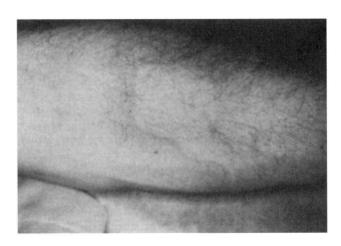

Figure 16–3. Positive ice cube test in a patient with cold urticaria demonstrating a wheal the shape of the cube and a track where ice water had dripped along the arm. (From Kaplan AP: Urticaria and angioedema. *In* Kaplan AP [ed]: Allergy, 2nd ed. Philadelphia, WB Saunders, 1997, p 575.)

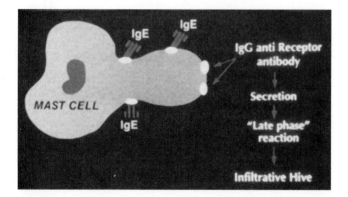

Figure 16–4. A possible mechanism of hive formation in a third of patients with chronic urticaria who also have circulating IgG antibody to the α subunit of the IgE receptor (Fc$_\epsilon$Rlα). (From Kaplan AP: Urticaria and angioedema. *In* Kaplan AP [ed]: Allergy, 2nd ed. Philadelphia, WB Saunders, 1997, p 586.)

eloma; and malignant tumors of the colon, rectum, liver, lung, ovary, and testicles. In children, rare reports of urticaria and angioedema have been associated with lymphomas. Lymphoma also has been associated with angioedema caused by an acquired deficiency of C1-esterase inhibitor. Affected patients have decreased C1q levels in addition to low C4 and C1 esterase inhibitor levels. Careful medical evaluation and laboratory screening will help to identify malignancies that are causing chronic urticaria.

Hereditary Angioedema

An uncommon but treatable type of angioedema involves the hereditary deficiency of C1-esterase inhibitor. The gene for C1-esterase is inherited as an autosomal dominant trait and it is common for hereditary angioedema (HAE) to display a familial history. Deficiency of this regulatory protein results in complement activation and recurrent mast cell degranulation (Fig. 16–5). There are actually two forms of HAE. Most patients have type I HAE with low levels of C1-esterase inhibitor; whereas approximately 15% have type II HAE with normal levels of a dysfunctional C1-esterase inhibitor protein. Patients with HAE have recurrent, circumscribed edema, typically affecting the extremities and face, brought about by minor tissue trauma such as dental work. As many as 25% of patients affected will die from laryngeal edema. Affected patients rarely have urticaria associated with their angioedema. A low C4 concentration serves as a good initial screening test. During acute attacks, patients may also have reduced levels of C2. Patients with reduced C4 levels should

have quantitative and functional levels of C1-esterase inhibitor measured.

Angioedema can also occur in patients with acquired C1-esterase inhibitor deficiency. As previously discussed, angioedema is found with autoimmune diseases, such as systemic lupus erythematosus or lymphoproliferative disorders.

Angiotensin-converting enzyme inhibitors also cause angioedema, especially in geriatric patients. Medications that have been implicated are benazepril, captopril, enalapril, fosinopril, lisinopril, moexipril, quinapril, ramipril, and trandolapril.

Differential Diagnosis

Typically, the diagnosis of urticaria and angioedema is straightforward. Finding the cause, however, may be more difficult. There are other dermatologic conditions that can mimic urticaria. Erythema multiforme has target-shaped, erythematous, macular, or papular lesions that may look similar to those seen in urticaria. A differentiating feature of erythema multiforme is that the lesions are fixed, last for several days, and do not respond to subcutaneous epinephrine. Other dermatologic diseases that may resemble urticaria and are quite pruritic include dermatitis herpetiformis and bullous pemphigoid. Another condition, mastocytosis, is characterized by mast cell infiltration of various organs, including the skin. Some patients will have skin lesions very similar in appearance to urticaria rather than the classic urticaria pigmentosa. Typically, urticaria pigmentosa appears as hyperpigmented, red-brown macules, which may coalesce. When these lesions are stroked, they will urticate,

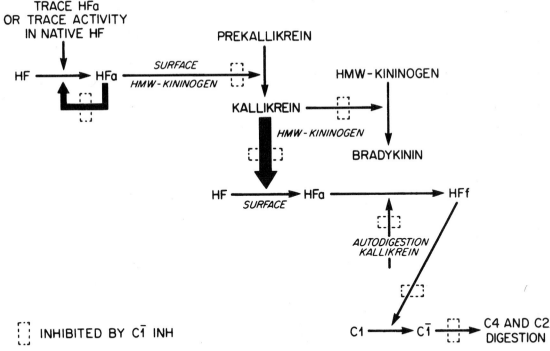

Figure 16–5. Pathway for bradykinin formation and linkage to the complement cascade indicating all steps that are inhibitable by C1 INH. (From Kaplan AP: Urticaria and angioedema. *In* Kaplan AP [ed]: Allergy, 2nd ed. Philadelphia, WB Saunders, 1997, p 584.)

which is called Darier's sign. A rare disorder that should be included in the differential diagnosis of childhood urticaria is Muckle-Wells syndrome. It is an autosomal dominant disorder characterized by episodic urticaria presenting in infancy, with sensorineural deafness, amyloidosis, arthralgias, and skeletal abnormalities. Another rare disease is Schnitzler's syndrome, which is characterized by chronic urticaria and macroglobulinemia. In addition, affected patients will have bone pain, anemia, fever, fatigue, and weight loss. And finally, urticarial vasculitis represents a small vessel vasculitis with histologic features of leukocytoclasis. The main distinguishing features of urticarial vasculitis are that the lesions last longer than 24 hours, may be tender, and leave behind skin pigmentation. Skin biopsy is required for definitive diagnosis.

DIAGNOSIS

For the patient with acute urticaria who is otherwise healthy, a detailed history and physical examination is usually sufficient for an initial evaluation. Perhaps half of the time this evaluation will yield a diagnosis. In the remainder of patients, treatment can be started and the course of the illness observed. Those cases that persist and become chronic usually require additional evaluation.

At this point, most allergists obtain a complete blood count and differential, a chemistry panel including liver function and thyroid function tests, an antinuclear antibody determination, a sedimentation rate, and a urinalysis. These tests are intended to look for a systemic disorder such as hypo- or hyperthyroidism, systemic lupus erythematosus, or vasculitis. If the clinical description or appearance of the urticarial lesions is suggestive of a cutaneous vasculitis, that is, lesions that persist for longer than 24 hours and leave purpura with resolution, then a skin biopsy may be useful (Fig. 16–6). The biopsy specimen should be taken at the edge of the wheal with a histologic examination. Direct immunofluorescence for perivascular deposition of immunoglobins and complement is rarely helpful.

Affected patients also should undergo skin testing with their own serum to look for autoantibodies to the IgE receptor on cutaneous mast cells. Testing is performed and interpre-

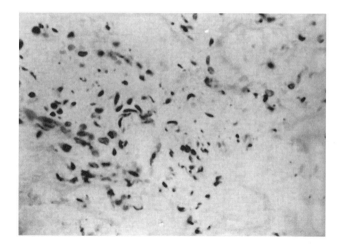

Figure 16–6. Skin biopsy of a patient with leucocytoclastic angiitis demonstrating necrosis of the vessel, neutrophilic infiltration, karyolysis, and nuclear debris. (From Kaplan AP: Urticaria and angioedema. *In* Kaplan AP: Allergy, 2nd ed. Philadelphia, WB Saunders, 1997, p 586.)

ted at 15 minutes as are all immediate skin tests, but sometimes the wheal-and-flare response may be slightly slower to develop, and therefore observation at 60 minutes is suggested. Should the history suggest dermatographism, this can be confirmed by stroking the skin with the wooden edge of a cotton swab, and cold urticaria can be confirmed by application of an ice cube. Other physical urticarias require more complex methods for confirmation and are rare.

If angioedema, especially affecting the face or airway, is predominant, hereditary or acquired C1-esterase deficiency should be strongly considered. The presence of C1-esterase deficiency is evaluated by measuring a C4 titer and the C1-esterase concentration. During an episode of C1-esterase deficiency angioedema these values will usually always be low. Even between attacks, the C4 level is usually low in this disease. A low level of C1-esterase is found in about 80% to 85% of affected patients, but in 15% to 20% the level is normal and the protein is nonfunctional; thus a functional C1-esterase assay is necessary to confirm the diagnosis. If the patient's history suggests cholinergic urticaria, in that the lesions are provoked by exercise, warmth, or heat exposure and are only a few millimeters in diameter with a large surrounding flare, a methacholine skin test can be performed. Intradermal injection of 0.02 ml of methacholine at 10 mg/ml will induce small, characteristic wheals in 30% of patients with a suggestive history.

TREATMENT

Elimination should be the first-choice treatment when appropriate. If a food or medica-tion is clearly identified as a causative or exacerbating factor or a physical stimulus is responsible, this factor should be avoided.

Pharmacologic treatment is usually started with antihistamines. Many first-generation antihistamines are effective for treating urticaria, but performance impairment and sedation are very common. For this reason, first-generation antihistamines are often used at night, and the dose is gradually increased as tolerated. Hydroxyzine (Atarax, Vistaril, Pfizer, Inc.), 50 to 200 mg/day, is a usual first choice; the dose is increased as needed and based on the severity of the symptoms. Hydroxyzine can be administered all at bedtime or in divided doses for patients who are tolerant of the somnolence effect. Diphenhydramine (Benadryl, Warner-Lambert Co.) can be used in a similar fashion except that its shorter duration of action requires repeated doses and it is not as useful if given only at bedtime. Cyproheptadine (Periactin, Merck & Co., Inc.), 4 mg, 4 times per day, can be tried in patients in whom hydroxyzine is not effective or added to hydroxyzine if relief is only partial. Doxepin (Sinequan, Pfizer, Inc.), a tricyclic antidepressant, is also a potent histamine H1 and H2 receptor blocker. It is another agent that is often beneficial, although it is usually quite sedating. It is best administered at bedtime, starting at 10 mg and increasing as needed to a maximum of 150 mg each night. It is perhaps best used in low doses in addition to other agents.

Second-generation, non- or less-sedating antihistamines are generally the first choice treatment for urticaria. Cetirizine (Zyrtec, Pfizer, Inc.) is often the first choice; it is started at 10 mg daily and increased as needed to a maximum of 60 mg per day. The benefit must be weighed against somnolence, as this agent becomes sedating at high doses. Loratidine (Claritin, Schering Corporation) can be used in a similar fashion and is less sedating even at high doses. Both drugs are available in syrup form for children; the starting pediatric dose is 5 mg per day. Fexofenadine (Allegra, Hoechst Marion Roussel), 60 mg, has a shorter half-life and requires twice a day dosing. Astemizole (Hismanal, Janssen Pharmaecutical), 10 mg, is nonsedating and is often very effective for chronic urticaria. However, it has been withdrawn from the market by the US Food & Drug Administration. Its onset of action is slower than that of other second-generation agents, and it may take 5 to 7 days to evaluate its effectiveness. Because of the remote risk of cardiac arrythymia, this drug should not be increased above 10 mg per day and should not be used in patients with cardiac or liver disease or in combination with drugs that inhibit cytochrome P450 liver enzymes, such as erythromycin or ketoconazole.

A small percentage of patients may benefit from histamine H2 receptor antagonists used in addition to H1 blockers. Cimetidine (Tagamet, SmithKline Beecham), 300 mg 4 times a day, or ranitidine (Zantac, Glaxo Wellcome, Inc.), 150 mg twice a day, may be added to an H1 blocker or combination of H1 blockers if they are inadequate alone.

If antihistamines are insufficient and for treatment of severe and extensive urticaria, corticosteroids are necessary and almost always effective. It is generally best to start with a sufficiently high dose to achieve control and then taper. In adults, generally 40 to 60 mg of prednisone or equivalent daily is given as one morning dosage with food. This dose may need to be continued for 5 to 10 days, depending on symptom severity, and tapered over a 2- to 4-week period. The goal is to induce a remission without continuing use of prednisone or at least achieve every-other-day dosing. Rare patients may responsed to prednisolone or methylprednisone and not prednisone.

Other immune modulating agents have been used in situations of resistant urticaria, autoimmune urticaria, or cutaneous vasculitis. Steroid-sparing agents often used in rheumatologic conditions, in particular hydroxychloroquine (Plaquenil, Sanofti) or methotrexate (Immunex), have been found to be of some benefit in a proportion of these patients. Other drugs that have been used with some success include the calcium channel blocker, nifedipine, and the mast cell stabilizer and antihistamine-blocking agent, ketotifen.* There are reports that the immunosuppressant agent cyclosporin and even intravenous immunoglobulin (IVIG) have been used with some success. These modalities require intensive monitoring, and IVIG is very costly; however, in severe, resistant cases, these therapies may be warranted.

Treatment for C1-esterase deficiency angioedema differs from treatment for other forms of angioedema and urticaria. In acute attacks, epinephrine is given subcutaneously or intramuscularly, and intravenous fluids may be needed if hypotension occurs or if the patient cannot eat or drink. If laryngeal edema occurs, a tracheostomy or intubation may be needed. Preventive therapy is generally initiated with attenuated androgens such as stanozolol (Winstrol) or danazol (Danocrine). These agents not only prevent attacks of swelling but also induce synthesis of C1-esterase and cause C4 levels to increase. Second-choice agents for prophylaxis are antifibrinolytic agents such as aminocaproic acid or tranexamic acid.

KEY POINTS

▶ Acute urticaria and angioedema are defined as lasting for 6 weeks or less and have an apparent cause in about 50% of cases.
▶ Chronic urticaria is of longer duration and is usually idiopathic or autoimmune in etiology.
▶ Hidden food or food additive allergies rarely cause chronic urticaria.
▶ Patients with angioedema without urticaria, especially with airway involvement, should be evaluated for C1-esterase deficiency.
▶ Nonsedating antihistamines are the treatment of choice for most cases of urticaria.

Suggested Reading

Beltrani VS: Urticaria and angioedema. Dermatol Clin 14:171–198, 1996

*Not available in the United States.

Champion RH, Roberts SO, Carpenter RG, Roger JH: Urticaria and angioedema: A review of 554 patients. Br J Dermatol 81:588–597, 1969

Charlesworth EN (ed): Urticaria. Immunol Allergy Clin North Am 15:641–821, 1995

Charlesworth EN: Urticaria and angioedema: A clinical spectrum. Ann Allergy Asthma Immunol 76:484–496, 1996

Fisher AA: Contact urticaria. *In* Fisher AA (ed): Contact Dermatitis. Philadelphia, Lea & Febiger, 1986, pp 686–709

Greaves MW: Chronic urticaria. N Engl J Med 332:1767–1772, 1995

Hide M, Francis DM, Grattan CEH, et al: Autoantibodies against the high-affinity IgE receptor as a cause of histamine release in chronic urticaria. N Engl J Med 328:1599–1604, 1993

Kaplan AP: Urticaria and angioedema. *In* Middleton E Jr, Reed CE, Ellis EF, et al (eds): Allergy: Principles and Practice, 5th ed. St. Louis: Mosby-Year Book, pp 1104–1122, 1998

Orfan NA, Kolski GB: Physical urticarias. Ann Allergy 71:205–215, 1993

Ormerod AD: Urticaria: Recognition, causes, and treatment. Drugs 48:717–730, 1994

Chapter 17

Contact Dermatitis

Marshall P. Welch

DEFINITIONS AND PATHOPHYSIOLOGY

Contact dermatitis may be caused by irritants, allergic sensitizers, or a combination of both. The major types of contact dermatitis, irritant contact dermatitis (ICD) and allergic contact dermatitis (ACD), are compared and contrasted nicely by Sherertz and Storrs (Table 17–1). ACD and ICD may be clinically indistinguishable from one another, even when initially confronted by dermatologists with experience in evaluating contact dermatitis. Consequently, this chapter emphasizes common clinical situations that the primary care physician is most likely to encounter in the ambulatory setting, and offers some general practical guidelines for the diagnostic and therapeutic approach. Often it is most time-effective and cost-effective to refer acute cases of contact dermatitis that are refractory to initial treatment, and cases of chronic dermatitis, especially when there is a question of occupational causation or aggravation, to a physician with extensive experience in evaluation and management of these problems.

ICD is a nonallergic reaction that is caused by exposure to substances or physical conditions that irritate the skin. The mechanism of action appears to be by a direct effect on the epidermal keratinocytes and cells in the superficial dermis. At present there is no known specific immune sensitization involved in ICD. Despite this difference between the underlying initiating signals in ICD versus ACD, there is an enlarging body of evidence suggesting that ACD and ICD share many common characteristics in their pathophysiology, including similarities in phenotypes of the inflammatory cells and in the cytokine profiles present in the cutaneous infiltrates.

In general, the skin of any person can eventually react to an irritant if the concentration and duration of contact with the skin are sufficient. However, atopic individuals as a whole appear to have skin that is more susceptible to irritants than the skin of nonatopic individuals. Irritants include mildly irritating substances such as soaps or organic solvents and also strongly irritating substances such as strong acids or alkali. ICD arising after a single exposure to a strong irritant is known as single exposure dermatitis or a chemical burn. In addition, physical conditions such as heat, cold, repeated frictional exposure, or low humidity may result in ICD. Overall, ICD is thought to account for about 80% of cases of contact dermatitis.

Allergic contact dermatitis (ACD) occurs as a result of skin exposure to allergens to which an individual has become sensitized previously. It is a delayed-type (Gell and Coombs type IV) cellular-mediated hypersensitivity. The sequence of sensitization is that a hapten, which is usually a small, lipid-soluble molecule, is able to penetrate the stratum corneum and contact epidermal cells. It then binds to a protein, is taken up by an antigen-presenting cell (APC) such as an epidermal Langerhans cell, is processed into an antigen and presented to precursor T-cells in the context of major histocompatibility complex (MHC) molecules. If the exposed individual possesses populations of T-cells that specifically recognize the antigen, these cells can be stimulated to expand in a clonal fashion. Evidence suggests that at least some of this activity occurs in regional lymph nodes (Fig. 17–1).

241

Table 17–1.   **Generalizations About Contact Dermatitis**

Variables	Irritant	Allergic
Who	Many people	Few people
Where	Localized	Spreads
When	Rapid with strong irritants (minutes to hours); delayed with weak irritants (months)	24 to 72 hours
Job relatedness	Improves with long (3 wks) vacations	May improve even on weekends
Atopy	Predisposes	No known predisposition
Morphology	Erythema, scale, fissures	Vesicles; may be indistinguishable from irritant
Distribution	Hands-90%	Hands-90%
Intermittent & frequent water exposure	May cause and perpetuate	May perpetuate
Immune system	No specific immune response	Type IV (cell-mediated immunity/delayed hypersensitivity)
Histology	Spongiosis or upper epidermal damage, some lymphocytes	Spongiosis with lymphocytic cellular infiltrate; may be indistinguishable from irritant
Chronicity	Often	If diagnosed early, clears; can be chronic
Diagnosis	History and physical examination	History and physical examination; patch testing
Examples	Hair dressers and machinists, chronic hand dermatitis	Poison oak or ivy, nickel, chrome

Adapted from Sheretz E, Storrs FJ: Contact dermatitis. *In* Rosenstock L, Cullen MR (eds): Textbook of Clinical Occupational and Environmental Medicine, Philadelphia, WB Saunders Company, 1994, pp 514–530, with permission.

IRRITANT CONTACT DERMATITIS

Clinical Findings

Exposure to mild irritants to an extent sufficient to produce ICD results in a dermatitis that is characterized by burning, pain, and

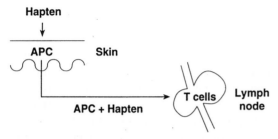

Figure 17–1. Induction phase of cellular-mediated (type IV) delayed contact hypersensitivity. For a chemical to serve as a contact allergen, it must (1) be able to penetrate the stratum corneum, thereby reaching living epidermal cells; (2) interact with and activate antigen-processing cells in skin, and (3) be capable of stimulating proliferation of T cells in an antigen-specific (clonal) manner. (From Cruz Jr PD: Basic mechanisms underlying contact allergy. *In* Guin JD (ed): Practical Contact Dermatitis: A Handbook for the Practitioner. New York, McGraw-Hill, 1995, p 4, used with permission.)

pruritus. On examination, the affected skin is erythematous, dry, scaly, and may either be glazed-appearing and thinned or thickened and fissured secondary to cracking of the stiff skin. In more severe cases there may be vesicles, oozing, and swelling that can be indistinguishable from allergic contact dermatitis.

Diagnosis

The diagnosis of ICD is largely made on clinical grounds, taking into account the history of exposure to irritants, subjective complaints, and physical findings. In cases involving the hands, ICD frequently involves the web spaces, especially if the patient is involved in wet work (Fig. 17–2). A complete skin examination should be done to gather additional diagnostic clues; other diagnostic studies are sometimes warranted as well. These may include potassium hydroxide (KOH) wet mount examinations of scale to rule out dermatophyte infection, and possibly diagnostic testing for latex allergy (see Chapter 22) or patch testing (discussed later in this chapter) to rule out ACD. Biopsy studies are not routinely done, because they are often not helpful unless another der-

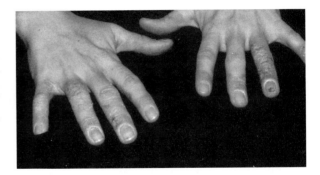

Figure 17–2. Irritant contact dermatitis (ICD) superimposed on atopic hand dermatitis in a machinist. There is predominantly involvement of the dorsal aspects of the fingers, and also web space involvement, typical of ICD. The palms are relatively spared. All patch test results, including a panel of antigens specific for machinists, were negative.

matosis such as psoriasis is in the differential diagnosis.

Treatment and Prevention of ICD

Minimization of contact with the irritant is of utmost importance. Contact reduction often can be accomplished by measures such as wearing gloves or applying thick ointments or creams that serve as barriers to irritants and also help to maintain hydration of the skin.

Measures for the treatment and prevention of hand dermatitis (Table 17–2) are usually also applicable to ICD in general. With these measures alone, mild irritant contact dermatitis often will improve considerably.

For more severe cases with erythema and vesicles, treatment is similar to that for ACD, which is discussed in the next section. Cases of single-exposure ICD (chemical burns) should be treated first with prolonged, vigorous irrigation with water, followed by the appropriate treatment for a burn of that degree.

Table 17–2. **Principles of Treatment of Hand Dermatitis**

- Protect the hands from direct contact with soap, detergent, scouring powder, and similar harsh chemicals by wearing waterproof heavy-duty vinyl gloves, either lined or unlined. It is often beneficial to wear white cotton gloves under the vinyl gloves. The patient should have a sufficient number of white cotton gloves so that they can be washed frequently, and also a sufficient supply of heavy-duty vinyl gloves. Heavy-duty vinyl gloves are preferable to rubber gloves because patients occasionally become allergic to rubber gloves.
- Wear the gloves while cooking with acid foods, e.g., peeling or squeezing lemons, oranges, or grapefruit, peeling potatoes, and handling tomatoes.
- Wear leather or heavy-duty fabric gloves when doing dry work and especially when gardening. Dirty the gloves, not the hands. The patient should place a dozen pairs of cheap cotton gloves strategically about the home for dry housework. When dirty, put in the washing machine. Wash gloves, not hands.
- Dishwashers and automatic clothes washers are musts for people with hand dermatitis.
- Avoid direct contact with household products that contain irritating solvents, e.g., turpentine, paint, paint thinner, and various polishes (metal, floor, furniture, and shoe).
- Wear heavy-duty waterproof gloves when using them.
- Use lukewarm water and very mild soap when washing the hands. Rinse the soap off thoroughly and dry gently. All soaps are irritating.
- Lubricate the hands immediately after washing. Place a lubricant strategically near any sink you use. Petrolatum is best. The patient should carry a small tube or bottle of lubricant.
- The patient should remove rings when doing housework and before washing the hands because rings often worsen dermatitis by trapping irritating materials beneath them.
- When outdoors in cold or windy weather, wear gloves to protect the hands from drying or chapping.
- Use only prescribed medicines and lubricants on the hands. Do not use other lotions, creams, or medications because some of these may irritate the skin.
- Suspected bacterial superinfection (often manifested by fissures and honey-colored crusts) should be treated aggressively with antistaphylococcal antibiotics.
- Topical corticosteroid ointments are preferable to topical corticosteroid creams or lotions for treatment of inflammation.
- The hands should be protected for *at least* 4 months after the dermatitis has healed and maybe longer. It takes a long time for skin to recover, and unless one is careful the dermatitis tends to recur.
- There is no fast "magic" treatment for hand dermatitis. The skin must be given a rest from irritation. Follow the above-listed instructions carefully.

ALLERGIC CONTACT DERMATITIS

Clinical Findings

Mild cases of ACD may be indistinguishable from ICD on clinical grounds alone. In general, pruritus is the predominant symptom of ACD. On physical examination, vesicles are considered the hallmark of ACD. These may appear as linear or grouped tense vesicles. In more severe cases, there may be bullae. Edema may be present, especially if the involved area is the face, eyelids, ears, or genital region. Contrary to a common myth, the vesicle fluid itself is transudate and does not contain appreciable amounts of the antigen, and will not spread the eruption to other areas of the body or to other individuals.

Diagnosis

The anatomic distribution of the dermatitis and the often artifactual configuration are what clinically distinguish the eruption and lead to the suspicion of contact dermatitis. The eruption usually occurs on exposed or contacted areas, and there are often acute angles or straight lines or well-demarcated straight margins that suggest exposure to an extrinsic source as the cause of the eruption. Specific case examples of ACD are discussed subsequently. Bacterial superinfection of either ICD or ACD, usually with *Staphylococcus aureus,* occurs commonly. It may be worthwhile to confirm bacterial superinfection by sending a culture swab from underneath crusts or unroofed pustules for bacterial culture and sensitivity testing. Patch testing is the diagnostic test used for the confirmation of ACD.

Principles of Treatment and Avoidance

If acute exposure to an allergen is apparent, for example, poison ivy, oak, or sumac, avoidance immediately after exposure involves promptly washing the skin with soap and water with the goal of removing the antigen from the skin before it becomes bound to skin pro-

teins. Avoidance measures in cases of chronic, ongoing exposure to allergens are often complex and depend on the source or sources of antigen. If patch testing is anticipated to delineate the cause, it should be delayed until after the dermatitis is under control. Patients suspected of having bacterial superinfection should be treated with appropriate topical and systemic antibiotics, because untreated superinfection may impair response to the other treatments and delay recovery.

Treatment of Mild ACD

For relatively mild ACD, topical corticosteroids are usually beneficial and bring about relief within a few days. A moderate- to high-potency topical corticosteroid is often necessary. For dermatitis involving the face or intertriginous areas, a lower potency topical corticosteroid is often sufficient, because its effect is intensified by higher absorption in these anatomic regions. A moderate- to high-potency topical corticosteroid may used in these regions for a very brief period such as a few days to a week. The patient should be warned about risks and potential side-effects of using stronger corticosteroid preparations in these areas, including thinning of the skin, telangiectasia, and stretch marks; cataracts and glaucoma are potential side-effects if used around the eyes for prolonged periods.

For the initial few days of treatment of acute vesicular dermatitis, wet compresses with tap water or Burow's solution may be soothing, antipruritic, and also may promote vasoconstriction in the dermis, by evaporative cooling of the skin. This vasoconstriction may help reduce inflammation by lowering cutaneous blood flow. Additionally, compresses help debride crusts, and dry the skin slightly, which are usually desirable effects in acute vesicular contact dermatitis. Soothing baths in tap water with or without colloidal oatmeal (numerous OTC brands available) may bring temporary relief from pruritus. A topical corticosteroid in gel form may be good for initial treatment because the gel type of vehicle has a drying effect. The "drying" treatments should be discontinued after 2 or 3 days, however, because these treatments themselves can eventually cause ICD. Thereafter, the patient should discontinue wet compresses and should change to a more occlusive topical corticosteroid vehicle, usually an ointment. The topical corticosteroid may need to be continued for at least several weeks. For symptomatic relief of itching, an H1 antihistamine is often helpful. For most patients the classic sedating types of H1 antihistamines are more effective than the nonsedating H1 antihistamines, perhaps because much of the pruritus in ACD and ICD is not histamine-mediated, and because the soporific effect of the antihistamine dulls the perception of pruritus. Many dermatologists prefer to use hydroxyzine hydrochloride (Atarax, Pfizer Labs; generics available) or hydroxyzine pamoate (Vistaril, Pfizer Labs; generics available) for itching, 25–50 mg every 6 hours as needed; or cyproheptadine hydrochloride (Periactin, Merck & Co.; generics available) 4 mg every 8 hours as needed. Hydroxyzine or cyproheptadine often seems to be more effective for the pruritus associated with contact dermatitis than diphenhydramine.

Treatment of Moderate and Severe Acute ACD

If correctly diagnosed and adequately treated, moderate to severe cases of ACD usually respond dramatically to treatment over a period of 2 to 3 days. This improvement is tremendously relieving to the patient, and consequently, very gratifying to the treating physician.

The topical treatments previously outlined for mild to moderate contact dermatitis are also often indicated in cases of moderate to severe ACD. However, often systemic corticosteroids are necessary to control fully moderate to severe ACD. Indications for a course of systemic corticosteroids include severe localized dermatitis, especially when there is severe swelling of a limb, the face, or eyelids; genital involvement (which could lead to urinary tract obstruction); progressively spreading dermatitis (including autoeczematization, also known as an id reaction, discussed farther on); or widespread dermatitis. Of course, these indications should be weighed against whatever contraindications against a 2- to 3-week course of corticosteroids exist in the patient, such as

diabetes, hypertension, glaucoma, or a history of psychotic behavior. The initial starting dose is usually 0.5 to 1 mg/kg/day prednisone or equivalent, in one morning dose. In severe cases, at least for the initial few days of systemic corticosteroid therapy, some dermatologists give the systemic corticosteroid in several divided doses. Systemic corticosteroids should be given in a slowly tapering dose schedule over 2 to 3 weeks. Abrupt discontinuation of systemic corticosteroids after only a few days of treatment will likely result in a severe relapse of the dermatitis, and systemic corticosteroids will often need to be restarted. Consequently, the prescribing of blister-packaged dose packs containing corticosteroids such as methylprednisolone, with tapering schedules over 5 to 6 days, is discouraged for ACD. Systemic antibiotics also may be necessary in the case of suspected bacterial superinfection, as discussed previously. These patients also usually find symptomatic relief from the sedating H1 antihistamines.

It should be emphasized that patients suffering from moderate to severe acute ACD are often in severe discomfort from pruritus, so they may be severely sleep deprived by the time they seek medical attention. Consequently, it is important to give them explicit written instructions regarding their diagnosis and treatment, as they often cannot remember verbal instructions given to them in their state of distress. It may be worthwhile to give the initial dose of systemic corticosteroid during the initial visit, in either oral or parenteral form. Follow-up visits to monitor progress and, if possible, to taper the systemic corticosteroids to the lowest dose required to maintain control of the dermatitis, are strongly encouraged.

Common Contact Allergens, with Case Examples

A list of common contact allergens in North America is given in Table 17–3. This is a relatively abridged list, but it will likely appear daunting to the uninitiated. When confronting this information initially, the reader is encouraged to first consider the antigens in terms of categories or groups, and not worry as much about the names and details of each antigen. These and many other contact anti-

Table 17–3. **Commonly Encountered Contact Allergens**

Category (Antigen Name)	Patch Test Available*	Examples of Sources of Exposure
Plants		
Urushiols		Anacardiaceae family: poison ivy, poison oak, poison sumac, mango tree (mango rind), cashew nut shell oil, gingko tree, Japanese lacquer tree
Sesquiterpene lactones		Compositae family: chrysanthemum (mums), daisy, sunflowers, dandelion, lettuce; liverwort, *Frullania*
Adhesives, resins		
Epoxy resin	+	Plastics, paints, glues, composite resins
p-tert butylphenol formaldehyde resin	+	Neoprene, plastics, glues (i.e., shoes, automobiles)
Toluenesulfonamide formaldehyde resin		Nail polish, adhesives
Methyl methacrylate		Screening allergen for acrylates, e.g., dental materials
Ethyl acrylate		Screening allergen for acrylates used in artificial nails and in anaerobic sealants
Fragrances/flavorings		
Balsam of Peru	+	Fragrance screening antigen; plastics, medications
Cinnamic aldehyde		Plastics; perfumes; flavoring in toothpastes, mouthwash, candy, cola
Fragrances (fragrance mix)	+	Mix of 8 different fragrances/flavorings found in cosmetics/toiletries and foods; includes cinnamic aldehyde
Metals		
Nickel (nickel sulfate)	+	Numerous metal tools, devices, coins, clothing fasteners; jewelry; penetrates some gloves
Chromium (potassium dichromate)	+	Wet concrete/mortar, leather tanning, anticorrosion (chrome plating), paints
Cobalt (cobalt dichloride)	+	Nickel coreactor, animal feeds, photography, acrylates, paints
Formaldehyde-releasing preservatives		
Formaldehyde	+	Antimicrobial preservative, fabric finishes, plastics
Quaternium-15	+	Cosmetic and industrial antimicrobial preservative
Imidazolinyl urea		Cosmetic and industrial antimicrobial preservative
Diazolidinylurea		Cosmetic and industrial antimicrobial preservative
DMDM hydantoin		Cosmetic and industrial antimicrobial preservative
2-bromo-2-nitropane-1,3-diol (Bronopol)		Cosmetic and industrial antimicrobial preservative
Other preservatives		
Chloromethylisothiazolinone/ methylisothiazolinone (CMI/MI; Kathon CG)	+	Cosmetic and industrial antimicrobial preservative; present in shampoos, lotions
Parabens (Paraben mix)	+	Cosmetic and industrial antimicrobial preservative; a relatively rare sensitizer compared with other preservatives
Thimerosal	+	Antimicrobial preservative (e.g., vaccines); tincture of merthiolate; nasal sprays and drops; ophthalmic preparations; otic preparations; contact lens solutions. Thimerosal-allergic patients may have a photoallergic reaction to piroxicam

Table 17–3. **Commonly Encountered Contact Allergens** *Continued*

Category (Antigen Name)	Patch Test Available*	Examples of Sources of Exposure
Methyldibromoglutaronitrile/ phenoxyethanol (trade name, Euxyl K-400)		A 2-ingredient preservative for metalworking, cosmetics, latex paints, dispersed pigments, and detergents
Chloroxylenol (para-chloro-metaxylenol [PCMX])		Antimicrobial used in soaps.
Glutaraldehyde		Cold sterilization, e.g., dental instruments, endoscopy devices; leather tanning; some waterless hand cleansers; penetrates rubber and vinyl gloves
Propylene glycol		Antimicrobial; used as a vehicle/solvent in cosmetics and topical medicaments such as topical corticosteroids; used in foods as a solvent for colors and flavors and to prevent mold growth
Rubber chemicals		
Carbamates (*carba* mix)	+	Rubber additive, fungicide
Thiuram mix	+	Rubber accelerator (especially shoes and gloves), fungicides
Black rubber mix/*p*-phenylenediamine (PPD)	+	*p*-phenylenediamine-related chemicals; black or grey rubber
Mercapto mix and mercaptobenzathiazole (MBT)	+	Rubber curing accelerator (especially gloves); fungicide (veterinary products), anticorrosive
Fabric finish		
Ethyleneurea melamine-formaldehyde		Formaldehyde-containing fabric finish in clothing, draperies, and so forth. May cause clothing-area dermatitis in formaldehyde-allergic individuals
Topical medicaments/vehicles		
Bacitracin		Topical antibiotic; may occur as a co-sensitizer with neomycin, or as a sensitizer alone
Benzocaine		Widely used topical anesthetic; para-amino chemical cross-reactive (see paraphenylenediamine below)
Diphenhydramine		H-1 antihistamine—ethanolamine class. High sensitizing potential when used topically
Caine mix (patch test contains a mixture of benzocaine, tetracaine, and dibucaine)	+	Topical anesthetics
Neomycin	+	Topical antibiotic
Wool wax alcohols (lanolin)	+	Topical medications, emollients–emulsifier
Ethylenediamine dihydrochloride	+	Soldering fluxes; used as a stabilizer in topical medications; present in aminophylline; potentially cross-reactive with ethylenediamine class of H1 antihistamines
Quinoline mix	+	Topical antimicrobials, e.g., clioquinol
Other antigens		
Colophony (rosin)	+	Cosmetics, glues, soldering flux, antiskid preparation (athletes, violinists)
p-phenylenediamine (PPD)	+	A blue-black aniline dye, commonly used as a hair dye. Related to black rubber chemicals. Potentially cross-reacts with benzocaine, procaine, sulfa drugs, sulfonylureas, para-aminobenzoic acid (PABA) sunscreens

Adapted from Sheretz E, Storrs FJ: Contact dermatitis. *In* Rosenstock L, Cullen MR (eds): Textbook of Clinical Occupational and Environmental Medicine, Philadelphia, WB Saunders Company, 1994, pp 514–530.

*A (+) in this column indicates that this antigen is commercially available in the United States.

gens are discussed in detail in several excellent references on contact dermatitis listed.

A few case examples, all seen in the primary care and specialty outpatient clinics at the author's clinic over the past several years are presented below, with comments on diagnosis and treatment. These are quite representative of cases of ACD encountered in the primary care setting.

Plants

ACD caused by poison ivy, oak, or sumac is frequently encountered in individuals who come in contact with these plants at home, during outdoor leisure activities, and in occupational settings such as agriculture and forestry. This appearance is the prototype of severe acute ACD. Systemic corticosteroids are frequently needed, even in relatively localized cases if there is swelling or the possibility of urinary outlet obstruction. Fisher has stated that "edema of the prepuce may lead to urinary obstruction and is an indication for systemic corticosteroid therapy even in mild cases of poison ivy dermatitis." A representative case of poison oak dermatitis is shown in Figure 17–3. Because urushiol, the sap that drains

from these plants when injured, contains such strong sensitizers, patch testing is usually not performed with these antigens. Other plants that contain these antigens are listed in Table 17–3, and urushiol-sensitive patients should be cautioned to avoid these plants and plant products. Barrier creams may be helpful in preventing ACD to urushiol.

The sesquiterpene lactones are another group of antigens that occur in plants, including chrysanthemum (mums), daisies, and sunflowers, that can cause ACD. They may be encountered in occupational settings such as horticulture.

Adhesives and Resins

Many cases of ACD due to these substances occur in occupational settings. Epoxy resins are widely used in the manufacture of aircraft components, electronics, sports equipment, and in paints. Epoxy glues are sometimes used in the home. Toluenesulfonamide formaldehyde resin is usually the cause of ACD due to nail polish. This nail polish–caused ACD often occurs on the face, scalp, or eyelids, with relative sparing of the fingers. The acrylates also are used widely in occupational settings such

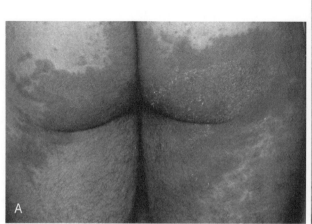
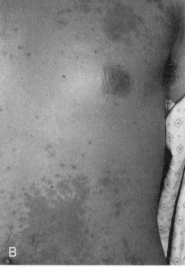

Figure 17–3. *A* and *B*, Widespread acute allergic contact dermatitis caused by poison oak. This patient had unintentionally used poison oak leaves as a substitute for toilet paper while on a camping trip. He was in severe discomfort. He improved dramatically over the 2 days following initiation of prednisone, 1 mg/kg/day. He was treated with a tapering dose schedule of prednisone for a duration of 3 weeks. Discontinuation of systemic corticosteroids before 2 to 3 weeks of treatment can lead to a rebound recurrence of the dermatitis in severe cases such as this.

as dentistry and electronics. Acrylate dermatitis can present as dermatitis involving the fingers.

Fragrances and Flavorings

Fragrances are a very common cause of dermatitis that is due to cosmetics and toiletries (Fig. 17–4). Individuals thought to have ACD possibly caused by a fragrance should be instructed to use personal care products labeled fragrance-free. Products labeled as unscented may contain masking fragrances; fragrance-free should be specified. Fragrance allergy also may present as an oral mucositis or perioral dermatitis if it is caused by substances such as cinnamic aldehyde, a flavoring agent used widely in foods and dentrifices.

Metals

Nickel remains one of the most common contact allergens in North America. Nickel is an

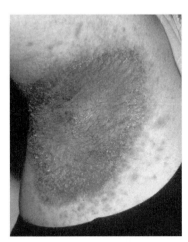

Figure 17–4. Allergic contact dermatitis occurring bilaterally in the axillae owing to fragrance in a deodorant. Note that the entire axilla is involved, including the axillary vault. In contrast, dermatitis caused by contact with clothing usually involves the axillary folds, with relative sparing of the axillary vault. There was also superinfection with *Staphylococcus aureus,* an indication for systemic antibiotics. This dermatitis was treated with topical corticosteroids and oral antibiotics. In severe cases, a course of systemic corticosteroids may hasten resolution. Patients with dermatitis caused by a deodorant should be instructed to use only fragrance-free personal care products. Patch testing can confirm fragrance allergy. Patch testing should not be performed until several weeks after acute dermatitis has resolved.

ubiquitous antigen, present on many metal objects, clothing, and jewelry. A list of nickel-containing objects is given in Table 17–4, as is information on the dimethylglyoxime test kit, which is used for testing metal objects for nickel release. Nickel can be solubilized by water or sweat and can then penetrate latex gloves, cloth gloves, or clothing and cause dermatitis on the underlying skin. In general, although stainless steel contains nickel, it usually does not liberate enough nickel to cause ACD in most nickel-allergic individuals. Two cases typical of nickel allergy are shown in Figure 17–5. Chromium (hexavalent chromium or chromate) is another common cause of ACD due to metals. It is used widely in industry, for example, in wet concrete and mortar (Fig. 17–6). It is also a strong irritant and can cause chemical burns.

Formaldehyde-Releasing Preservatives and Formaldehyde

Formaldehyde is used in tissue specimen processing and embalming. Formaldehyde-releasing preservatives, listed in Table 17–3, are used very widely in personal care products, and also in industry as antimicrobial preservatives in water-based coolants and cutting fluids. Quaternium-15 remains a very common cause of ACD related to personal care products such as moisturizers. Allergy to this and other formaldehyde-releasing preservatives in cosmetics or moisturizers often presents insidiously as a pruritic, patchy erythema involving sites where the product has been applied, and may spread beyond these sites as well. Patients who are allergic to either formaldehyde or to any one of the formaldehyde-releasing preservatives should be warned about the potential of their also being allergic to other members of this group. They should be given the name formaldehyde and the names of all of the formaldehyde-releasing preservatives listed in Table 17–3 and should be encouraged to become label-readers, checking the ingredient lists of all personal care products for any of these substances before using them.

Other Preservatives

Other preservatives also are common causes of ACD due to cosmetics and personal care

Table 17–4. **Nickel Avoidance Information**

Nickel contactants	Sources of dimethylglyoxime test kit for testing objects for nickel release
appliance dials	
clothing—snaps/buttons/rivets/zippers	Allerderm Laboratories
coins, medallions	P O Box 2070
doorknobs	Petaluma, CA 94953–2070
eyeglass frames	www.allerderm.com
eyelash curlers—bilateral eyelid dermatitis	
jewelry	Delasco
keys	608 13th Avenue
letter openers	Council Bluffs, IA 51501–6401
paper clips—fingertip dermatitis	www.delasco.com
pens	
refrigerator handles	
safety pins	
scissors	
table edges	
tools	
water faucet handles	
wheelchairs—frames and wheels	
wristwatches and watchbands/buckles	

products. Thimerosal, which has been used as a preservative in vaccines, is also present in many over-the-counter and prescription topical preparations (Fig. 17–7). Thimerosal-positive patch test results are observed frequently, but many affected patients do not appear to have presently relevant reactions. Even patients with a seemingly irrelevant thimerosal-positive patch test response should be given instructions on avoidance of thimerosal, as it remains widely in use.

Chloromethylisothiazolinone/methylisothiazolinone (CMI/MI) is present in many shampoos and other preparations designed to be rinsed off, such as cream rinses. Glutaraldehyde is used widely for cold sterilization of medical, surgical, and dental instruments. It is able to penetrate latex gloves and can cause

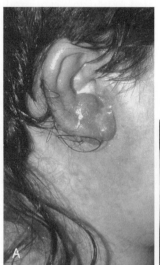
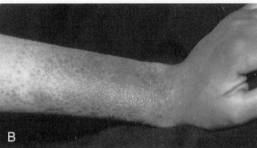

Figure 17–5. Allergic contact dermatitis caused by nickel. Patients shown in both *A* and *B* were wearing nickel-containing jewelry. *A,* Allergic contact dermatitis with *Staphylococcus aureus* superinfection caused by earrings. The condition improved following treatment with appropriate systemic antibiotics and moderate-potency topical corticosteroids. *B,* Chronic allergic contact dermatitis from a nickel-containing bracelet. Nickel exposure from items such as the bracelet can sometimes be avoided by painting the nickel-releasing object with a clear polyurethane varnish.

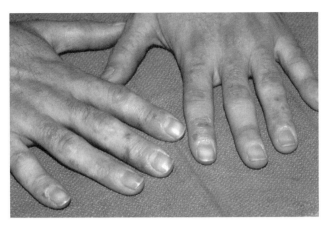

Figure 17–6. Hand dermatitis in a tile setter caused by acute contact with chromium salts in wet mortar. The diagnosis was confirmed by patch testing. In this case, wearing protective gloves was not feasible, and the patient changed occupations.

ACD of the fingertips in workers in medical and dental settings.

Rubber Chemicals

Rubber chemical substances are added to latex rubber for purposes such as acceleration of the rubber curing process (vulcanization) and to retard oxidation of the rubber product and therefore enhance its performance. They are widely encountered in clothing (e.g., elastic, shoes) and also are used in other applications such as pesticides, fungicides, and veterinary

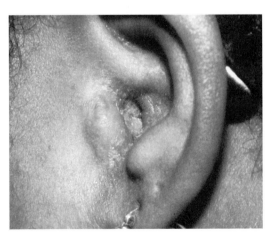

Figure 17–7. Allergic contact dermatitis complicating otitis externa. This patient had been treated with an otic suspension consisting of neomycin and triamcinolone. Patch testing showed strong positive reactions to nickel, neomycin, and also thimerosal, which was used in the otic suspension as a preservative. The otitis may have been initially related to the patient's nickel allergy; note the earring. Patch test results were negative to triamcinolone itself and also to a panel of other topical corticosteroids. The dermatitis completely resolved over 2 months following discontinuation of the otic suspension.

products. Table 17–5 lists the differential diagnoses of extrinsic causes of hand dermatitis associated with rubber gloves.

Fabric Finish

Ethyleneurea melamine formaldehyde is used in fabric finishes in clothing and draperies. It may cause allergic contact dermatitis involving skin in close contact with clothing, especially the permanent-press or easy-care varieties of clothes.

Topical Medicaments or Vehicles

Topical medicaments are widely used in many over-the-counter and prescription products. In general, these products should not be used on dermatitic skin, because of their high sensitization potential when used in this setting (Fig. 17–8). Only very bland topical agents should be used on dermatitic skin, such as topical corticosteroids in bland ointment vehicles such as petrolatum. Creams should be avoided if possible, as they contain substances such as lanolin (wool alcohols) and also preservatives and fragrances. Local anesthetics can cause severe ACD in individuals with contact allergy to these. They should not be applied to dermatitic skin. Neomycin is a very common sensitizer. Twelve percent of the over 3000 patients patch tested by the North American Contact Dermatitis Group (NACDG) from 1994 to 1996 were allergic to neomycin, and high percentages of these positive test results were clinically relevant. Mupirocin is a relatively safe

Table 17–5. **Causes of Hand Dermatitis Related to Gloves**

	Mechanism	Causative Agent(s)	Clinical Manifestations	Diagnostic Testing
Latex allergy	Type I (IgE-mediated, immediate) immunologic contact reaction	Allergens are proteins in natural latex rubber from the rubber tree *Hevea brasiliensis*	*Immediate* onset (minutes to hours) contact reactions—pruritis, urticaria to anaphylaxis. If exposures are repeated, may also manifest as *chronic* hand dermatitis	1) Serum assay for latex-specific IgE; 2) Wear test; 3) Immediate skin testing (2 and 3 are read in *15–30 minutes*)
Contact dermatitis from rubber	Type IV (cellular-mediated/delayed-type) contact hypersensitivity	*Additives* to rubber catalysts, antioxidants; i.e., carbamates, thiurams, mercapto compounds	Acute or chronic dermatitis in anatomic distribution of rubber contact. i.e., *acute* vesicular dermatitis or *chronic* hand dermatitis corresponding to the area covered by a rubber glove	Patch testing: readings done at 48 hours and at 3 to 7 days or longer after patch test application
ICD	No specific immune sensitivity	Irritants, glove powder, soaps, solvents, water	Acute or chronic dermatitis	History and physical; possibly testing for latex-specific IgE and patch testing to exclude allergic causes

alternative if a topical antibiotic is needed for dermatitic skin. Patients with allergy to ethylenediamine dihydrochloride should not be given aminophylline; this could result in severe generalized systemic contact dermatitis (Table 17–3).

Other Antigens

Colophony (rosin) is used by athletes, and is also present in soldering fluxes. Paraphenylenediamine continues to be a common cause of ACD related to hair dyes (Fig. 17–9). Figure 17–10 shows likely sources of antigen exposure for contact dermatitis localized to various anatomic sites.

Patch Testing

Patch testing is carried out by placing standardized samples of antigens or antigen mixes in small chambers on the patient, usually on the back (Fig. 17–11). These are held in place by tape for 48 hours, and then readings are done after removal, and at least once again 3 to 7 days or longer after the date of patch application. A positive patch test response to a particular antigen is represented by a small

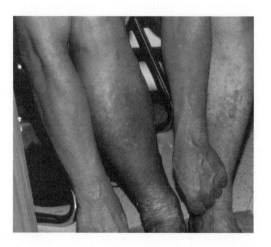

Figure 17–8. Allergic contact dermatitis with autoeczematization. This condition arose as a complication of stasis dermatitis that was caused by venous insufficiency. This patient had been applying an over-the-counter antibiotic cream containing neomycin and had become allergic to this common sensitizer. He had begun to develop dermatitis on the opposite leg and on the arms. The spread of dermatitis to remote anatomic regions such as this is known as autoeczematization or an *id reaction*. Because of the autoeczematization the treatment of choice was a once-a-day moderate dose of prednisone, along with support bandages for the stasis dermatitis, and discontinuation of all topical agents. Autoeczematization usually requires systemic corticosteroids for control. This patient's condition improved rapidly with this treatment, and avoidance measures.

Figure 17–9. Allergic contact dermatitis caused by a paraphenylenediamine-containing hair dye. As is often the case, there was relative sparing of the scalp; the ears, neck, and eyelids were more severely affected than the scalp. Systemic corticosteroids are usually necessary to control this dermatitis, as it is very difficult to deliver sufficient amounts of corticosteroids topically to the affected areas. Systemic corticosteroids should be continued for 2 to 3 weeks' duration in cases such as this. Affected patients are often superinfected with *Staphylococcus aureus,* so appropriate systemic antibiotics should be administered in addition to corticosteroids if superinfection is suspected.

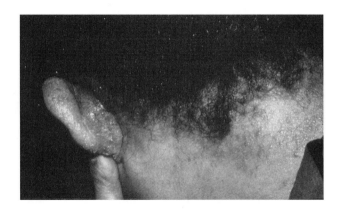

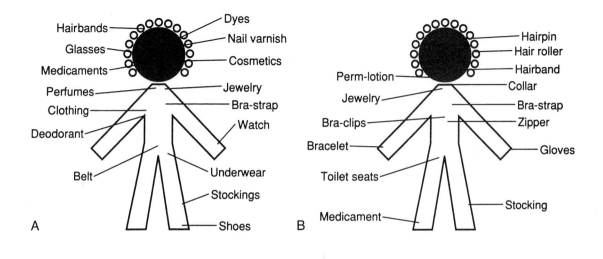

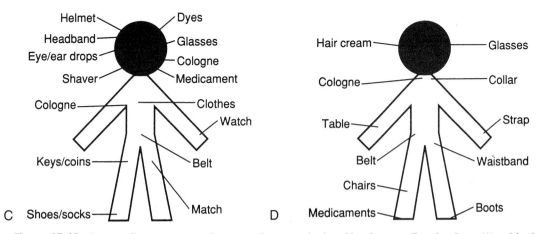

Figure 17–10. Contact allergen sources of exposure by anatomic site of involvement. Females: front *(A)* and back *(B)*. Males: front *(C)* and back *(D)*. (From Goh CL: Allergic contact dermatitis. *In* Guin JD [ed]: Practical Contact Dermatitis: A Handbook for the Practitioner. New York, McGraw-Hill, 1995, pp 22–23. Reproduced with permission of the McGraw-Hill Companies.)

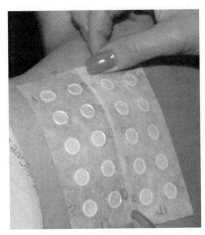

Figure 17–11. Patch testing. Samples (patches) of standardized allergens are placed on the patient's back and worn for 48 hours. The patches are then removed, and each patch test site examined on at least two occasions for dermatitis, which could represent a positive response. Patch testing has a central role in the diagnosis of allergic contact dermatitis.

area of dermatitis in the area corresponding to where the patch was located. It is of utmost importance to do an additional reading at a time beyond the initial 48-hour reading, to allow for irritant reactions to subside, and to allow additional time for the elicitation of any late positive allergic-type reactions. Some antigens also are irritants even at the standardized patch test concentrations that are used, for example, carba mix and potassium dichromate.

Additionally, some antigens such as metals and neomycin are known to appear as positive reactions relatively late, for example, after 3 days, and may be missed if only a 48-hour reading is performed. It should be stressed that there are many nuances to performing and reading patch tests, and therefore patch testing should only be carried out by physicians who are experienced in their reading and interpretation. A disservice is done to a patient by having positive patch test reactions missed because of readings being carried out at improper time points. It is also a problem for the patient, and possibly for their employer, if the patient is told that they are allergic to a substance when in reality the reaction merely represented an irritant reaction. Patch testing is not useful in confirming whether a substance is a cause of ICD.

Once an allergic-type patch test response

is obtained, further investigation is often warranted. If the source of the antigen exposure is not apparent, the patient may need to be further questioned about any possible exposures to that antigen both within and outside of the workplace, in the present and in the past. It may be wise to repeat patch testing several weeks later to confirm positive or negative results, particularly if results during the initial testing are unexpected. Often if there is no known present exposure to an antigen, a positive patch test response is considered to be of unknown relevance or relevant in the past (e.g., a past history of dermatitis from costume jewelry in a patient with a positive patch test response to nickel). After completion of patch testing, the patient should be given a listing of the names of the antigens that gave positive, allergic-type responses and written instructions for avoiding each of them. Several readings listed at the end of this chapter contain excellent patient instructions for allergen avoidance.

IMMEDIATE CONTACT REACTIONS

Definitions

Immediate contact reactions include contact urticaria, a localized wheal and flare; they also may manifest as itching, stinging, or burning, accompanied by erythema but without whealing. The contact urticaria syndrome, which is characterized by both local and systemic immediate reactions caused by contact urticaria agents, is the most severe manifestation in this group. When obtaining a history, it is important to obtain a time course of onset from the patient; to make the diagnosis the onset should be immediate, within minutes to an hour after contact with the offending agent.

Nonimmunologic Immediate Contact Reactions

Nonimmunologic immediate contact reactions occur without prior sensitization in many if not most individuals who are exposed to a causative agent. It can be a useful point in the history as to whether other individuals who may have been exposed were affected. These reactions are rarely of a severe, life-threatening nature. The causative agents include many fragrances and flavorings. The mechanisms of many of these reactions are not fully understood; possible mechanisms include a direct pharmacologic effect on blood vessel walls, or a nonantibody–mediated release of mediators such as prostaglandins, leukotrienes, or substance P. Nettles are a well-known cause of nonimmunologic urticaria, which is due to direct contact of histamine with the skin. Consequently, antihistamines may be useful in these types of reactions when histamine is a mediator. Some of these reactions, such as those caused by benzoic acid, cinnamic acid, or cinnamic aldehyde, can be suppressed by nonsteroidal anti-inflammatory drugs. The diagnosis can be confirmed by studies such as a rub test on the skin, or a use test, in which the patient repeats the exposure to the suspected agent under medical supervision. Management consists mainly of patient education regarding avoidance of the causative agent.

Immunologic Immediate Contact Reactions

Immediate contact reactions are IgE-mediated reactions that occur in individuals who have been previously sensitized. These reactions have been known for quite some time to occur after contact with many different foods, and have been the subject of considerable interest during the past decade due to the problem of latex allergy (see Chapter 22). They can range from mild itching, burning, and stinging accompanied by erythema, to full-blown anaphylaxis. If exposures occur repeatedly, these types of reactions can develop into a chronic eczematous dermatitis that can resemble ACD or ICD. Again, the time course of onset of symptoms after contact is important to note. The diagnosis can be made either by the studies mentioned previously for nonimmunologic contact reactions or by prick skin testing. However, caution should be exercised when performing diagnostic skin testing when there is a history of a severe reaction. Management

includes antihistamines, topical corticosteroids if an eczematous dermatitis is present, patient education on avoidance, and personal protection.

PHOTOCONTACT DERMATITIS

Photoallergic Contact Dermatitis

Photoallergic contact dermatitis (Photo-ACD) is an allergic contact dermatitis arising from conversion of a chemical by light exposure into a hapten, which causes an allergic contact dermatitis. Photo-ACD often has many features of ACD such as severe pruritus and a vesicular dermatitis. It occurs on light-exposed areas of the skin in a so-called photodistribution involving the face, ears, and anterior V area of the neck, and also the backs of the hands and the forearms. The submental region and upper eyelids tend to be spared. The diagnosis is confirmed by photopatch testing, in which patch testing is carried out, but ultraviolet light exposures of the patch test sites also are done. An airborne ACD (e.g., to epoxy resins) is often in the differential diagnosis. Some causes of Photo-ACD are shown in Table 17–6.

Phototoxic Contact Dermatitis

Phototoxic reactions have nonimmunologic mechanisms in which a chemical absorbs a specific wavelength of light and causes cellular damage. These reactions are often characterized more by a burning sensation or pain than by itching, and they appear similar to an exaggerated sunburn and develop bullae (Fig. 17–12). Often a characteristic post-inflammatory hyperpigmentation develops that may persist for several months. Plants containing psoralen compounds (furocoumarins) are common causes of phototoxic contact dermatitis (Table 17–7), for example the "Club Med" dermatitis that occurs in bartenders and their clientele whose skin becomes exposed to juice from

Table 17–6. **Causes of Photocontact Dermatitis**

Photo-ACD	Source of Exposure
Antigen	
Para-aminobenzoic acid (PABA)	Sunscreens
Sulisobenzone	Sunscreens, lip balms, moisturizers, shampoos/ hair care products
Oxybenzone	Sunscreens
Musk ambrette	Men's aftershaves, colognes
Sandalwood oil	Soaps, aftershaves, colognes, cosmetics
Chlorhexidine	Surgical scrubs, hand cleansers, dentifrices, eye drops, wound care
Phototoxic Contact Dermatitis	
Phototoxic substance	
Tars	Pitch, creosote, therapeutic tar (psoriasis)
Furocoumarins	Fragrances (oil of Bergamot); plants (see Table 17–7)
Eosin, methylene blue	Dyes
Sulfonamides	Drugs: medical, pharmaceutical

lime peels and then to sunlight. This type of reaction also has been reported to occur secondary to aromatherapy oils. Other causes of phototoxic contact dermatitis are shown in Table 17–6.

HAND DERMATITIS

As the reader has certainly already surmised, most cases of contact dermatitis involve the hands. This condition can be very debilitating, particularly in occupational settings, and it may take many months for the hands to recover from contact dermatitis. The differential diagnosis of hand dermatitis includes ACD, ICD, atopic hand dermatitis, id reactions secondary to dermatitis or dermatophyte infections of the feet, dermatophyte infections (2-foot/1-hand disease), bacterial infections, and other chronic dermatoses such as psoriasis and lichen planus. Topical corticosteroids usually should be given in ointment form for dermatitis involving the hands, and high-potency topical corticosteroids may be needed at least initially. Principles of management of hand

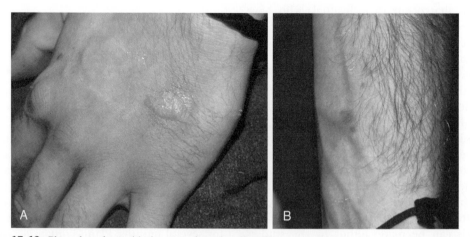

Figure 17–12. Phytophotodermatitis in a produce handler. This type of dermatitis is a phototoxic localized sunburn caused by contact of the skin with any of a number of plants, fruits, or vegetables containing furocoumarin compounds (see Table 17–7). This case was caused by contact with celery, followed by exposure of the contacted skin to sunlight. This type of dermatitis is not immune-mediated, but instead is due to phototoxicity. It is sometimes confused with allergic contact dermatitis. Unlike allergic contact dermatitis, it is usually not severely pruritic. Note the characteristic localized bullae and hyperpigmentation. Treatment is the same as for a localized burn. Protective clothing to avoid contact with the offending plants is often the most practical avoidance measure.

Table 17–7. **Plants Containing Furocoumarin Compounds**

Angelica	Dill
Bergamot	Fennel
Bitter orange	Giant hogweed
Carrot (garden, wild)	Lemon
Celery	Lime
Citron	Masterwort
Common rue	Parsnip (garden, wild)
Cow parsley	Persian lime

dermatitis are outlined in Table 17–2. A method of removal of a ring from a severely swollen finger has been discussed by Exner and also by Leider (Fig. 17–13). This method involves the winding of the string around the finger, starting distally near the DIP joint, and then winding the string around the finger

proximally. This serves to drive the edema proximally, and under the ring. When the string has been wound proximally to the ring, it is then slipped under the ring, and then the string is slowly unwound from behind the ring, pushing the ring distally down the swollen finger, much to the patient's relief. Leider advises that this should not be attempted if infection is present.

Occupational Contact Dermatitis

As seen in some of the case examples presented, contact dermatitis often occurs in occupational settings. It is sometimes necessary

Table 17–8. **Leading Causes of Contact Dermatitis in High-Risk Occupations**

Occupation	Leading Causes
Agricultural/forestry/horticulture	Plants Pesticides, usually irritant contact dermatitis
Construction/masonry	Chromate salts—concrete, leather, wood preservative Irritants—dirt, wet concrete, friction, hand cleansing
Dentistry	Glutaraldehyde: cold sterilization Rubber additives, latex allergy (gloves) Acrylic resins Irritants: handwashing, soaps
Food service	Contact urticaria—fish, shellfish most common Contact dermatitis—garlic, onions Irritants—wet work
Hairdressers	Glyceryl monothioglycolate salon perms Paraphenylenediamine Nickel
Housekeeping personnel	Rubber additives, latex allergy (gloves) Antimicrobial preservatives (skin care, cleansers)
Machinists	Antimicrobial preservatives (coolant and cutting fluids) Corrosion inhibitors: mercaptobenzothiazole Nickel Colophony
Mechanics	Irritants: solvents, fuel, oil, hand cleansing Rubber additives Chromium salts—cleaners Colophony—soldering flux Acrylates—anaerobic sealants
Medical	Irritants: handwashing, soaps, glove powder Rubber additives, latex allergy (gloves) Glutaraldehyde: cold sterilization Formaldehyde: lab specimens Antimicrobial preservatives—skin care, soaps
Printers	Chromium salts (inks) Ink and printing plate resins

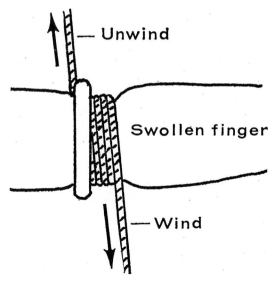

Figure 17–13. Procedure for removal of a ring from swollen finger. (From Exner FB: Removal of ring from swollen finger (letter). JAMA 210:558, 1969; Copyright 1969 American Medical Association.)

to remove the patient from work or request a change of work duties until an evaluation can be completed. A list of occupations at high risk for contact dermatitis and the most frequent causes of contact dermatitis in these settings is given in Table 17–8.

Suggested Reading

Arndt K, Bowers KE, Chuttani A: Manual of Dermatologic Therapeutics, 5th Ed. Boston, Little, Brown, 1995

Guin JD (ed): Practical Contact Dermatitis: A Handbook for the Practitioner. New York, McGraw-Hill, 1995

Lahti A, Maibach HI: Immediate contact reactions: Contact urticaria and the contact urticaria syndrome. *In* Marzulli FN, Maibach HI (eds): Dermatotoxicology. New York, Hemisphere Publishing, 1991, pp 473–495

Leider M: Removal of a ring from a swollen finger without injuring the ring. J Derm Surg Oncol 6:298–299, 1980

Marks JG, DeLeo VA: Contact and Occupational Dermatology. St. Louis, Mosby–Year Book, 1997

Marks JG Jr, Belsito DV, DeLeo VA, et al: North American Contact Dermatitis Group patch test results for the detection of delayed-type hypersensitivity to topical allergens. J Am Acad Dermatol 38(Pt 1):911–918, 1998

Rietschel RE, Fowler JF (eds): Fisher's Contact Dermatitis. Baltimore, Williams & Wilkins, 1995

Sherertz EF, Storrs FJ: Contact dermatitis. *In* Rosenstock L, Cullen MR (eds): Textbook of Clinical Occupational and Environmental Medicine, Philadelphia, WB Saunders, 1994, pp 514–530

Chapter 18

Adverse Reactions to Food

Clifton T. Furukawa

From a patient's point of view *any* abnormal response attributed by that patient to the ingestion of food or drink is an adverse reaction to food. It is the time-relationship between food or drink ingestion and response that is most often focused on. It is up to the physician to determine the mechanisms and assure the appropriate recommendation. In the process of determining what mechanisms are involved it has been helpful to categorize food reactions into two major groups: allergy and intolerance (Table 18–1).

A food allergy reaction is any immunologically mediated adverse food reaction; most commonly it is IgE-mediated. A food intolerance is a nonimmunologic reaction and includes toxicity or poisoning, pharmacologic reactions to chemicals present in the food, metabolic reactions from enzyme deficiencies, and idiosyncratic and psychological reactions. The prevalence of adverse food reactions in adults is perceived to be very common, but actual IgE-mediated food allergy occurs in about 1% of the population. Adverse food reactions occur in about 8% of children, with IgE-mediated food allergy accounting for the majority of these reactions.

Patients who have an allergic reaction to food usually can relate what food or drink may have caused it. The most common causes are egg, milk, legumes (especially soy and peanut), tree nuts, shellfish, fish, and wheat. Although any food may cause anaphylaxis, the offending food is usually obvious because the reaction is so intense and occurs within minutes of ingestion (Table 18–2). Patients may develop laryngeal edema, difficulty in breathing, and urticaria, the latter of which usually occurs rapidly although the onset may be delayed up to several hours. Eczema or atopic dermatitis, the other cutaneous reaction affected by foods, occurs slowly. It is thought to be related to histamine-releasing factors, and affected patients have more difficulty identifying causative foods. The food triggers an allergic reaction, and the itching induced by the food results in scratching, which causes the characteristic dermatitis.

Respiratory symptoms, including asthma, may occur as part of the immediate anaphylactic reaction. Asthma caused by foods more often results from inhalation of the food allergen from cooking or food processing than from ingestion. Gastrointestinal symptoms from food allergy may include pruritus around the mouth, nausea, vomiting, diarrhea, abdominal pain, or chronic malabsorption and failure to thrive.

FOOD ALLERGY

In children, 90% of food allergy (listed in decreasing prevalence) is caused by egg, peanut, milk, soy, wheat, or fish. In adults, peanuts, nuts, fish, and shellfish predominate. Persons sensitive to peanuts, tree nuts, fish, and shellfish are less likely to lose their sensitivity than persons allergic to other foods. About one third of adults and children with a history of a food allergy are no longer sensitive when re-challenged using double-blind food

Table 18–1. **Categories of Adverse Food Reactions**

Category	Mechanism	Examples
Food allergy	Immunologic	Anaphylaxis (IgE)
		Atopic dermatitis (IgE histamine releasing factor)
		Oral allergy syndrome (IgE)
		Urticaria/Angioedema (IgE)
		Heiner's syndrome (IgG)
		Cow protein enterocolitis (Type IV cell-mediated)
		Gluten enteropathy (Type IV cell-mediated, IgA, IgE)
Food intolerance	Nonimmunologic	Anaphylactoid syndrome
		Toxicity
		Poisoning
		Enzyme deficiency
		Idiosyncratic
		Pharmacologic

challenge tests after they eliminate the food from their diet for several years.

Patients with food hypersensitivity may lose their symptomatic reaction, possibly through development of immunologic tolerance. With children, bowel permeability and enzymatic maturation may allow tolerance of foods that still could otherwise elicit an allergic (IgE) reaction. Therefore, an offending food that has been eliminated from the diet should be reintroduced cautiously and gradually to see if it can be tolerated. These regular interval challenges must be carefully controlled, using very small amounts of the food and gradually increasing the challenge. In this instance the physician should be adequately prepared to treat anaphylaxis. Patients with proved anaphylaxis to a specific food should not be rechallenged.

Many persons with an allergy to pollens (birch, ragweed, grass, mugwort) may react to raw foods such as melons, apples, peaches, and celery. Such cross-reaction may also be experienced by latex-sensitive persons (see Table 18–3 and Chapter 22). Symptoms usually are oral itching and swelling, which is known as oral allergy syndrome. Heat or cooking denatures the profilin proteins that are responsible.

DIAGNOSIS

Diagnosis of food allergy is initiated by obtaining a detailed dietary history. Patients who present with urticaria, eczema, or gastrointestinal symptoms may require diagnostic tests. The most useful test for IgE-mediated disease is a percutaneous test with the suspected food allergen (see Chapter 5 on Food Allergens). Positive skin test responses have a predictive accuracy of 30% to 50% when compared with double-blind food challenge tests, and negative test results have a predicative accuracy of greater than 90%. Intradermal testing is associated with high false-positive rates and, therefore, is not an accurate predictor of clini-

Table 18–2. **Anaphylaxis and Anaphylactoid Food Reactions**

IgE-mediated
  IgE to specific food allergen (e.g., egg, peanut)
  IgE to a contaminant in the food (e.g., penicillin)
Histamine-induced
  Fish with high histamine content (e.g., contaminated scombroid fish)
  Bacterial contamination (e.g., cheese or canned fish overgrown with *Proteus* or *Klebsiella*)
Miscellaneous/unknown mechanisms
  Sulfites
  Monosodium glutamate
  Ethanol
  Idiopathic and exercise-induced anaphylaxis associated with ingestion of specific foods

Table 18–3. **Cross-Reacting Allergens with Food**

Allergen	Food Cross-Reactions
Birch pollen	Apple, carrot, celery, hazelnut, kiwi, pear, potato
Ragweed pollen	Bananas, melon
Mugwort pollen	Celery
Grass pollen	Celery, peach, tomato
Latex	Avocado, banana, chestnut, kiwi

cal sensitivity. Radioallergosorbent test (RAST) results correlate with positive percutaneous skin test results but are more expensive and give false-positive results in patients with high serum IgE levels. The gold standard for food testing is the oral, double-blind challenge test. This test is conducted by administering opaque capsules containing the suspected food or a placebo or by concealing the suspected food in another food to which the patient is not sensitive or administering unaltered food. The results of a single-blind challenge test with the suspected food concealed in a drink, cookie, or capsule may reflect the bias of the observer. A diary of all food and drink ingested and symptoms may be useful for some patients, but is also subject to biased interpretation by the patient or physician. An elimination diet also can be used; however, there are many uncontrolled variables. Open challenge tests are subject to bias by the observer and the patient; however, a lack of reaction during an open challenge test can be convincing to both the patient and the observer. Thus open challenge tests have a role in confirming that a certain food is safe to consume.

THERAPY AND PREVENTION

Food allergy in infants can be minimized by restricting the ingestion of the major food allergens by the infant, by prescribing elemental formulas, and by restricting the foods the breastfeeding mother ingests, such as milk and egg, the allergenic proteins of which can be transmitted to the infant in breast milk. Peanuts, nuts, and wheat also should be avoided under similar circumstances. Such a restricted diet has been associated with less severe and later onset of allergic symptoms in the infant. Mothers who breastfeed and do not restrict their diets or the use of cow's milk–derived hypoallergenic formulas for infants do not prevent food allergy.

Treatment consists of avoiding the offending food, modifying the food protein with heat or enzymatic action, and appropriately treating the food-induced allergic reaction. The use of oral cromolyn to prevent food allergy has never been shown to be effective in well-controlled trials. Immunotherapy with

food allergens is considered experimental, although there is a report of successful treatment of peanut-sensitive patients with rush immunotherapy. Antihistamines can help reduce the severity of reactions to foods, particularly eczema and the oral allergy syndrome. The treatment of choice for an acute reaction to food (i.e., anaphylaxis) is epinephrine, available as Epi-pen, Epi-pen Jr (for children 45 pounds or less), and Anaguard.

NON–IgE-MEDIATED IMMUNE REACTIONS

NonIgE-mediated immunologic reactions to food include Heiner's syndrome, food-induced enterocolitis, celiac disease, dermatitis herpetiformis, allergic eosinophilic gastroenteritis, protein-losing enteropathy, and infantile colic. Heiner's syndrome is a form of pulmonary hemosiderosis. Affected patients have rhinitis, pulmonary infiltrates with hemosiderosis, iron deficiency anemia secondary to gastrointestinal bleeding, and failure to thrive. Most cases have been related to hypersensitivity to cow's milk protein, but the same syndrome has been reported with soy, egg, and pork. Patients with this syndrome have serum precipitins to milk, soy, egg, or pork and have peripheral blood eosinophilia. The syndrome resolves with avoidance of the causative allergens.

Infants with enterocolitis from cow's milk or soy milk protein sensitivity present with protracted diarrhea, projectile vomiting, and occult blood, leukocytes, and eosinophils in their stools. In older patients, this type of enterocolitis also has been associated with the ingestion of eggs. The colitis resolves within days of allergen elimination. Malabsorption disorders, which have been reported with cow's milk, soy, egg, and wheat hypersensitivity, are associated with diarrhea, steatorrhea, flatulence, nausea, vomiting, and weight loss. The small bowel biopsy specimen usually shows patchy villus atrophy with a cellular infiltrate.

Gluten-sensitive enteropathy or celiac disease may be associated with more severe intestinal symptoms; the small bowel biopsy specimen shows severe atrophy of the villi and extensive cellular infiltration. Patients with dermatitis herpetiformis, which is associated with gluten-sensitive enteropathy, present with a very pruritic rash. Treatment consists of avoidance of gluten and prescription dapsone or other sulfones. A skin biopsy specimen usually shows an infiltration of leukocytes and deposits of IgA around the dermal papillae. Infants with eosinophilic gastroenteritis present with nausea, vomiting, abdominal pain, diarrhea, and failure to thrive. Older children and adults develop the same symptoms with weight loss. Affected patients often have allergic diseases with elevated serum IgE levels, positive skin test reactions to foods and airborne allergens, peripheral blood eosinophilia, and hypoalbuminemia and anemia associated with a protein-losing enteropathy. Part of the treatment is removal of food allergens for several months.

Infantile colic can be associated with certain foods. Some 2- to 4-week-old infants cry, develop abdominal distention, and assume the fetal position when they ingest certain foods, particularly cow's milk. This reaction occurs more commonly in formula-fed than breastfed infants and usually resolves on withdrawal of the offending food.

FOOD INTOLERANCE

Categories of food intolerance include toxic and pharmacologic reactions, metabolic reactions from enzyme deficiencies, and idiosyncratic and psychological reactions.

Toxic and Pharmacologic Reactions

Toxic reactions may occur as a consequence of naturally occurring toxic substances or because of microbial or chemical contamination of foods. Many common foods contain toxic substances but in very low amounts, so that adverse reactions from these chemicals are rare. Poisoning occurs from these toxic substances when (1) foods generally recognized as unsafe are eaten intentionally or accidentally, for example, *Psilocybe* or *Amanita* mushrooms, herbal teas, or puffer fish; (2) foods containing toxic chemicals are eaten, for example, green potatoes, which contain sola-

nine, or raw red kidney beans, which contain lectins and hemagglutinins and cause severe gastroenteritis; (3) some foods are eaten in large quantities, for example, beans, which cause increased flatulence from the lectins that are not removed by washing and cooking, or ingestion of large amounts of goitrogens from foods in the cabbage family in iodine-poor areas resulting in goiters; and (4) foods are ingested by persons taking monoamine oxidase inhibitors or isoniazid who may experience an anaphylactic-like reaction to contaminated fish or cheese because of a decreased ability to metabolize vasoactive substances.

Microbial and chemical contamination is the leading cause of adverse reactions to foods, and most of these reactions are to naturally occurring toxins. Other sources of chemicals that cause reactions to foods include insecticides, fungicides, fertilizers, preservatives, and flavor, or appearance enhancers. Aside from the chemical agents used to produce quality food products, the most common chemicals include sulfites, tartrazine, and monosodium glutamate.

Sulfites are used to control fermentation in wine, beer, and vinegar and to enhance the natural appearance of foods. Sulfites are also used in the processing of mushrooms, potatoes, and other foods. Patients with asthma who are sensitive to sulfites react with acute bronchospasm, but sulfites also have been implicated as a cause of anaphylaxis, urticaria, and angioedema. Tartrazine dye (FD&C yellow #5) has been implicated in triggering wheezing in some patients with asthma, particularly those who are aspirin-sensitive, and causing urticaria in other patients. Some studies have not confirmed these associations. Monosodium glutamate, a flavor enhancer, can cause headaches, a burning sensation along the back of the neck, chest tightness, nausea, and sweating. It has been reported to aggravate asthma in some patients. Aspartame, an artificial sweetening agent, may rarely cause urticaria and angioedema. The mechanism for this reaction is unknown.

Microbial contamination may result in poisoning because of the action of the microbial toxin or the microbial infection. Reactions from the toxins produced by microbes occur within minutes to several hours after ingestion, whereas infection may take several days to become evident. The most immediate reaction that occurs from microbial contamination results from high histamine levels in a food, for example, in canned fish or naturally fermented cheeses or in raw fish contaminated by *Proteus* or *Klebsiella* species. The bacteria decarboxylate the amino acid histidine, resulting in high levels of histamine in the food, which, when ingested, causes an anaphylaxis-like reaction. Fish typically involved are in the scromboid family and include tuna, skipjack, and mackerel. Reactions that occur several hours after ingestion, which consist primarily of vomiting and diarrhea, are more typical of staphylococcal food poisoning. Late but fatal reactions can occur with the ingestion of canned goods contaminated by *Clostridium botulinum.* Seafoods account for many toxins including ciguatera, an algal neurotoxin present in some reef fishes that ingest algae. Paralytic shellfish poisoning is caused by saxitoxin. Neurotoxic shellfish poisoning is associated with the ingestion of clams and oysters contaminated with brevitoxins of the algae *Ptychodiscus brevis.* These toxins become airborne when the algae bloom on the water surface and cause asthma by stimulating vagal nerve sodium channels causing release of acetylcholine at the neuromuscular junction. In addition to producing toxins, microbial agents may themselves reproduce and cause infections that resemble an adverse reaction to food. An example is *Campylobacter jejuni,* which causes diarrhea, gastroenteritis, and secondary lactase deficiency.

Many foods contain active pharmacologic agents, usually in sufficiently small quantities that ingestion causes no significant reaction. In patients susceptible to relatively small doses, various clinical syndromes have been recognized, however. Persons who are sensitive to vasoactive amines, which may be present in naturally fermented cheeses, wines and other fermented beverages, and chocolate, may be affected. Persons taking monoamine oxidase inhibitors are at particular risk. Chocolate contains theobromine and the vasoactive amine, phenylethylamine, which may cause headaches in some patients. Mothers who are breastfeeding and who ingest large amounts of chocolate may induce theophylline-like side-effects in their infants. Methylxanthines also are present in cola beverages, coffee, and tea, but patients may not fully appreciate the adverse effects of nervousness and insomnia that can occur from large amounts or prolonged use.

Taking large doses, especially megadoses, of vitamins can produce adverse effects. Excessive ingestion of vitamin A from any source can result in irritability, vomiting, increased intracranial pressure, and occasionally death. Excessive vitamin D intake can cause anorexia, nausea, vomiting, diarrhea, headaches, polyuria, and polydipsia. Vitamin K excess in pregnancy can result in hyperbilirubinemia in the premature infant. Broccoli in large quantity can provide enough vitamin K to counteract the pharmacologic effects of warfarin sodium.

Metabolic Disorders

The most common and significant metabolic reactions to food are caused by disaccharidase deficiencies. The symptoms of carbohydrate malabsorption, which include bloating, cramps, flatulence, and diarrhea, occur within a few hours of eating the food and can be erroneously attributed to food hypersensitivity. The most common defect is lactase deficiency, which occurs with the ingestion of milk (including human milk) or milk products that contain lactose. The small intestine cannot absorb a disaccharide, so the lactose passes unchanged to the large intestine. The fermentation of the lactose by bacteria and the osmotic effect in the bowel result in malabsorption. Normal persons have lower lactase levels after the third year of life, but approximately 80% of North American blacks, most Africans and Asians, Greenland Eskimos, and Israeli-area Arabs have a problem with lactase deficiency. This is in contrast to a 3% prevalence in the Danish population and 5% to 20% prevalence in North American whites. Lactase deficiency also can occur in otherwise normal individuals secondary to chronic bowel dysfunction or acute infectious diarrhea. In severe states, a secondary sucrase or maltase deficiency also may occur. Sucrase, fructase, and isomaltase deficiencies are much less common than primary lactase deficiency.

Tryptophan, an essential amino acid, is used by some persons as a food supplement. More than 1000 cases of eosinophilia–myalgia syndrome have developed in persons using tryptophan supplements. This syndrome of fatigue, myalgia, scleroderma-like skin changes, fasciitis, and eosinophilia is thought to be caused by an unknown contaminant in the tryptophan produced by one pharmaceutical manufacturer.

Idiosyncratic Reactions

Idiosyncratic food reactions are those that are reproducible even under blind circumstances but their mechanism is unknown. Ethanol causes immediate flushing and erythema in some Asians and even non-Asians may be affected rarely. Some affected patients may even have symptoms and signs that resemble an anaphylaxis-like syndrome. Although direct mast cell degranulation has been suggested as a cause, histamine has not been demonstrated as a mediator. Instead, the reaction may be related to an unusual metabolism of ethanol and the accumulation of acetaldehyde. As with most idiosyncratic reactions, once the mechanism is determined it will be reclassified.

Psychological Reactions

Psychological aversions to food are common, and such aversions can be associated with various symptoms including nausea, vomiting, and diarrhea. Food fads can be a particular problem and may stem from misinformation or poor education. Anxiety and depression can present as food allergy. The physician has to remain open-minded and objective in assessing patients with complaints associated with the ingestion of food. The physician also has to be cognizant that gastrointestinal symptoms that appear to be psychological sometimes can be caused by gastrointestinal illnesses such as gastroesophageal reflux, peptic ulcer, gallbladder or inflammatory bowel disease, pancreatic insufficiency, and neoplasias. Referral to an allergist may be needed to either rule in or to rule out specific food allergy versus adverse reactions on another causative basis. Avoidance and restrictive diets without sound evidence for such restriction is difficult for patients. There are potential problems of malnutrition if these diets are maintained

without adequate supplementation. In particular, children need to have the diagnosis confirmed to appropriately justify a restricted diet.

RESOURCES

- The Food Allergy Network
  10400 Eaton Place
  Suite 107
  Fairfax, VA 22030
  Tel: 703–691–3179
  Fax: 703–691–2713
  Web site: www.foodallergy.org

- American Academy of Allergy and Immunology (AAAAI)
  611 East Wells Street
  Milwaukee, WI 53202
  Tel: 414–272–6071
  Fax: 414–276–3349
  Web site: www.aaai.org

- American College of Allergy
  85 West Algonquin Road
  Suite 550
  Arlington, IL 60005
  Tel: 847–427–1200
  Fax: 847–427–1294
  E-mail: mail@acaai.org
  Web site: www.allergy.mcg.edu

Suggested Reading

Bock SA, Atkins FM: Patterns of food hypersensitivity during sixteen years of double-blind, placebo-controlled food challenges. J Pediatr 117:561–567, 1990

Ferguson A: Food sensitivity or self-deception? N Engl J Med 323:476–478, 1990

Jewett DL, Fein G, Breenberg MH: A double-blind study of symptom provocation to determine food sensitivity. N Engl J Med 323:429–433, 1990

Joint Task Force on Practice Parameters: Diagnosis and management of anaphylaxis. J Allergy Clin Immunol 101:S465–S528, 1998

Sampson HA: Peanut anaphylaxis. J Allergy Clin Immunol 86:1–3, 1990

Sampson HA, Broadbent KR, Bernhisel-Broadbent J: Spontaneous release of histamine from basophils and histamine-releasing factor in patients with atopic dermatitis and food hypersensitivity. N Engl J Med 321:228–232, 1989

Sampson HA, Scanion SM: Natural history of food hypersensitivity in children with atopic dermatitis. J Pediatr 115:23–27, 1989

Takeshi Y, Sato M, Nakamura A, et al: Plant defense-related enzymes and latex antigens. J Allergy Clin Immunol 101:379–385, 1998

Workshop on experimental methodology for clinical studies of adverse reactions to foods and food additives. J Allergy Clin Immunol 86:421–442, 1990

Chapter 19

Anaphylaxis

Mark M. Millar and Roy Patterson

Anaphylaxis is a severe systemic reaction caused by mediator release from immune system cells. Classically, the term anaphylaxis has been applied to the clinical manifestations of an IgE-mediated, immediate hypersensitivity reaction. A similar clinical picture, however, can be induced by other mechanisms, such as aspirin sensitivity, and has been termed an anaphylactoid reaction or a pseudoanaphylactic reaction. These reactions are clinically indistinguishable from IgE-mediated reactions, as they often involve many of the same mediators. The primary difference between the reactions is the mechanism of activation. In common practice, however, all these reactions are often called anaphylaxis, regardless of the mechanism.

The term anaphylaxis was created by Portier and Richet in 1902 after experiments in which they attempted to immunize dogs to toxin of the Portuguese man-of-war. They discovered that sensitized dogs developed fatal reactions with subsequent toxin exposure. This outcome was in contrast with the process of immunization they had hoped to achieve, and they applied the term anaphylaxis (Greek: *ana* meaning backward, *phylaxis* meaning protection).

The true incidence and prevalence of anaphylaxis are not known. In an emergency room setting estimates range from 1 per 1500 to 1 per 2300 patients. In hospitalized patients estimates of anaphylaxis range from 1 per 1400 to 1 per 5100 patients. For the general populace, estimates cover a wider range. A population in Denmark was found to have an incidence of anaphylaxis of 3.2 cases per 100,000 people per year, whereas a population in Canada had 0.04 cases per 100,000 people per year. The mortality rate of anaphylaxis also is not exactly known, but it has been estimated to cause approximately 500 deaths per year.

Anaphylaxis is a medical emergency that requires immediate treatment. Evaluation of a patient with anaphylaxis requires a thorough history to determine if an external inciting factor is involved, as future avoidance measures are essential. In some patients an external agent is not involved, and these patients have idiopathic anaphylaxis.

PATHOPHYSIOLOGY

Anaphylaxis and anaphylactoid reactions are the final clinical manifestations that can result when different aspects of the immune system are activated. The reactions appear similar, because common mediators can ultimately be involved. The immune system cells that release these mediators, and the mechanisms through which they are activated, however, can be very different. Mast cells and IgE antibody play a major role in allergen-induced *anaphylactic* reactions. A variety of different mechanisms can be involved in *anaphylactoid* reactions. Table 19–1 lists the mechanisms of activation in anaphylactic and anaphylactoid reactions.

Anaphylactic Reactions

IgE-Mediated, Immediate Hypersensitivity

IgE-mediated hypersensitivity is synonymous with type I, or immediate, hypersensitivity reactions. In these reactions a foreign substance is recognized by the immune system and binds

Table 19–1. **Mechanisms of Anaphylactic and Anaphylactoid Reactions**

Anaphylaxis

Immediate/type I/IgE-mediated
  hypersensitivity
  Foods
  Medications
  Latex
  Venom
  Allergen immunotherapy

Anaphylactoid Reactions

Direct, nonspecific stimulation of mast cells
  Opiates
  Radiocontrast media
  Exercise
  Physical factors
Irregular metabolism of arachidonic acid
  Aspirin
  Nonsteroidal anti-inflammatory drugs
Complement activation
  Cytotoxic reactions
  Immune aggregate reactions
  Alternative complement pathway activation
Other mechanisms
  Contact (kallikrein-kinin) system

to IgE antibody. Cross-linking of IgE antibody with the foreign substance can lead to activation of IgE receptors on mast cells, with subsequent internal activation of mast cell mechanisms. The mast cell, once activated, can release pre-formed and newly synthesized mediators, as well as a variety of cytokines. Preformed mediators include histamine, heparin, tryptase, and chymase. Newly generated mediators include leukotrienes (LTB4, LTC4) and prostaglandins (PGD2). These mediators act on target tissues to produce the symptoms and signs seen in anaphylaxis.

Foreign substances that can interact with IgE antibodies include proteins, haptens, and polysaccharides. Over 100 different agents have been reported to cause anaphylactic reactions. A partial list of some of these agents, by category, is presented in Table 19–2. Some commonly recognized offending agents include foods, medications, Hymenoptera venom, and latex.

Anaphylactoid Reactions

Direct, Nonspecific Mast Cell Stimulation

Although mast cells can be triggered by specific sensitivity to immunologically recognized substances, mast cells can also be triggered in a nonspecific manner. Although the exact mechanism is not known, it is thought that mast cells can be activated to release their contents by direct stimulation, without the presence of IgE. This type of reaction can occur on first exposure and does not require prior sensitization. Possible causes for direct mast cell activation include the following:

- Activation of IgE receptor (Fc ε RI) without IgE
- Cytokines
- Drug effects (e.g., radiocontrast media)
- Physical factors (e.g., cold temperature)

Table 19–2. **Agents That Can Induce IgE-Mediated Anaphylactic Reactions**

Foods
  Milk
  Egg
  Tree nuts
  Legumes (peanut)
  Seafood (fish, crustaceans, mollusks)
  Soy
  Wheat

Medications
  Antibiotics
    Penicillins
    Cephalosporins
    Tetracycline
    Clindamycin
    Nitrofurantoin
  Hormones
    Insulin
    Parathyroid hormone
    Adrenocorticotropic hormone
  Enzymes
    Chymotrypsin
    Chymopapain
    Penicillinase

Venoms
  Hymenoptera venoms
    Apid venoms (bumblebee, honeybee)
    Vespid venoms (hornet, wasp, yellow jacket)
    Fire ant venom

Blood Products
  Foreign serum
  Intravenous immunoglobulin
  Antithymocyte globulin

Latex

Other
  Dextran
  Ethylene oxide (dialysis membranes)
  Vaccines
  Vitamins

Irregular Arachidonic Acid Metabolism

Some individuals develop an anaphylactoid reaction after exposure to aspirin, or related nonsteroidal anti-inflammatory drugs (NSAIDs). The normal effect of aspirin is to block the cyclooxygenase pathway of arachidonic acid metabolism. Other NSAIDs can also block the cyclooxygenase pathway (Fig. 19–1). In certain individuals, disrupting this pathway can lead to adverse events. When the cyclooxygenase pathway is blocked in these individuals, arachidonic acid metabolism is shunted to the lipoxygenase pathway. This shift leads to the production of leukotrienes (LTC4, LTD4, LTE4), which can produce bronchoconstriction and increased vascular permeability. These effects are clinically identical to an anaphylactic reaction. They do not involve specific immune recognition and IgE antibody, however, so they are termed anaphylactoid reactions.

Complement Activation

A variety of stimuli can lead to complement system activation. Activation in certain cases can lead to the production of complement fragments called anaphylatoxins, so named because of their ability to produce reactions mimicking anaphylaxis. The anaphylatoxins include the complement components C3a and C5a. These components have the ability to activate mast cells and cause mediator release independent of IgE.

One situation in which this release can occur is in cytotoxic reactions. In these reactions, other types of antibodies besides IgE bind to antigen fixed to a cell wall. The antigen–antibody immune complexes can lead to complement activation, production of anaphylatoxins, and subsequent mast cell activation. An example is a transfusion reaction, in which patients react to foreign blood cells. These blood cells bear antigen that is fixed to the cell wall and can be recognized by circulating antibodies. It should be noted, however, that this is only one possible mechanism involved in transfusion reactions.

Another situation leading to complement activation occurs in the presence of immune aggregates. Antigens and antibody molecules also can bind to one another independent of cells and form immune complexes. These free-

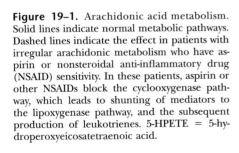

Figure 19–1. Arachidonic acid metabolism. Solid lines indicate normal metabolic pathways. Dashed lines indicate the effect in patients with irregular arachidonic metabolism who have aspirin or nonsteroidal anti-inflammatory drug (NSAID) sensitivity. In these patients, aspirin or other NSAIDs block the cyclooxygenase pathway, which leads to shunting of mediators to the lipoxygenase pathway, and the subsequent production of leukotrienes. 5-HPETE = 5-hydroperoxyeicosatetraenoic acid.

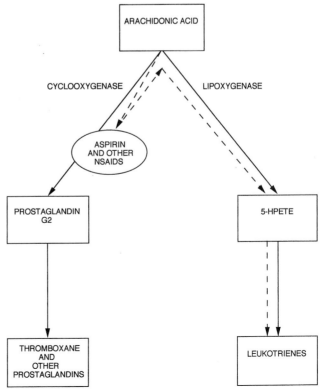

floating antigen–antibody immune complexes can later deposit on cell walls and result in complement activation and the production of anaphylatoxins. This is another mechanism through which transfusion reactions can occur.

A third possible mechanism involving complement is through the alternative complement pathway. Although immune complexes can activate the classical complement pathway and production of anaphylatoxins, other agents may stimulate the alternative complement pathway. Anaphylactoid reactions to dialysis membranes may occur through this mechanism.

Other Mechanisms

It should be noted that all the mechanisms leading to anaphylactic or anaphylactoid reactions are not known. Other mechanisms and mediators may be involved. Some other mechanisms may involve neuropeptides, the contact (kallikrein–kinin) system, or mediators involved in the coagulation cascade.

It should also be noted that any one agent may cause a reaction through different mechanisms in different individuals. For example, radiocontrast material may cause direct mast cell release, complement activation, or contact (kallikrein-kinin) system activation. Dialysis membranes may be involved in IgE-mediated reactions against the ethylene oxide sterilizing agent or may cause activation of the complement system. Foreign serum may cause an IgE-mediated anaphylactic reaction, a cytotoxic anaphylactoid reaction, or an immune aggregate anaphylactoid reaction.

Not only can a single agent lead to a reaction through multiple potential mechanisms, but conversely, a single anaphylactic event may have multiple potential inciting agents. An example is intraoperative anaphylaxis. During a surgical procedure with anesthesia, a patient is exposed to a wide variety of agents. The first step is to determine if anaphylaxis has indeed occurred. Shock, rashes, or cardiac and pulmonary dysfunction can occur for other reasons in the surgical patient. For example, shock can occur because of hypovolemia or sepsis, and rashes may occur because of infection or cutaneous drug reactions. The second step involves identifying all the agents the patient has received. The list of possible inciting agents is extensive. This list includes induction agents, anesthetics, antibiotics, blood products, plasma volume expanders, protamine, opiates, and latex. Exposure to these products and their temporal relation to the event can help in identifying the causative agent. Further diagnostic testing may be necessary to determine the causative agent.

Finally, it should be noted that patients can have idiopathic anaphylaxis. In these cases, patients do not have an apparent external trigger. Although the mechanism is not known, an internal problem is speculated to cause reactions in these patients. One theory postulates that affected patients have autoantibodies to IgE, which leads to IgE cross-linking and mast cell activation. Another theory is that affected patients have autoantibodies to the IgE receptor (FcεRI), which could cause activation of the receptor and subsequent mast cell activation. A third theory speculates on the involvement of histamine releasing factors (HRF) and histamine release inhibitory factors (HRIF). These substances are known to affect mediator release from basophils and mast cells and are thought to regulate the intrinsic reactivity of these cells. As their names imply, HRF can lead to mediator release, particularly histamine, from basophils and mast cells, and conversely, HRIF can inhibit these cells from releasing mediators. Patients with idiopathic anaphylaxis may have an imbalance between HRF and HRIF and be susceptible to mast cell activation.

Mediators

Mediators released in an anaphylactic or anaphylactoid reaction may originate from a variety of cell types. Cell types involved include mast cells, basophils, monocytes or macrophages, eosinophils, neutrophils, and platelets. Mediators involved include histamine, leukotrienes, prostaglandins, bradykinin, platelet activating factor (PAF), anaphylatoxins, and others.

The mediators released act on smooth muscle cells, blood vessels, nerves, and other immune system cells ultimately to produce the

Table 19–3. **Mediators, Their Actions, and Their Target Site Manifestations**

Mediators	Actions	Manifestations
Histamine Leukotrienes Prostaglandins Platelet activating factor (PAF) Anaphylatoxins Bradykinin	Vasodilatation Vascular permeability	Airway edema Gastrointestinal edema Hypotension Urticaria
Histamine Leukotrienes Prostaglandins Thromboxane PAF Anaphylatoxins Bradykinin	Smooth muscle contraction	Bronchospasm Gastrointestinal motility
Histamine Leukotrienes Prostaglandins Anaphylatoxins Bradykinin	Mucus production	Rhinorrhea Bronchorrhea
Tryptase Kallikrein-kinin	Complement activation (anaphylatoxins)	Propagation of reaction
Leukotriene (LTB4) PAF Anaphylatoxin (C5a) Cytokines Eosinophil chemotactic factor (ECF) Neutrophil chemotactic factor (NCF)	Chemotaxis (cell recruitment)	Propagation of reaction

clinical manifestations of anaphylaxis. The primary effects include the following:

- Smooth muscle contraction leading to bronchoconstriction
- Vasodilatation leading to hypotension
- Vascular leakage leading to tissue swelling and hypotension

Table 19–3 lists a variety of mediators, their actions, and their subsequent target site manifestations.

CLINICAL PRESENTATION

Anaphylaxis is a systemic process and can affect virtually any organ system. The presenting symptoms and signs may vary in different individuals, and may vary in subsequent reactions in the same individual. Possible symptoms and signs, with the organs affected, are listed in Table 19–4. The most common signs are urticaria and angioedema. Not all patients develop cutaneous findings, however, and severe reactions may still occur without cutaneous manifestations.

Timing

Symptoms can occur within minutes, and the majority of reactions occur within 1 hour.

Table 19–4. **Symptoms and Signs in Anaphylaxis**

Site	Symptoms	Signs
Integument	Itching Burning	Flushing Rash Urticaria Angioedema
Oropharynx	Dysphagia Dysarthria Dyspnea	Lip edema Tongue edema Pharyngeal edema Laryngeal edema
Respiratory system	Cough Dyspnea Wheeze	Bronchospasm Pulmonary edema
Cardiovascular system	Chest pain Dyspnea Dizziness	Hypotension Arrhythmia Syncope
Gastrointestinal system	Nausea Abdominal pain	Vomiting Diarrhea
Neurologic system	Dizziness Headache	Syncope Seizure

Symptoms may not appear until 2 to 4 hours with some routes of exposure. It has been speculated that the more immediate the reaction, the more severe the reaction. Late reactions, however, still have the potential to be severe and life threatening.

Although the initial event may occur quickly and resolve with treatment, patients can have a recurrence of symptoms hours later. This occurrence is termed the biphasic effect. It is known that the immune cells originally involved in the reaction can release mediators and cytokines. These agents may have a prolonged effect on the original cells or recruit other cells and activate them to become involved in perpetuating the reaction. The continued effect of these agents can lead to a recurrence of symptoms and the second part of the biphasic response. Resolution of the immediate event, either spontaneously or with treatment, should not be taken as definite completion of the event. The patient should continue to be monitored for several hours owing to the possibility of return of symptoms.

It is also important to consider that patients may have protracted anaphylaxis. Some patients develop symptoms that do not respond immediately to treatment and may last for hours. These patients require hospitalization, close monitoring, and intensive therapy.

Severity

Factors influencing the severity of the reaction include underlying medical conditions and concomitant medication use. Regarding medical conditions, patients with underlying pulmonary or cardiac disease will not tolerate the insult of anaphylaxis as well as normal individuals. Examples include patients with underlying asthma or coronary artery disease.

Regarding concomitant medication use, patients who take certain medications may have more difficulty tolerating anaphylaxis or the standard treatments for anaphylaxis. Examples of such medications include beta-adrenergic blocking medications, angiotensin-converting enzyme inhibitors, and monoamine oxidase inhibitors. Beta-adrenergic blocking medications are problematic because they can interfere with the actions of epinephrine, a standard treatment for anaphylaxis.

Beta-adrenergic blocking medications should be used cautiously in patients receiving immunotherapy and in those at high risk for anaphylaxis.

Angiotensin-converting enzyme inhibitors also can be problematic. These agents prevent formation of angiotensin II, a substance that normally acts to help compensate cardiovascular conditions during an anaphylactic event. As a result, patients taking angiotensin-converting enzyme inhibitors may not tolerate anaphylaxis as well. It has been noted that patients receiving Hymenoptera immunotherapy who are also on these agents may be at increased risk for anaphylaxis. The newer class of related medications, the angiotensin II receptor antagonists, also block angiotensin II action. Although experience with these agents is limited, in theory they also may pose a risk for patients with a history of anaphylaxis.

Finally, monoamine oxidase inhibitors are another class of medications that can be problematic. These medications interfere with the metabolism of epinephrine and can increase its effects beyond those desired, or needed, in treating anaphylaxis.

Fatal Reactions

Patients with severe reactions can progress to fatality. Death in most cases is due to airway obstruction or cardiovascular failure. In regard to airway obstruction, it may be due to upper or lower airway narrowing. In the upper airway, extravasated fluid accumulation in the submucosal tissues can produce laryngeal edema or pharyngeal edema and can lead to total closure. Airway obstruction also can occur in the lower airway at the level of the bronchial passages. Smooth muscle spasm, submucosal swelling, and collection of mucous secretions can combine to block these passageways.

In regard to cardiovascular failure, system collapse can occur for several reasons. First, mediator release can lead to extreme vasodilatation and fluid extravasation, depleting intravascular volume. This can produce profound hypotension. Second, stress on the myocardium can lead to myocardial hypoxia, myocardial infarction, or dysrhythmia. Any of these could lead to a drop in cardiac output. It is also possible for a combination of these events to occur and lead to collapse of the cardiovascular system.

Risk Factors

There are no specific associations between race, geography, or season with risk for anaphylaxis. A definite risk factor is repeat exposure to a known offending agent. Also, parenteral administration of a known offending agent is more likely to produce a reaction, when compared with oral administration. Further, repeated and interrupted exposures to an agent may increase the likelihood of developing sensitivity.

DIAGNOSIS

Anaphylaxis is usually a dramatic event and easily diagnosed. This is not true in all cases, however, and physicians need to use the patient's history, objective physical findings, and appropriate laboratory testing.

The history should be consistent with the typical symptoms, as listed in Table 19–4. Patients may describe sudden itching or the sudden appearance of a rash. They may experience wheezing or shortness of breath. They may have swelling of the lips, tongue, or throat and may describe difficulty speaking, swallowing, or breathing. Patients can have episodes of chest pain or chest tightness. They may describe abdominal pain, nausea, vomiting, or diarrhea. They also may experience dizziness or frank loss of consciousness.

In addition to a patient's subjective report of complaints, it is important to examine him or her for objective findings and to document such findings. These findings can include rash or urticaria; visible lip, tongue, or throat swelling; decreased blood pressure; increased respiratory rate or heart rate; abnormal pulse oximetry or arterial blood gas findings; wheezing on respiratory examination; and altered mental status.

Once a diagnosis of anaphylaxis is made, it is important to search for a possible causative agent. The history should explore for involvement of the following agents:

- Medications, both prescription and over-the-counter preparations
- Foods
- Insect stings
- Latex exposure
- Exercise
- Physical factors

For any of these factors to be the causative agent it must be temporally related to the event. Exposure should be within several hours before the event for it to be considered a causative agent. Further evidence supporting causation is the presence of verifiable sensitivity to the agent. Verification can be done through radioallergosorbent testing (RAST), skin testing, or test dose challenge. RAST is a serum test that can identify the presence of IgE antibody to a specific agent. A correlating history is needed to warrant its use. Its validity is limited by the fact that it is an *in vitro* test and does not give absolute information on clinical sensitivity.

Another approach is skin testing. Skin testing is done by prick or intradermal application. In skin prick testing a drop of extract containing the antigen in question is placed on the skin, and the skin surface is punctured with a needle. In skin intradermal testing a small quantity of extract (usually 0.02 ml) is injected under the very top layer of skin to form a bubble. Test sites are interpreted after 15 to 20 minutes. A wheal-and-flare reaction is consistent with the presence of IgE-mediated hypersensitivity. These test results must be interpreted in the presence of positive and negative controls (usually histamine and saline, respectively). Causes for false-positive skin test responses include dermatographism or latex exposure (in latex-allergic individuals exposed to latex during testing). Causes for false-negative skin test results include recent antihistamine use or improper testing technique with failure to puncture the skin. Standardized skin testing is available for foods (prick test), Hymenoptera venoms (prick and intradermal tests), fire ant venom (prick and intradermal tests), and penicillin (prick and intradermal tests). It should be emphasized that skin testing should only be pursued if the history reasonably suggests the agent as a possible cause. Random skin testing in search of positive reactions, without a correlating history, is of little value. When skin testing is available, it is preferred over RAST testing as it is more sensitive. Further, it is an *in vivo* test and is considered more valid in determining clinical sensitivity.

The other testing method to consider is provocative test dosing. This method entails administering gradually increasing doses of the suspected agent in an attempt to provoke a reaction. Although this type of testing is the most clinically useful, it is also the most dangerous. It may provoke a repeat anaphylactic reaction and has the potential for fatality. The risks and benefits must be carefully examined, and if the risk–benefit ratio argues against test dosing, its use is discouraged. When available and warranted, skin testing is the test of choice to verify sensitivity to an agent.

In some patients the history and objective findings support a diagnosis of anaphylaxis, but no external agent can be found. These patients are suspected of having an internal cause and have idiopathic anaphylaxis.

In other patients, the diagnosis of anaphylaxis is in doubt either because of an inconsistent history or lack of objective findings. One strategy is to require the patient to go to the emergency room for any event in an effort to obtain objective evidence. Another strategy is to use further laboratory testing. Laboratory tests that can help confirm a mast cell–mediated event include histamine and tryptase levels. Histamine is released quickly and has a short half-life. As a result it is difficult to detect in serum but may be found in urine collection after the event. Tryptase is another mediator that is released and can be measured. Tryptase peaks 60 to 90 minutes after the event and can persist to 12 hours. These tests are not universally available and are typically not done except in confounding cases. In such complex cases it is also helpful to explore the differential diagnosis.

DIFFERENTIAL DIAGNOSIS

Other conditions can mimic or give the appearance of anaphylaxis. Because anaphylaxis can be a fatal condition, it is important to determine the correct diagnosis. Table 19–5 lists other conditions to be considered in patients with symptoms suggestive of anaphylaxis.

Table 19–5. Differential Diagnosis of Anaphylactic Symptoms

Flushing Syndromes
> Carcinoid syndrome
> Postmenopausal
> Alcohol-sulfonyreal reaction
> Medullary carcinoma of the thyroid
> Red-man syndrome (vancomycin)
> Idiopathic flushing

Histamine Syndromes
> Systemic mastocytosis
> Basophilic leukemia

Syncope
> Vasovagal reaction
> Cardiac disease
> Neurogenic disease
> Cerebrovascular disease
> Situational syncope
> Psychogenic

Shock
> Cardiogenic
> Neurogenic
> Hypovolemic

Restaurant Syndromes
> Scromboid and other fish poisoning
> Sulfites
> Toxigenic

Nonorganic
> Hyperventilation or panic attacks
> Vocal cord dysfunction
> Munchausen's stridor
> Undifferentiated somatoform idiopathic anaphylaxis (US-IA)

Other Diseases
> Pheochromocytoma
> Hereditary angioedema
> Acute myocardial infarction
> Pulmonary embolism
> Epilepsy
> Foreign body aspiration
> Urticaria and asthma
> Hypoglycemia
> VIPoma

In determining a diagnosis in a confusing case, several avenues can be explored. Additional past history can be helpful. History of any previous events can help to determine if a pattern of exposure exists. Reports from witnesses of previous events or medical professionals involved in previous events can be helpful. Objective findings from the current event, or previous events, are also important. This often entails obtaining prior emergency room or hospitalization records.

Laboratory testing may be helpful in identifying other conditions. Examples include the following:

- Patients with carcinoid can have an elevated blood serotonin level or elevated urinary 5-hydroxyindoleacetic acid (5-HIAA) level
- Patients with systemic mastocytosis can have an increased number of mast cells on skin biopsy specimens of urticaria pigmentosa lesions or on bone marrow biopsy
- Patients with pheochromocytoma can have elevated urinary metanephrine, catecholamine, or vanillylmandelic acid (VMA) levels
- Patients with hereditary angioedema can have abnormal complement results, with a decreased C4 level and decreased C1-esterase inhibitor level
- Patients with vocal cord dysfunction can have inappropriate adduction of the vocal cords during bronchoscopic evaluation

It should be noted that these conditions are relatively rare, and testing for these conditions should be prompted by a plausible history.

TREATMENT

Anaphylaxis is a medical emergency and requires immediate treatment. The cornerstone of treatment is epinephrine. Although some patients and even physicians are fearful of using epinephrine, withholding it in a case of anaphylaxis is more dangerous than administering it. The adult dose of epinephrine is 0.3 ml of a 1:1000 concentration. In a child, the dose is typically 0.15 ml for ages 12 and under (or 0.01 ml/kg). It should be administered subcutaneously (SQ) or intramuscularly (IM), in a large muscle group such as the deltoid, quadriceps, or gluteus. If anaphylaxis is caused by an injection or sting and it is in a large muscle group, epinephrine can be given at the site of the sting to help slow antigen absorption. Also, a tourniquet can be applied proximal to the injection or sting site to further slow antigen absorption.

Patients should be assessed according to standard cardiopulmonary resuscitation protocol. The patient should be evaluated for the ABCs (airway, breathing, circulation), and vital signs should be measured. Emergency personnel should be notified. Further measures include supine positioning of the patient with legs elevated, intravenous fluid administration, oxygen supplementation, and use of antihistamines such as diphenhydramine.

Patients who have sustained symptoms should receive repeat doses of epinephrine and antihistamine. Patients also should be given corticosteroids. This is for two reasons. First, although corticosteroids will not act immediately, they may help prevent prolongation of the reaction by inhibiting further mediator release and inhibiting further mediator action. Second, some patients can have a biphasic response, as discussed earlier, and corticosteroids may help prevent a recurrence that can be seen several hours later.

Patients who do not improve or who show progression of their symptoms require treatment in an intensive care unit. Patients may require aminophylline for bronchospasm. In extreme cases, they may require intubation or tracheostomy. Further, venous access may be needed for fluid administration, and in severe cases, patients may require pressors for support of blood pressure.

Patients who are taking a beta-adrenergic blocking medication may require additional treatment. Glucagon can be used in an emergency for patients taking beta-adrenergic blockers. For bradycardia, atropine can be used in an emergency situation. A summary of the treatment for anaphylaxis is presented in Table 19–6.

For patients with limited reactions, these extreme measures may not be needed. Patients should still seek medical attention and proceed to the nearest emergency room. Patients should be treated with epinephrine and an antihistamine to counter the acute symptoms. They should receive corticosteroids to counter any prolonged effect and a possible biphasic response. Patients should be monitored for several hours at minimum and be considered for overnight observation in a hospital setting. Patients may require a short course of prednisone at discharge.

FURTHER MANAGEMENT

The continued management of a patient after an anaphylactic event depends on a variety of factors, including the severity of the reaction, the cause of the reaction, the age and medical

Table 19–6.   **Treatment of Anaphylaxis**

Epinephrine

Epinephrine 1:1000 as 0.3 ml dose SQ or IM
(in children 0.15 ml or 0.01 ml/kg)

General Measures

ABCs (airway, breathing, circulation)
Measure vital signs
Alert emergency services
Lay patient flat and raise legs
Intravenous fluid
Oxygen
Prepare for intubation

Medications (Adult Doses)

Diphenhydramine 25 to 50 mg po or IM or IV
Hydrocortisone sodium succinate 200 mg IV
Epinephrine repeated every 15 minutes as
needed, for 2 doses

For Bronchospasm

Epinephrine, if not already done
Hydrocortisone, if not already done
Aminophylline 6 mg/kg IV up to 500 mg, over
20 minutes
Intubation or tracheostomy, as required

**For Hypotension (Systolic Blood Pressure <90
mm Hg)**

Two IV lines with IV fluid wide open
Dopamine 400 mg in 500 ml D5W, infuse to
systolic blood pressure of 90 mm Hg—then
titrate
Norepinephrine 4 mg in 1000 ml D5W, infuse
to systolic blood pressure of 90 mm
Hg—then titrate

**For Patients on Beta-Adrenergic Blocking
Medications**

Glucagon 1 mg bolus IV; then 1 to 5 mg/hour
IV infusion
Atropine for bradycardia—0.3 to 0.5 mg IV
every 10 minutes to maximum of 2 mg

---

condition of the patient, and additional factors.

The basics of further management include education regarding avoidance measures to prevent further exposure and chance of a repeat reaction. It also includes instructions on the self-administration of epinephrine for emergency situations. Epinephrine comes in two commercial preparations, which the patient can keep at home or carry when traveling. One is the EpiPen (Dey Labs; Napa, Ca), a prefilled automatic injection device that delivers 0.3 mg epinephrine (1:1000 as a 0.3 ml dose) for EpiPen regular, and as a 0.15 mg dose for EpiPen Jr. The other preparation is the AnaKit (Bayer; West Haven, CT), which includes a prefilled syringe containing epinephrine 1:1000 and contains enough for two doses of 0.3 ml.

Other efforts to help reduce the risk of a fatal outcome include the following:

- Medical records should be clearly labeled noting the patient's sensitivity
- The patient should carry identification noting the sensitivity, either by emergency bracelet or medical card
- Management of other medical conditions should be optimized, particularly cardiac and respiratory conditions
- Complicating medications, such as beta-adrenergic blocking medications or angiotensin-converting enzyme inhibitors, should be replaced with alternatives

While these general rules apply to all patients, individual patients will also require individualized advice based on their specific sensitivity.

Food Allergy

Patients with food allergies must practice strict avoidance of the food. They must learn to read labels of food products diligently. They must become knowledgeable on the alternate names foods can be given to help in avoidance measures. For example, milk-allergic patients need to be aware that milk protein can also be listed as casein, caseinate, lactalbumin, lactose, or whey.

Patients must also be careful when eating away from home, where they have less control over preparation of the food. At restaurants they must read menus carefully and be prepared to ask questions regarding ingredients. Patients also need to recognize that they can still be exposed to a food even if it is not in the food they ordered. Utensils and cookware at restaurants can be used in the preparation of different dishes, and there can be cross-contamination of foods through this shared hardware. Patients need to carry emergency medications with them at all times.

Counseling with a dietician is helpful, especially in patients who have trouble meeting their nutritional requirements. Patients may wish to become involved in local or national food allergy associations. These organizations can help with updates on changes in manufactured food products and mislabelings. They also can provide social support and help with nutrition ideas.

Younger patients with food allergies will

require special instructions while attending school. School personnel need to be informed regarding the patient's sensitivity and educated on avoidance strategies. An emergency plan should also be reviewed with school personnel.

Medication Allergy

Patients with medication allergies need to be educated on the multiple names of the medication to which they are sensitive. They also need education on any possible combination drugs that could contain the medication. They need to be aware of other medications that can be cross-reactive so they can avoid these medications as well. For example, patients with penicillin allergy need to be aware of the multiple drug names for penicillin derivatives and of their potential cross-reactivity with cephalosporins.

It should be stressed that patients should have some form of notification regarding their medication sensitivity in the case of an emergency. This notification can be in the form of an emergency alert bracelet or wallet card.

Hymenoptera Allergy

Patients with venom sensitivity require skin testing to confirm the species of Hymenoptera to which they are allergic. Suspects include not only flying insects such as bees, wasps, and hornets but also fire ants. Patients should receive immunotherapy because it can significantly reduce the risk of anaphylaxis with subsequent exposure. The risk of anaphylaxis with subsequent venom exposure is approximately 50% without immunotherapy; the risk is decreased to 5% to 10% after immunotherapy. Immunotherapy also has been shown to be beneficial for patients with fire ant sensitivity. Patients should be educated on avoidance techniques. These techniques include the following:

- Destroying any insect nests near the home (this should not be done by sensitive individuals themselves to avoid inadvertent exposure)
- Wearing protective clothing (long sleeves, pants, protective footwear)
- Avoiding brightly colored clothing and clothing with floral prints
- Avoiding perfumes, cologne, and fragrant cosmetics
- Using caution near parks, woods, picnic areas, and garbage collection areas
- Using insect repellant

Avoidance techniques for fire ants are similar and include the following:

- Destroying fire ant mounds
- Wearing protective footwear (avoid going barefoot)
- Wearing gloves when gardening

Latex Allergy

Patients with latex allergy require education on the products that contain exposed latex. These products include medical devices and some toys. Patients need to notify all medical personnel they interact with of their sensitivity, and latex allergy should be clearly labeled on their medical records. Dental and surgical procedures need to be performed in latex-free environments.

Radiocontrast Media Sensitivity

Patients with radiocontrast media sensitivity need to alert all medical personnel of their sensitivity any time they have a procedure performed. Their sensitivity should be clearly marked in their medical records. In some individuals, repeat administration of radiocontrast media is medically necessary for diagnostic testing. In such cases, patients should receive nonionic contrast, if possible. These patients should also receive preprocedure treatment. The regimen for preprocedure treatment is as follows:

- prednisone 50 mg orally
  13 hours prior to procedure
  7 hours prior to procedure
  1 hour prior to procedure
- diphenhydramine 50 mg, orally or intramuscularly
  1 hour prior to procedure
- ephedrine 25 mg orally, or albuterol 4 mg orally 1 hour prior to procedure (withhold

either if patient has a history of cardiac disease or hypertension)

Patients who have reactions even with preprocedure treatment require consultation with an allergy-immunology specialist.

Patients with radiocontrast media sensitivity are often suspected of having shellfish or iodine sensitivity. The opposite association also has been suspected. This association is erroneous. Patients with radiocontrast media sensitivity are not necessarily shellfish- or iodine-sensitive, and patients with shellfish sensitivity are not necessarily sensitive to radiocontrast media.

Aspirin or Nonsteroidal Anti-Inflammatory Drug Sensitivity

Patients with aspirin or NSAID reactivity need to be aware of the multiple names of the medication to which they are sensitive. They also need to be educated on any possible combination drugs that contain the agent. For example, patients sensitive to aspirin need to avoid aspirin and the multiple brand name versions of the medication. They also must avoid combination medications that contain aspirin. Aspirin is often found in cold remedies and other over-the-counter preparations. Some patients with aspirin sensitivity or NSAID sensitivity may have cross-reactivity with other NSAIDs. This is not the case for most patients, but as a precaution patients should avoid this entire class of medications because of the possibility of cross-reactivity. If a related medication is essential, patients can undergo test dosing to determine if they are also sensitive to that particular medication. This test should be done by an allergy-immunology specialist experienced with test dosing protocols.

Allergen Immunotherapy

Patients receiving allergen immunotherapy have the potential to develop reactions after injections. Risk factors for a reaction include the following:

- History of previous reactions
- Starting a new vial

- Excessively rapid increase in dose
- Unstable asthma

Although systemic reactions to allergen immunotherapy are rare, efforts must be made to minimize the risk involved. Appropriate safety measures include the following:

- Allergen immunotherapy should be administered only by trained personnel in a medical facility
- A system of checks should be in place to avoid any clerical or dosage errors
- Patients should have an evaluation of their general medical condition and a review of their medication list for any possible complicating medications before starting immunotherapy
- Patients with asthma should be questioned before receiving an injection as to their respiratory status. If the patient is symptomatic or has abnormal lung function, the injection may need to be withheld until better control of asthma is achieved
- Emergency medications should be available to treat a possible systemic reaction
- After an injection, patients must wait in the clinic for 20 to 30 minutes, to be observed for any reaction
- In the case of local or systemic reactions, immunotherapy dosage and frequency schedules must be reviewed and adjusted appropriately

Exercise-Induced Anaphylaxis

Patients may develop episodes of anaphylaxis after exercise or in situations of eating before exercise. In some patients this reaction occurs if any food is eaten before exercise, whereas in other patients it is relevant only with a particular food before exercise.

Patients must be evaluated to ensure that they do not have other exercise-induced disorders. Other possible problems associated with exercise include cholinergic urticaria, exercise-induced asthma, and arrhythmias or heart failure in patients with cardiovascular disease.

Patients with exercise-induced anaphylaxis must carry emergency medications with them. They should exercise with a partner in case of an event. They also should carry identification noting their condition. Often patients will have early symptoms heralding the onset of a

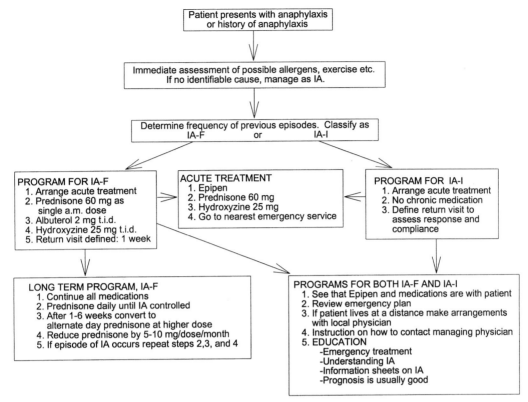

Figure 19–2. Algorithm for assessment and initiation of management of idiopathic anaphylaxis (IA) of the frequent (F) or infrequent (I) types when seen at first patient visit. (From Patterson R [ed]: Idiopathic Anaphylaxis. Providence, RI, OceanSide, 1997, p 22; with permission.)

systemic reaction. In such cases, patients must know to stop exercising with the appearance of symptoms. For patients with food-associated exercise-induced anaphylaxis, they must not exercise for 4 to 6 hours after eating.

Idiopathic Anaphylaxis

A subset of anaphylaxis patients can have isolated or recurrent episodes of anaphylaxis with no apparent cause. These patients have no identifiable external agent triggering their reactions. These patients have idiopathic anaphylaxis. An internal cause is suspected in these patients, as reviewed earlier. This entity has been well documented, and the incidence of the disease is estimated at 20,000 to 30,000 cases in the United States. Protocols for management of idiopathic anaphylaxis have been developed and have been used successfully. Figure 19–2 reviews the protocols for treatment of patients with idiopathic anaphylaxis.

Because patients with idiopathic anaphy-laxis have no obvious trigger, they can develop episodes unpredictably. It is essential for these patients to carry emergency medication at all times in the event of an episode. These patients are instructed on the use of emergency medications and are instructed to proceed directly to an emergency room after using the medications.

Some patients, and even some physicians, are reluctant to believe these reactions are not triggered by an external agent. They may pursue analysis of unlikely external agents. Taken to the extreme, this can be detrimental to the patient and to the other physicians involved in the patient's care. Although all patients should be evaluated for external triggers, this should be done within reason, to prevent further delay in treatment.

WHEN TO REFER

Patients with a definite diagnosis of anaphy-laxis and a convincing triggering agent that is temporally related to the event can be managed by a primary care physician. These patients, as with all anaphylaxis patients, need education on avoidance measures and education on emergency treatment measures.

Other cases may not be as simple and may require consultation with an allergy-immunology specialist. More complex cases can include the following:

- Patients with an unclear diagnosis
- Patients who require RAST, skin testing, or test dosing to determine sensitivity to a possible offending agent
- Patients with Hymenoptera venom sensitivity, to discuss immunotherapy
- Patients who have not responded to standard therapies
- Patients who have been noncompliant
- Patients who have coexisting pulmonary or cardiac disease
- Patients with anaphylaxis during surgery

Patients with idiopathic anaphylaxis should be evaluated by an allergy-immunology specialist at least once, to review for any external agents as a cause. If the diagnosis of idiopathic anaphylaxis is confirmed, patients may be managed by primary care practitioners. Management would require that the primary care practitioner has reviewed literature on the topic.

KEY POINTS

- ▶ Patients with allergen-induced *anaphylactic* reactions have an IgE antibody-mediated hypersensitivity. Patients with *anaphylactoid* reactions have similar reactions due to other external exposures, but they are mediated through different mechanisms.
- ▶ Some patients have definite anaphylaxis but no clear external cause. These patients have idiopathic anaphylaxis, and an internal cause is suspected.
- ▶ Patients with anaphylaxis can present dramatically and require emergent treatment.
- ▶ Even after emergent treatment with epinephrine and antihistamines, patients can still have a late recurrence. Patients should be monitored for this possible recurrence and should receive corticosteroids to help prevent it.

- ▶ For patients with a clear external cause, avoidance measures to prevent further exposures are the focus of management.
- ▶ Since reactions cannot always be predicted, patients with a history of anaphylaxis must carry emergency medication, such as an EpiPen, with them at all times.

Resources

The American Academy of Allergy, Asthma & Immunology
611 East Wells Street
Milwaukee, WI 53202
(414) 272–6071
website—www.aaaai.org

The American College of Allergy, Asthma & Immunology
85 West Algonquin Road
Suite 550
Arlington Heights, IL 60005
(708) 427–1200
website—www.acaai.org

The Food Allergy Network
10400 Eaton Place
Suite 107
Fairfax, VA 22030–2208
(703) 691–2713
website—www.foodallergy.org

Texts

Patterson R, DeSwarte RD, Greenberger PA, et al (eds): Drug Allergy and Protocols for Management of Drug Allergies. Providence, RI, OceanSide Publications, 1995

Patterson R (ed): Idiopathic Anaphylaxis. Providence, RI, OceanSide Publications, 1997

Suggested Reading

Portier P, Richet C: De l'action anaphylactique due certain venins. C R Soc Biol (Paris) 54:170–172, 1902

Stewart AG, Ewan PW: The incidence, aetiology and management of anaphylaxis presenting to an accident and emergency department. Q J Med 89:859–864, 1996

Boston Collaborative Drug Surveillance Program: Drug-induced anaphylaxis. JAMA 224:613–615, 1973

International Collaborative Study of Severe Anaphylaxis: An epidemiological study of severe anaphylaxis and anaphylactoid reactions among hospital patients: Methods and overall risks. Epidemiology 9:141–146, 1998

Sorensen HT, Nielsen B, Ostergaard Nielsen J: Anaphylactic shock occurring outside hospitals. Allergy 44:288–290, 1989

Orange RP, Donsky GJ: Anaphylaxis. *In* Middleton E, Reed CE, Ellis EF (eds): Allergy: Principles and Practice. St. Louis, Mosby, 1978

Marquardt DL, Wasserman SI: Anaphylaxis. *In* Middleton E, Reed CE, Ellis EF (eds): Allergy: Principles and Practice. St. Louis, Mosby–Year Book, 1993

Hakim RM, Breillatt J, Lazarus JM, Port FK: Complement activation and hypersensitivity reactions to dialysis membranes. N Engl J Med 311:878–882, 1984

Patterson R, Harris KE: Idiopathic anaphylaxis: Management and theories of pathogenesis. Clin Immuno Therapeutics 4:265–268, 1995

Grant JA, Alan R, Lett-Brown MA: Histamine-releasing

factors and inhibitors: Historical perspectives and possible implications in human illness. J Allergy Clin Immunol 88:683–693, 1991

Grammer LC: Potential mechanisms of idiopathic anaphylaxis. *In* Patterson R (ed): Idiopathic Anaphylaxis. Providence, RI, OceanSide Publications, 1997, pp 59–64

Stark BJ, Sullivan TJ: Biphasic and protracted anaphylaxis. J Allergy Clin Immunol 78:76–83, 1986

Douglas DM, Sukenick E, Andrade WP, Brown JS: Biphasic systemic anaphylaxis: An inpatient and outpatient study. J Allergy Clin Immunol 93:977–985, 1994

Tunon-de-Lara JM, Villanueva P, Marcus M, Taytard A: ACE inhibitors and anaphylactoid reactions during venom immunotherapy [letter]. Lancet 340:908, 1992

Kemp SF, Lieberman P: Inhibitors of angiotensin II: Potential hazards for patients at risk for anaphylaxis? Ann Allergy Asthma Immunol 78:527–529, 1997

Golden DBK, Kwiterovich KA, Kengey-Sobotka A, Lichtenstein LM: Discontinuing venom immunotherapy: Extended observations. J Allergy Clin Immunol 101:298–305, 1998

Stafford CT: Hypersensitivity to fire ant venom. Ann Allergy Asthma Immunol 77:87–99, 1996

Joint Task Force on Practice Parameters: The diagnosis and management of anaphylaxis. J Allergy Clin Immunol 101(part 2):S465–S528, 1998

Lieberman P, Taylor WW Jr: Recurrent idiopathic anaphylaxis. Arch Intern Med 139:1032–1034, 1979

Wiggins CA, Dykewicz MS, Patterson R: Idiopathic anaphylaxis: Classification, evaluation, and treatment of 123 patients. J Allergy Clin Immunol 82:849–855, 1988

Patterson R, Hogan MB, Yarnold PR, Harris KE: Idiopathic anaphylaxis: An attempt to estimate the incidence in the United States. Arch Intern Med 155:869–871, 1995

Patterson R, Stoloff RS, Greenberger PA, et al: Algorithms for the diagnosis and management of idiopathic anaphylaxis. Ann Allergy 71:40–44, 1993

Ditto AM, Harris KE, Krasnick J, et al: Idiopathic anaphylaxis: A series of 335 cases. Ann Allergy Asthma Immunol 77:285–291, 1996

Patterson R (ed): Idiopathic anaphylaxis. Providence, RI, OceanSide Publications, 1997

Chapter 20

Adverse Reactions to Drugs

Michael E. Weiss

Adverse drug reactions are important and frequent complications of medication therapy. Estimates are that 5% to 15% of patients develop adverse reactions to medications during treatment. As many as 30% of hospitalized patients experience at least one adverse drug reaction. Approximately 3% of all acute care medical admissions and 0.3% of all hospital admissions are attributed to adverse medication reactions. Fatal drug reactions occur in 0.1% of medical inpatients and 0.01% of surgical inpatients. Drug sensitivity has been implicated in 5.6% of cerebral damage cases and 4.3% of deaths from anesthetic mishaps reported in the United Kingdom. The first step in properly diagnosing adverse drug reactions is to understand the different types of adverse drug reactions that can occur.

There are certain adverse drug reactions that may occur in all individuals. These include overdoses, which are toxic reactions caused by excessive doses or impaired excretion or metabolism of a medication; side-effects, which are undesirable effects but potentially unavoidable because of the pharmacologic action of the particular medication such as tremors with use of beta-agonists; secondary effects, which are undesirable effects that are unrelated to the primary pharmacologic action of the medication such as oral candidiasis secondary to use of inhaled steroids; and drug interactions, which involve the interaction of two or more drugs causing toxicity that otherwise would not be present, such as cardiotoxicity from the interaction of terfenadine and erythromycin. Other adverse drug reactions occur only in susceptible patients in an unpredictable manner. These include drug intolerance, which is caused by a lower threshold to the normal pharmacologic action of a particular medication, such as tinnitus seen at low doses of salicylates in selected patients; idiosyncratic reactions, which usually result from a genetically determined metabolic or enzyme deficiency that is not expressed under normal situations such as hemolytic anemia occurring in patients with glucose-6-phosphate dehydrogenase deficiency after receiving an oxidant drug; drug allergies, which, by definition, involve immunologic mechanisms such as IgE-mediated penicillin anaphylaxis; and pseudoallergies, which are reactions that have clinical manifestations similar to those of allergic reactions but in which immune mechanisms are not involved. Allergic or immunologic drug reactions account for only 5% to 10% of adverse drug reactions.

Properly diagnosing an offending medication as a cause of an adverse drug reaction is often difficult. Often multiple medications are in use at the same time, and the clinical symptoms of adverse drug reactions may overlap with symptoms of the underlying disease. A common example is a patient who develops an exantham. It is often unclear if the cutaneous reaction is related to the antibiotic prescribed or to the underlying infectious process.

Our general lack of knowledge of the immunochemistry of drug metabolism and immunoreactive metabolites also greatly hampers our ability to accurately use diagnostic tests to evaluate allergic drug reactions. Except for penicillin and, to a lesser degree, anticonvulsant medications and sulfonamides, our understanding of the immunoreactive metabolites and immunochemistry of medications is quite limited. At times we employ tests for drug-specific immune responses without knowledge of the positive and negative predictive values of these tests. This lack of knowledge is understandable because there are only a few studies in which large numbers of patients with negative and positive diagnostic tests have been rechallenged with the suspected medication.

Despite these difficulties, it is worth attempting to diagnose immunologic drug reactions. It is important to define the causal agent to help guide the selection and use of future medications for a given patient and to properly manage the present adverse drug reaction. Labeling a patient inaccurately as allergic to a medication may cause the future use of less effective or more toxic medications as substitutes for the preferred medication.

Gell and Coombs classified immunopathologic reactions into four categories: immediate, cytotoxic, immune complex (Arthus reaction), and cell mediated. Some drug reactions have an obscure immunologic pathogenesis and do not fit in the Gell and Coombs classification system. Levine, using penicillin as a model, proposed classifying adverse reactions according to their time of onset (Table 20–1). Allergic reactions also can be classified according to their predominant clinical manifestations as shown in Table 20–2.

DETERMINING THE CAUSE OF ALLERGIC DRUG REACTIONS

Detailed History

The evaluation of allergic drug reactions starts with a detailed medical history. To properly diagnose an allergic drug reaction, meticulous history taking is often required. The detailed history should include all medications both regularly and intermittently used by the patient, including doses, indications, when initiated, and duration of therapy. The detailed history of the clinical manifestations of the reaction including associated symptoms is like-

***Table* 20–1. Classification of Allergic Reactions Based on Their Time of Onset**

Reaction Type	Onset	Clinical Manifestations
Immediate	0–1 hr	Anaphylaxis Hypotension Laryngeal edema Urticaria/angioedema Wheezing
Accelerated	1–72 hrs	Urticaria/angioedema Laryngeal edema Wheezing
Late	> 72 hrs	Morbilliform rash Interstitial nephritis Hemolytic anemia Neutropenia Thrombocytopenia Serum sickness Drug fever Stevens-Johnson syndrome Exfoliative dermatitis

Table adapted from data published in Levine BB: Immunologic mechanisms of penicillin allergy. A haptenic model system for the study of allergic diseases of man. N Engl J Med 275:115, 1966.

wise extremely valuable. Ongoing medical problems and conditions also should be inquired about in detail. Equally important information includes prior exposure to the same or structurally related medications, the effect of drug discontinuation, the treatment of the reaction to date, and the patient's response to the treatment. It is important to ascertain if any diagnostic tests or rechallenges have already been done and their results. Knowledge of the medical literature with particular reference to a medication's known propensity for causing reactions is paramount. The proximity of drug administration to the onset of the reaction should be determined because, in general, agents that have been used for long, continuous periods of time before the onset of an acute reaction are less likely to be implicated than are agents recently introduced or re-introduced. Patients with a history of prior allergic reactions appear to have an increased risk of subsequent adverse drug reactions. It is often useful to do a MEDLINE search concerning all medications being considered as culprits for allergic reactions. It also may be useful to contact the pharmaceutical manufacturers about the medications in question because they may have unpublished information concerning post-marketing reports of adverse reactions to their particular products. In com-

Table 20–2. **Classification of Allergic Reactions According to Their Predominant Clinical Manifestations**

Reaction Type	Clinical Manifestations
Anaphylaxis	Laryngeal edema
	Hypotension
	Bronchospasm
Cutaneous reactions	Urticaria/angioedema
	Vasculitis
	Stevens-Johnson syndrome
	Exfoliative dermatitis
	Contact sensitivity
	Fixed drug eruption
	Toxic epidermal necrolysis
	Pruritus
	Maculopapular (morbilliform) rash
	Erythema multiforme
	Erythema nodosum
	Photosensitivity reactions
Destruction of formed elements of blood	Hemolytic anemia
	Neutropenia
	Thrombocytopenia
Pulmonary reactions	Interstitial/alveolar pneumonitis
	Edema
	Fibrosis
Hepatic reactions	Cholestatic reactions
	Hepatocellular damage
Renal reactions	Interstitial nephritis
	Glomerulonephritis
	Nephrotic syndrome
Serum sickness	
Drug fever	
Systemic vasculitis	
Lymphadenopathy	

plicated scenarios, it is often useful to prepare a flow diagram to better see the reaction in relationship to medications received and ongoing therapy and treatment.

Recent studies have shown that when charts are reviewed by either physicians or hospital pharmacists that there are significant inaccuracies in hospitalized patients' records concerning histories of medication allergies. This underscores the need for a personally obtained, detailed, and accurate history about medication reactions.

IN VIVO TESTS

Skin Testing for Immediate Hypersensitivity Reactions

Although standardized skin tests are commonly used by allergists in the diagnosis of aeroallergen and *Hymenoptera* allergy, the evaluation of drug allergy is hampered by the relative unavailability of relevant drug metabolites or appropriate multivalent testing reagents. Skin testing has an established role in the evaluation of IgE-mediated penicillin allergy and also is useful in the evaluation of allergy to muscle relaxants, barbiturates, chymopapain, streptokinase, insulin, latex, and other miscellaneous drugs, and most biologicals. Specific protocols for skin testing have been published in detail.

For safety, a scratch or puncture (epicutaneous) test should be performed before the more definitive intradermal test. When skin tests are performed with drugs or reagents that have not been previously validated, all positive skin test responses should be confirmed by skin testing three to five normal individuals as appropriate controls to rule out irritative, false-positive skin responses. If normal controls are skin-test negative using the same concentration, then the positive skin test response in the patient can be considered to be immunologically valid. Skin testing cannot be done in the presence of medications that will affect the skin test response (e.g., H1 antihistamines, tricyclic antidepressants, and high-dose sympathomimetic agents). Appropriate positive (histamine) and negative (diluent) controls should be used. Immediate skin testing is a bioassay that detects the physiologic response to mediators released from cutaneous mast cells when drug-specific IgE antibodies bound to skin mast cells are cross-linked by the drug in question. Preferably, skin testing should be performed 4 to 6 weeks after a drug reaction. Skin tests for drug allergy are primarily used for the confirmation of adverse reactions mediated by type I hypersensitivity.

Tests for drug-specific immune response are hindered because we rarely know the drug's immunochemistry. As most drugs are small–molecular-weight chemicals, they are haptenic and must first combine with larger carrier molecules to stimulate an immune response and subsequently an allergic reaction.

In the case of most drugs other than penicillins, we have little or no information about the predominant specificity of the drug-specific immune responses. Without such information, a negative skin test response with the native drug may not indicate a true lack of allergy. If the skin test responses are positive at concentrations at which normal subjects have a negative test result, the patient may be presumed to be at significant risk for an acute allergic reaction if the drug is readministered. Without information concerning the drug's immunochemistry, a negative skin test response to the native drug may not truly indicate a lack of immunologic sensitization, as has been shown for sulfonamide allergy. If the medication needs to be readministered it would be prudent to do so under a physician's supervision.

Interest and research in allergic drug reactions during the perioperative period has greatly increased. In patients with allergic reactions during surgery, studies have shown that skin testing with nonirritative concentrations of medications used during the induction phase of anesthesia may help in determining which medication caused the allergic reaction.

Patch Testing

Patch testing is a form of drug challenge applicable at times in diagnosing drug-induced contact dermatitis. Patch testing is performed by applying a nonirritating concentration of the agent in question to an absorbent pad, which is then attached to the skin under hypoallergenic occlusive tape. At 48 and 72 hours, the sites are inspected; a positive reaction is characterized by pruritus, vesiculation, and erythema. Interpretation of patch test results should be done carefully and by personnel well versed in the nuances of reading patch test results. To date, patch testing has been relegated to a minor role in diagnosing allergic contact reactions to medications.

Provocative Drug Challenge

The ultimate or gold standard of in vivo tests is the provocative drug challenge. At times, the drug challenge is the only diagnostic approach that can demonstrate adverse reaction potential with certainty. Provocative drug challenge obviously poses certain risks to the patient that should not be taken lightly. Patients often are reluctant to undergo provocative drug challenge when they are convinced that a medication has caused them adverse effects. Individu-

als who have had toxic epidermal necrolysis, Stevens-Johnson syndrome, and severe anaphylactic reactions should probably never undergo provocative drug challenge.

If provocative drug challenge is undertaken, it should be done using incremental dose challenges. A decision to challenge a potentially sensitive patient involves careful assessment of the risks and benefits derived from the drug challenge. Provocative drug challenges have recently increased with the acquired immunodeficiency syndrome (AIDS) epidemic. Approximately 40% of AIDS patients have had adverse reactions to trimethoprim/sulfamethoxazole, which is one of the most useful medications to both prevent and treat *Pneumocystis carinii* pneumonia. Faced with the knowledge that trimethoprim/sulfamethoxazole is the agent of first choice for this problem and with the high incidence of adverse reactions in human immunodeficiency virus (HIV) positive patients, clinicians have developed various desensitization protocols in which doses of trimethoprim/sulfamethoxazole are incrementally increased. Using trimethoprim/sulfamethoxazole desensitization protocols, approximately 50% of patients with prior reactions tolerate trimethoprim/sulfamethoxazole therapy. This approach is not risk-free, and serious adverse reactions have occurred using desensitization protocols. A drug challenge should only be conducted by experienced health care personnel under controlled circumstances.

IN VITRO TESTING

Radioallergosorbent Test

The radioallergosorbent test (RAST) is a solid-phase radioimmunoassay (RIA) that was first developed in 1967. The RAST measures circulating allergen-specific IgE antibody. The RAST and RAST analogs are performed by linking the allergen (drug) in question to a solid-phase (carbohydrate particle, paper disk, or the wall of polystyrene test tubes or plastic microtiter wells). The drug attached to the solid-phase is incubated with the patient's serum, during which time specific antibodies of all immunoglobulin isotypes are bound. After washing, a second incubation is done with a radiolabeled, highly specific anti-IgE antibody. Following washes, the bound radioactivity is directly related to the drug-specific IgE antibody content in the original patient's serum. When appropriately done, RAST correlates well with skin test end-point titration, basophil histamine release, and provocation test results. Results from the serum under study are compared with a positive reference serum and negative control serum. Application of the RAST for the diagnosis of a drug allergy is unfortunately limited owing to incomplete knowledge of the conformation of most drugs and their metabolites. A RAST has been developed to measure IgE antibody to the major penicilloyl determinant of penicillin, insulin, chymopapain, muscle relaxants, thiopental, protamine, and latex. False-positive test response may occur because of high nonspecific binding, high total serum IgE levels, or poor technique. False-negative tests may occur due to interference from high levels of IgG-specific antibodies or an inability to maximize assay sensitivity. RAST offers the advantage of measuring IgE-specific antibodies when patients cannot undergo skin testing. The use of RAST to diagnose penicillin allergy is limited by the fact that a RAST for the penicillin minor determinants is not currently available. If a RAST assay has not been developed to maximize sensitivity, false-negative results may give a false sense of security.

Measurement of Drug-Specific IgG or IgM Antibodies

Medications may stimulate drug-specific IgG or IgM antibody responses, but these usually have no associated pathologic consequences. With the exception of some cases of drug-induced thrombocytopenia, hemolytic anemia, and agranulocytosis, there often is no correlation between the presence or titers of drug-specific IgG or IgM antibodies and pathologic allergic drug reactions. Recent evidence suggests that certain protamine reactions may be mediated through protamine-specific IgG antibodies. Drug-specific IgG and IgM antibodies can be measured using solid-phase RIA or enzyme-linked immunosorbent assay (ELISA) tests.

Assays to Measure Complement Activation

Assays to assess complement activation include assays of serum complement components (i.e., C4, C3) or total hemolytic component (CH50), and measurements of products of complement activation (e.g., C3a, C4a, C5a). These assays, if positive, implicate complement activation in specific reactions but generally do not distinguish drug allergies from other adverse reactions or pinpoint a specific drug as the culprit.

Release of Histamine and Other Mediators from Basophils

Washed leukocytes that contain basophils with IgE antibody on their cell surface will release histamine and other mediators when incubated with relevant antigens. In general, results appear to correlate with those of direct immediate skin tests. Haptenic drug allergens are often quite weak stimulants, and therefore as a diagnostic test, leukocyte–histamine release has a low sensitivity. The assay is relatively laborious, requires whole blood drawn immediately before the test, and is limited in availability to research labs.

Measurement of Mediators in Serum and Urine

During and for a short time after allergic reactions, blood can be analyzed for the release of various inflammatory cell mediators such as histamine, prostaglandin D2, chemotactic factors, and serum tryptase. Urine also can be analyzed for metabolites of histamine or prostaglandin D2. Plasma histamine and prostaglandin D2 levels remain elevated for only brief periods of time, limiting their clinical utility. Bioassays to measure chemotactic factor activity are cumbersome to perform and suffer from large interassay variability. Assays to measure serum tryptase (a protease released specifically from mast cells) are more promising in the clinical assessment of mast cell–

mediated allergic reactions (anaphylaxis) because serum tryptase remains elevated for
hours rather than minutes after mast cell degranulation. Positive test results are more valuable than negative results because there are
many false-negative tryptase results.

Lymphocyte Transformation Assays

Lymphocyte transformation tests measure blas-
togenesis of lymphocytes by measuring the uptake of the DNA precursor, tritiated thymidine,
after a sample of the patient's peripheral
blood lymphocytes is cultivated with nontoxic
concentrations of the suspected drug. An enhanced proliferative response in the presence
of the suspected drug is interpreted as a sign
of a drug-specific T-cell sensitization. The clinical value of these tests is hindered by the complexity of the procedure, the delay in obtaining results, the significant interlaboratory
variability, and the poor reproducibility over
time. Considerable disagreement exists about
the value of the procedure in the diagnosis of
drug allergy. At present, these tests need further validation before they have defined clinical utility.

Leukocyte Toxicity Assay for Drug Hypersensitivity

It has been shown recently that reactive drug
metabolites may have a causative role in some
serum-sickness–like drug reactions in susceptible patients. In the leukocyte toxicity assay, the
drug in question is incubated with hepatic
microsomes prepared from mice as a source of
oxidative enzymes, primarily cytochrome P450.
Peripheral blood lymphocytes from the patient
in question are incubated with this drug–
microsome mixture, and the percentage of
dead lymphocyte cells is measured and used
as an index of toxicity of the drug metabolites
generated (Table 20–3).

This approach, first pioneered by Spiel-
berg, demonstrated that acetaminophen could
be metabolized in vitro to a metabolite that,
under appropriate conditions, was toxic to human peripheral blood mononuclear cells.

Table 20–3. **Diagnostic Tests for Drug Hypersensitivity**

Detailed history
Skin testing for immediate hypersensitivity reactions
Patch testing
Provocative drug challenge
Radioallergosorbent test (RAST)
Measurement of drug-specific IgG or IgM antibodies
Assays to measure complement activation
Release of histamine and other mediators from basophils
Measurement of mediators (histamine, prostaglandins, leukotrienes, tryptase)
Lymphocyte transformation
Leukocyte toxicity assay
Computer-assisted evaluation of adverse events using a bayesian approach

These observations were subsequently applied
to understand further the problem of severe
hypersensitivity reactions to sulfonamides and
aromatic anticonvulsants such as phenytoin,
phenobarbital, and carbamazepine. These hypersensitivity reactions are often characterized
by the development of high fever and severe
skin rash after 10 to 14 days of therapy. The
rash is often severe, being either toxic epidermal necrolysis, which is life-threatening, or erythema multiforme. Approximately 25% of patients also have involvement of the heart, liver,
kidney, or bone marrow. These reactions have
been associated with 30% to 50% mortality,
often secondary to infectious complications of
exfoliative dermatitis. This assay has also been
used to study serum-sickness–like reactions to
cefaclor.

This assay appears to reliably identify individuals genetically at risk for cytotoxic drug
reaction syndromes. It is critical to use appropriate positive and negative controls. The
assays are currently research tools and are not
widely available. The specificity, sensitivity, and
predictive value of these assays are presently
unknown.

Computer-Assisted Evaluation of Adverse Events Using a Bayesian Approach

Computerized decision aids have been developed recently and are under investigation for
diagnostic and therapeutic decision making.
With the understanding that the differential
diagnosis of adverse drug reactions is complex

because for each adverse event there are many possible drug and nondrug causes, a computerized, user-friendly diagnostic aid for bayesian assessment of adverse drug events has been developed.

The bayesian adverse reaction diagnostic instrument (BARDI) is explicit in the information that is used and how each piece of information is weighted; it uses bayesian statistics to combine factors coherently. The bayesian method can include any relevant information and can consider multiple possible causes. Testing has shown that BARDI is valid.

A prototype computer program called Mac BARDI-Q&A has been developed to calculate the odds in favor of a particular drug causing an adverse event compared with an alternative cause. These odds are referred to as the posterior odds. This computer-assisted evaluation of adverse drug events needs further study and validation, but results to date look encouraging. As further information is gained, it can be entered into existing data banks, in the hope of improving the accuracy of the computer-assisted diagnosis of adverse and immunologic drug reactions.

SPECIFIC DRUG REACTIONS

Penicillin and Cephalosporin Antibiotics

The immunochemistry of penicillins has been very well studied; we know that the beta-lactam ring opens up under physiologic conditions to form a covalent amide linkage with epsilon amino groups of lysine residues in serum and possibly membrane-bound proteins. The resulting antigenic configuration, known as the penicilloyl determinant, elicits the dominant immune response in patients receiving penicillin. The penicilloyl group has been designated the major determinant because approximately 95% of the penicillin molecules that irreversibly combine with proteins form penicilloyl moieties. This reaction occurs with the prototype benzylpenicillin and virtually all semisynthetic penicillins. Multiple penicilloyl determinants have been synthetically coupled to a weakly immunogenic polylysine carrier molecule to form penicilloyl-polylysine (PPL). Coupling multiple penicilloyl moieties to the poly-

lysine carrier molecule increases the sensitivity of detecting IgE antibodies to this antigenic determinant four- or five-fold. Penicillin also can be degraded by other metabolic paths to form additional antigenic determinants. These derivatives are formed in small quantities and stimulate a variable immune response and hence have been termed the minor determinants.

The penicilloyl-polylysine reagent is commercially available in the United States as PRE-PEN (Bayer, Spokane, WA). Because the minor determinants are labile and cannot be synthesized readily in multivalent form, skin testing for minor determinant allergens is usually accomplished using a mixture of native benzylpenicillin, its alkaline hydrolysis product (benzylpenicilloate), and its acid hydrolysis product (benzylpenilloate), collectively called the minor determinant mixture (MDM). Currently, an MDM is not commercially available in the United States. If one uses benzylpenicillin diluted to a concentration of 10,000 units per ml [10 M] as the sole minor determinant reagent, approximately 5% to 10% of skin test–reactive patients will be missed. However, some of those missed may be at risk for serious, anaphylactic reactions. It is generally acceptable to test patients with suspected penicillin allergy with penicilloyl-polylysine and benzylpenicillin at 10,000 units per ml.

Unlike many diagnostic tests for drug allergies, both the positive and negative predictive values of skin tests using penicillin reagents have been studied. When therapeutic doses of penicillin are given to patients with histories of penicillin allergy, but with currently negative skin tests to PPL and MDM, IgE-mediated reactions occur very rarely and are almost always mild and self-limited. Approximately 1% of skin test–negative patients will experience accelerated urticarial reactions, and approximately 3% will have other mild cutaneous reactions (Fig. 20–1). Patients with histories of penicillin allergy and negative skin test reactions may become re-sensitized after subsequent uneventful penicillin administration, and repeat skin testing before future penicillin administration may be prudent. In general, with increasing time from the allergic reaction to penicillin administration the prevalence of skin test positivity to penicillin determinants decreases, although for some patients

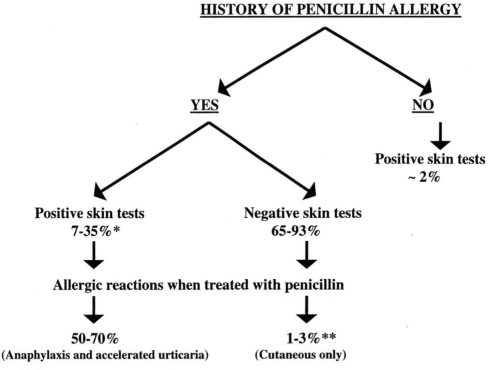

Figure 20–1. Prevalence of positive and negative penicillin skin test results and subsequent allergic reactions in patients treated with penicillin (based on studies using both penicilloyl-polylysine [PPL] and minor determinant mixture [MDM] as skin test reagents). *One study found 65% positive results. **Amoxicillin and ampicillin have higher rates of cutaneous reactions. (Adapted from Weiss ME, Adkinson NF Jr: Beta-lactam allergy. *In* Mandell LG, Douglas RG Jr, Bennett JE [eds]: Principles and Practice of Infectious Disease, ed 3. New York, Churchill Livingstone, 1989, p 264; with permission.)

penicillin-specific IgE antibodies persist indefinitely.

Recent studies have suggested that skin testing with major and minor determinants of benzylpenicillin may not detect all individuals with ampicillin- or amoxicillin-specific allergy. Some have advocated performing additional skin tests with native ampicillin or amoxicillin (20 mg/ml) or an aminopenicillin MDM if available. For reasons that are currently unclear, the diaminopenicillins (ampicillin and amoxicillin) induce nonurticarial rashes with greater frequency than other penicillins.

A limited number of patients with positive penicillin skin test responses have been treated with therapeutic doses of penicillin. The risk of an anaphylactic or accelerated allergic reaction ranges from 50% to 70% in such patients (see Fig. 20–1). If skin test results are positive, equally effective, noncross-reacting antibiotics should be substituted when available. If alternative drugs fail, induce unacceptable side-effects, or are less effective, the administration of penicillin can be considered using a desensitization protocol (Tables 20–4 and 20–5).

With the increasing use of cephalosporins, the risk of cross-reactivity between cephalosporins and penicillins is an increasingly important question. In the case of first-generation cephalosporins, there does appear to be an increased risk of adverse reactions to cephalosporins among patients with a history of penicillin allergy. The exact incidence of clinically relevant cross-reactivity between penicillins and first-generation cephalosporins is unknown and although probably small, cannot be dismissed on statistical grounds alone because life-threatening anaphylactic cross-reactivity has occurred. The newer, second- and third-generation cephalosporins appear to have much lower cross-reactivity with penicillins, but this could be in part due to less prevalent clinical use due to more recent availability.

Sulfonamides

Sulfonamides are frequently responsible for drug-induced skin eruptions and drug fever, often appearing between the seventh and tenth day of treatment. Less common reactions include vasculitis, the Stevens-Johnson syndrome, and urticaria. The introduction of trimethoprim-sulfamethoxazole, which is effective in treating a variety of infections, has been responsible for the resurgence of the widespread use of sulfonamides. The incidence of reactions from trimethoprim-sulfamethoxazole in hospitalized patents is between 3% and 6%. The incidence of reactions is approximately 10 to 15 times higher among patients with AIDS. The reason for the increased incidence of reactions in patents with AIDS is unknown. Although the immunochemistry of sulfonamide allergy in humans is not completely understood, recent evidence suggests that some sulfonamide reactions are mediated by hepatocyte-generated toxic drug metabolites in genetically susceptible patients.

Local Anesthetic Agents

Although patients commonly report adverse reactions to local anesthetics and that they have been advised that they are allergic to these agents, true allergic reactions to injected

Table 20–4. Protocol for Oral Desensitization of β-Lactam Antibiotic–Allergic Patients

Step	β-Lactam Drug (mg/ml)	Amount (ml)	Dose Given (mg)	Cumulative Dose (mg)
1	0.5	0.1	0.05	0.05
2	0.5	0.2	0.10	0.15
3	0.5	0.4	0.20	0.35
4	0.5	0.8	0.40	0.75
5	0.5	1.6	0.80	1.55
6	0.5	3.2	1.60	3.15
7	0.5	6.4	3.20	6.35
8	5.0	1.2	6.00	12.35
9	5.0	2.4	12.00	24.35
10	5.0	4.8	24.00	48.35
11	50.0	1.0	50.00	98.35
12	50.0	2.0	100.00	198.35
13	50.0	4.0	200.00	398.35
14	50.0	8.0	400.00	798.35

Next: Observe patient for 30 minutes. Then administer 1 g of same agent intravenously.

Drug suspension diluted in 30 ml of water for ingestion. Interval between doses, 15 minutes.
From Sullivan TJ: Drug allergy. *In* Middleton E, Reed C, Ellis E, et al (eds): Allergy: Principles and Practice, 4th ed. St. Louis, CV Mosby, 1993, pp 1523–1534.

Table 20–5. Protocol for Parenteral Desensitization of β-Lactam Antibiotic–Allergic Patients

Step	β-Lactam Drug (mg/ml)	Amount (ml)	Dose Given (mg)	Cumulative Dose (mg)
1	0.1	0.1	0.01	0.01
2	0.1	0.2	0.02	0.03
3	0.1	0.4	0.04	0.07
4	0.1	0.8	0.08	0.15
5	1.0	0.16	0.16	0.31
6	1.0	0.32	0.32	0.63
7	1.0	0.64	0.64	1.27
8	10	0.12	1.20	2.47
9	10	0.24	2.40	4.87
10	10	0.48	4.80	10
11	100	0.10	10	20
12	100	0.20	20	40
13	100	0.40	40	80
14	100	0.80	80	160
15	1000	0.16	160	320
16	1000	0.32	320	640
17	1000	0.64	640	1280

Next: Observe patient for 30 minutes. Then administer 1 g of same agent intravenously.

Doses administered subcutaneously (or intramuscularly or intravenously).
Interval between doses, 15 minutes.
From Sullivan TJ: Drug allergy. *In* Middleton E, Reed C, Ellis E, et al (eds): Allergy: Principles and Practice, 4th ed. St. Louis, CV Mosby, 1993, pp 1523–1534.

local anesthetics are exceedingly rare. Reactions to local anesthetics are often the result of vasovagal reactions, toxic reactions (probably because of inadvertent intravenous injection), side-effects from epinephrine, or psychomotor responses, including hyperventilation. Toxic symptoms often involve central nervous and cardiovascular symptoms and may produce slurred speech, euphoria, dizziness, excitement, nausea, emesis, disorientation, or convulsions. Vasovagal reactions are usually associated with bradycardia, sweating, pallor, and rapid improvement in symptoms when the patient is supine. Sympathetic stimulation, either from epinephrine or anxiety, may result in tremor, diaphoresis, tachycardia, and hypertension. Rarely are symptoms of reactions to local anesthetics consistent with IgE-mediated reactions, such as urticaria, bronchospasm, and anaphylactic shock. Valid documentation of IgE-mediated reactivity against local anesthetics is extremely rare.

The evaluation of a patient with a history of an adverse reaction to a local anesthetic should include a complete history of the epi-

Table 20–6. **Protocols for Evaluation of Local Anesthetic Allergy**

Step	Route	Volume (ml)	Dilution
Protocol A*			
1	Intradermal	0.02	1:1000
2	Intradermal	0.02	1:100
3	Intradermal	0.02	1:10
4	Intradermal	0.02	Undiluted
5	Subcutaneous	0.3	Undiluted
Protocol B*			
1	Puncture		Undiluted
2	Subcutaneous	0.1	Undiluted
3	Subcutaneous	0.5	Undiluted
4	Subcutaneous	1.0	Undiluted
5	Subcutaneous	2.0	Undiluted

*Administer at 15-minute intervals.
If history is strongly suggestive of IgE-mediated reaction, start with puncture at 1:1000 dilution.

sode, skin testing, and drug challenge. Two protocols are listed in Table 20–6; one uses skin testing and challenge, and the other follows an incremental drug challenge. Preparations without epinephrine should be used for skin testing, because epinephrine may mask a positive skin test response and induce toxic effects.

Radiocontrast Media

The incidence of reactions induced by conventional high-osmolar radiocontrast media (HORCM) injections is between 5% and 8%, with vasomotor reactions (nausea, vomiting, flushing, or warmth) most common. Anaphylactoid reactions to HORCM (urticaria, angioedema, wheezing, dyspnea, hypotension, or death) occur in 2% to 3% of patients receiving intravenous or intra-arterial infusions. Fatal reactions following the administration of radiocontrast media occur in approximately 1:50,000 intravenous procedures, and it has been estimated that as many as 500 deaths per year are caused by these agents. Most reactions begin 1 to 3 minutes after intravascular administration. Atopic patents appear to have about twice the risk of reactions to contrast media compared with nonatopic individuals. Patients with a previous reaction to HORCM have approximately a 33% (range, 17% to 60%) chance of a repeat reaction on re-exposure.

The etiology of adverse reactions to contrast media is not fully understood. Histamine

liberation appears to be a feature of most reactions. In vitro studies suggest that the hypertonicity of conventional HORCM (seven times the osmolality of plasma) results in nonimmunologic mediator release from mast cells and basophils. There is no evidence that IgE-mediated mechanisms have a role in radiocontrast media reactions.

A patient who requires the administration of radiocontrast media and who has had a previous reaction to this material has an increased (17% to 60%) risk for a reaction on re-exposure (Table 20–7). Pretreatment of these high-risk patients with oral prednisone (50 mg) 13 hours, 7 hours, and 1 hour before the administration of the contrast material along with oral diphenhydramine (50 mg) 1 hour before administration of the contrast medium reduces the risk of reactions to 9%. Almost all reactions in pretreated patients are mild. The addition of ephedrine (25 mg) 1 hour before the administration of radiocontrast media (in patients without angina, arrhythmia, or other contraindications for ephedrine administration) resulted in a reaction rate of 3.1% in one study (see Table 20–7). The addition of an H2-receptor antagonist, such as cimetidine or ranitidine, might further decrease the incidence of reactions to radiocontrast media, although studies to verify such a benefit have not been done.

Recently, newer low-osmolality radiocontrast media (LORCM) have been developed. The LORCM have only about twice the osmolality of plasma and appear to induce fewer adverse reactions. In patients with a history of a prior reaction to conventional HORCM, the incidence of an adverse reaction when contrast

Table 20–7. **Reaction Rate to Contrast Media in Patients with Previous Radiocontrast Media Reactions**

HORCM and no premedication	33% (range, 17% to 60%)
HORCM and premedication*	3.1% to 9%
LORCM and no premedication	2.7%
LORCM and premedication*	0.7%

Abbreviations: HORCM, high-osmolality radiocontrast media; LORCM, low-osmolality radiocontrast media.
*Premedication: prednisone (50 mg po) 13, 7, and 1 hr before radiocontrast media; diphenhydramine (50 mg IM or po) 1 hr before radiocontrast media; and ephedrine (25 mg po) 1 hr before radiocontrast media, if no contraindication to its use. Some have recommended pretreatment with ranitidine also.

media are readministered is lower with LORCM (2.7%) than with conventional HORCM (33%) (see Table 20–7). Unfortunately, LORCM cost 20 times more than conventional HORCM, and substituting LORCM for all procedures in which HORCM are now used would increase the cost from $100 million annually to $1.5 billion in the United States alone. A recent study using historical controls showed that combining premedication with LORCM is most beneficial (a reaction rate of only 0.7%) in preventing reactions in high-risk individuals (those with a prior reaction to HORCM) (see Table 20–7). It would seem prudent and cost-effective to limit the use of LORCM (with premedication) to patients who have had prior reactions to HORCM.

Aspirin

Reactions to aspirin appear to be limited either to the skin (urticaria with or without angioedema) or to the respiratory system (bronchospasm, rhinitis, and sinusitis). Aspirin-induced bronchospasm is rare in nonasthmatic individuals. It occurs in approximately 10% of asthmatic persons who are older than 10 years of age, in 30% to 40% of asthmatic persons with nasal polyps, rhinitis, and sinusitis, and in 60% to 85% of asthmatic persons who give a history of aspirin-induced reactions. These reactions may be severe, difficult to treat, and may cause death.

Reactions to aspirin are not IgE mediated, and the mechanism is incompletely understood. A working hypothesis is that aspirin, and other nonsteroidal anti-inflammatory drugs (NSAIDs) that inhibit cyclooxygenase, lead to a decrease in bronchodilating prostaglandins and shunt arachidonic acid metabolism through the 5-lipoxygenase pathway, producing increased amounts of the vasoactive and bronchoconstrictive leukotrienes C4, D4, and E4. Recent evidence suggests that aspirin-sensitive asthmatic individuals are 1000-fold more sensitive than asthmatic persons without aspirin sensitivity to the bronchoconstrictive effects of leukotriene E. Essentially all NSAIDs cross-react with aspirin and should be avoided in aspirin-sensitive asthmatic individuals. If aspirin or another NSAID is required for treatment of a disease in a patient with a history of aspirin sensitivity, aspirin desensitization may be indicated. Leukotriene antagonists may be used before aspirin desensitization is attempted, but should not be used in lieu of desensitization, because severe reactions can occur. Most aspirin-sensitive patients tolerate sodium or choline salicylate and acetaminophen in moderate doses without adverse reactions.

SUMMARY

Proper diagnosis of adverse drug reactions, although often complicated and difficult, is important for the patient and clinician. Often the question of whether it is safe to re-administer a medication is an important clinical judgment that needs to be made. Alternative medications may be less effective or have greater toxicities, cost, or both.

Areas of ongoing active research to improve diagnostic precision for allergic drug reactions include further understanding the immunochemistry of allergenic medications, improving the reproducibility and sensitivity of relevant in vitro assays, and further validating computer-assisted evaluation of adverse drug events. The positive and negative predictive values for these diagnostic tests need to be better defined where possible. At present, the primary diagnostic tool for properly assessing immunologic drug reactions remains a meticulous and detailed history obtained by an astute, knowledgeable, and motivated physician.

Suggested Reading

Adkinson NF Jr: Tests for immunological drug reactions. *In* Rose NF, Friedman H (eds): Manual of Clinical Immunology, ed 3. Washington, DC, American Society for Microbiology 1986, p 692

deShazo RD, Nelson HS: An approach to the patent with a history of local anesthetic hypersensitivity: Experience with 90 patients. J Allergy Clin Immunol 63:387, 1989

DeSwarte RD: Drug Allergy. *In* Patterson R (ed): Allergic Diseases: Diagnosis and Management, ed 3. Philadelphia, J.B. Lippincott, 1989, p 505

Gadde J, Spence M, Wheeler B, et al: Clinical experience with penicillin skin testing in a large inner-city STD clinic. JAMA 270:22456, 1993

Greenberger P, Patterson R: The prevention of immediate generalized reactions to radiocontrast media in high-risk patients. J Allergy Clin Immunol 87:867, 1991

Lanctot KL, Naranjo CA: Computer-assisted evaluation of adverse events using a bayesian approach. J Clin Pharmacol 34:142, 1994

Levine BB: Immunologic mechanisms of penicillin allergy: A haptenic model system for the study of allergy diseases of man. N Engl J Med 275:1115, 1966

Schwartz LB, Metcalfe DD, Miller JS, et al: Tryptase levels as an indicator of mast cell activation in systemic anaphylaxis and mastocytosis. N Engl J Med 316:1622, 1987

Stevenson DD: Diagnosis, prevention, and treatment of adverse reactions to aspirin (ASA) and nonsteroidal anti-inflammatory drugs (NSAIDs). J Allergy Clin Immunol 74:617, 1984

Weiss ME: Drug allergy. The Clinics of North America: Clinical allergy. 76:857, 1992

Weiss ME, Adkinson NF Jr: Beta-lactam allergy. *In* Mandell LG, Bennett JE, Dolin R (eds): Principles and Practice of Infectious Disease, ed 4. New York, Churchill Livingstone, 1994, 272–277

Chapter 21

Insect Allergy

Maité de la Morena and Richard F. Lockey

Many individuals throughout the world are stung by bees, wasps, hornets, yellow jackets, and fire ants. In the United States, approximately 400,000 visits per year to emergency rooms and 40 reported fatalities per year occur because of sequelae from insect stings. Stinging insect immunotherapy is used to prevent future systemic allergic reactions. One can expect a 60% systemic reaction rate on re-sting in untreated individuals versus less than a 5% rate in individuals treated with stinging insect immunotherapy.

This chapter focuses on the identification and care of individuals with reactions primarily to insect stings but also secondary to insect bites. The history, epidemiology, taxonomy, venom composition, clinical presentations, and diagnosis of stinging insect hypersensitivity are reviewed. The chapter concludes with a short discussion on protection and prevention of insect stings.

HISTORICAL PERSPECTIVE

The death of King Menses of Egypt after being stung by a stinging insect is believed to be the first reported case of insect sting allergy. In 1925, Braun used an extract prepared from honey bee bodies to confirm the diagnosis of honey bee allergy in a woman who had experienced anaphylaxis after being stung by a honey bee. The same extract was used to desensitize the patient by injecting increasing amounts at specific time intervals. Subsequently, Loveless showed in uncontrolled studies that the injection of increasing amounts of venom prepared from the venom sacs of vespids protected the sensitive individual from both field and controlled deliberate stings. It took another 30 years before a double-blind controlled study was done to prove that venom immunotherapy was effective to treat Hymenoptera hypersensitivity. In 1978, Hunt and colleagues demonstrated that venom immunotherapy and whole body vaccines, and not placebo, prevented the re-occurrence of insect sting–mediated systemic reactions in 95% of sensitive individuals. The 5% of patients who were treated with venom and still reacted had only mild and not life-threatening systemic reactions. In 1979, the Food and Drug Administration approved Hymenoptera venoms to diagnose and treat insect sting reactions. However, only 5% to 10% of insect sting allergic individuals in the United States receive this potentially life-saving therapy, and surveys indicate that patients seen in emergency rooms for insect sting allergic reactions are often not referred to appropriate specialists, many times because of lack of knowledge by the physician about venom immunotherapy. Fire ant sting-induced anaphylaxis is common in the southeastern and south central United States, in certain Caribbean islands, and in parts of South America. Fire ant whole body vaccines contain venom proteins and are used to treat fire ant sting-induced anaphylaxis.

EPIDEMIOLOGY

Between 0.4% and 4% of the United States population has a history of a systemic reaction to an insect sting. Data from the National Center of Health Statistics in the United States indicate that from 1982 to 1991 approximately 40 deaths per year occurred from insect stings.

These numbers are probably low because many deaths from stinging insects go unreported. Schwartz et al showed that of 94 sera obtained from subjects who died unexpectedly during the summer months, 22 (23%) contained elevated levels of IgE to at least one venom as compared to 6% of sera from 92 living blood donors. There is a 2:1 male:female ratio, and a history of atopy may be a potential risk factor for stinging insect-induced anaphylaxis. Insect reactions occur most commonly in rural rather than urban populations and take place primarily during the spring and summer months. Adults usually experience more serious reactions than do children, and the incidence of severe systemic reactions to subsequent stings in subjects with a history of a systemic reaction is lower in children than in adults. Adults with cardiovascular diseases appear to be at higher risk for death from insect sting-induced anaphylaxis. The incidence of allergic reactions to insect stings varies with geographic location. For example, in parts of the southeast United States, hypersensitivity to imported fire ant venom accounts for 42% of all visits to a clinic for Hymenoptera hypersensitivity and for 59% of all Hymenoptera immunotherapy. Honey bees and yellow jackets are most commonly incriminated as the cause of systemic allergic reactions in the northeast, whereas wasps cause most systemic allergic reactions in the western United States.

TAXONOMY

There are over 16,000 Hymenoptera insects in North America. The following information will assist the physician in determining which stinging insect is responsible for an insect sting reaction.

The Hymenoptera insects which account for most systemic allergic reactions belong to the following families: Vespidae (wasps), Apidae (bees), and Formicidae (ants) (Fig. 21–1). The family Vespidae is divided into seven subfamilies, two of which are most important: subfamily Vespinae, which includes yellow jackets and hornets, and the subfamily Polistinae, which includes the paper wasp (genus *Polistes*). The Apidae family include the *Apis mellifera* (honey bees) and the species *bombus* (bumble bees). Finally, the family Formicidae includes the subfamily, Myrmicinae, genus *Solenopsis,* species *richteri* and *invicta,* and genus *Pogonomyrmex* (harvest ants). Both *Solenopsis* species *richteri* and *invicta* are known as imported fire ants.

Yellow jackets are black and have yellow markings (Fig. 21–2). The queen measures approximately three-quarter of an inch long; the males and workers are approximately a half-inch long. Although they are most common in the northeastern and north central areas of the United States, they are also found in many

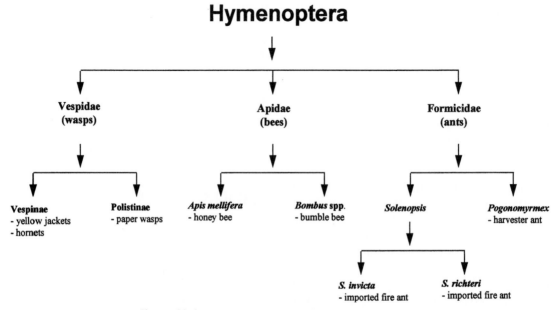

Figure 21–1. Taxonomy of medically important *Hymenoptera.*

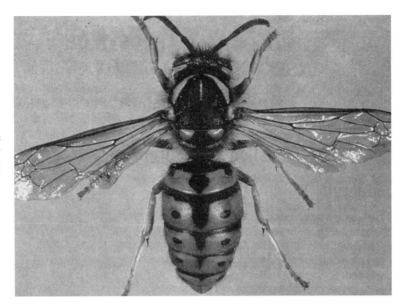

Figure 21–2. *Vespula germanica* (yellow jacket). (From The American Academy of Allergy, Asthma & Immunology: Insect Allergy, 3rd ed., 1995; with permission.)

areas of the world, including the Arctic. Their colonies are found in concealed locations and wall cavities, and their nests are made of paper-maché–like material. They scavenge for meats and sweets found near garbage bins and become more aggressive during the late summer and autumn months when colony populations are large and the colony life cycle is in a declining phase. Hornets are usually black or brown with white, orange, or yellow markings and are generally larger than yellow jackets. Their nests are usually found in tree hollows or in wall cavities (Fig. 21–3).

Wasps have slender, elongated bodies, are a half-inch to one inch long and may be black, brown, or red in color, usually with yellow markings (Fig. 21–4). Their nests are usually located under eaves, behind shutters, or in shrubs or woodpiles. They are slow flyers and feed on nectar and arthropods.

Honey bees are approximately a half-inch long and have round hairy bodies with dark brown coloring and yellow markings. They have barbed stingers that are commonly left behind in the skin after a sting. Because they are eviscerated when they fly away, they die after a sting. They are usually not as aggressive as are the Vespid species. Bees build nests in cavities found in the exteriors of homes, in discarded tires or holes in the ground, or in any partially protected site. They primarily live in manufactured hives, feed on nectar and pollens, and are commercially managed for honey production and pollination of fruit-bearing trees. Most stings from bees occur in individuals who walk barefooted on clover-covered lawns. The "killer bees" or Africanized honey bees are found in the southwestern United States and in South and Central America. They are more aggressive and may sting in swarms. Bumble bees also live on pollen and nectar; their nests resemble bunches of grapes and they are seldom responsible for human stings.

Imported fire ants are reddish-brown to black, approximately 1/8 of an inch long and include the genus *Solenopsis*, species *invicta* (Fig. 21–5) and *richter*. Imported fire ants are common in the southeastern and south central United States. Other species of the genus *Solenopsis, S. xyloni, S. aurea,* and *S. geminata,* also can sting and induce human anaphylaxis. The latter species also inhabit the southeastern United States. The imported fire ants (and harvester ants) attach to the skin by their mandibles and rotate, stinging repeatedly. Fire ants build their colonies in the ground, sometimes with prominent mounds. These fire ant nests can be found anywhere, but are often found along the borders of sidewalks, driveways, and along roadsides.

VENOM COMPOSITION

Hymenoptera venoms contain many allergenic and nonallergenic substances. Nonallergenic

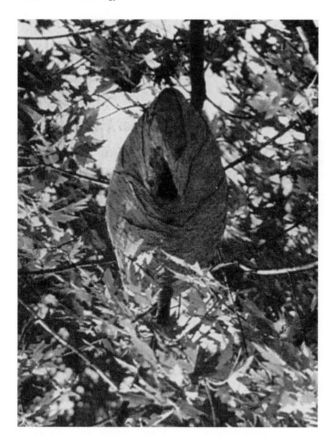

Figure 21–3. *Dolichovespula arenaria* nest (aerial yellow jacket or yellow hornet). (From The American Academy of Allergy, Asthma & Immunology: Insect Allergy, 3rd ed., 1995; with permission.)

substances include histamine, dopamine, serotonin, mast cell degranulation substances, kinins, adrenaline, noradrenaline, and chemoattractant peptides. These chemicals are primarily responsible for the vasoactive and toxic effects, which result in localized pain, swelling, erythema, and itching.

Hymenoptera venom proteins are responsible for the allergic or IgE-mediated reactions. The major honey bee allergens are two

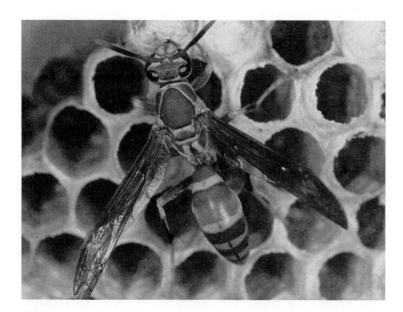

Figure 21–4. *Polistes exclamans* worker on nest (paper wasp). (From The American Academy of Allergy, Asthma & Immunology: Insect Allergy, 3rd ed., 1995; with permission.)

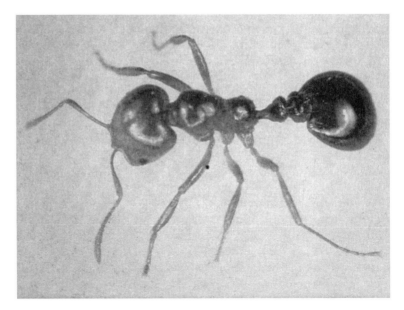

Figure 21–5. *Solenopsis invicta* worker (red imported fire ant). (From The American Academy of Allergy, Asthma & Immunology: Insect Allergy, 3rd ed., 1995; with permission.)

enzymes, phospholipase A2 and hyaluronidase. Other honey bee allergens include allergen C and mellitin. When mellitin is injected into the skin, pain, pruritus, and inflammation develop. Vespid venoms have three major allergens: (1) phospholipase A1, (2) hyaluronidase, and (3) a protein, antigen 5. Twenty-one proteins have been found in imported fire ant venom. Phospholipase A, phospholipase B, and hyaluronidase are among these. However, 90% to 95% of imported fire ant venom consists of water-insoluble *n*-alkyl and *n*-alkenyl piperidine alkaloids, which are responsible for the hemolytic, antibacterial, and insecticidal properties of the venom. Cross-reactivity among the different venom proteins occurs. For example, there is evidence for immunologic cross-reactivity between the phospholipase A1 of vespids and wasps and the phospholipase enzyme sol i 1, isolated from imported fire ant venom venom, *Solenopsis invicta.*

Honey bee, wasp, yellow jacket, and hornet venoms are commercially available as standardized diagnostic and therapeutic vaccines. Honey bee venom is collected by placing an electrically charged grid beneath a honey bee hive. The bees land on the grid, receive an electric shock, and sting on a latex membrane after which the venom is collected. Vespid venom vaccines are prepared by extracting venom sacs from frozen wasps. These sacs are then crushed, centrifuged, filtered, lyophilized, and stored until used, under vacuum at

−30°C. All licensed venom vaccines are analyzed and standardized by protein content. The Division of Allergenic Products and Parasitology of the Food and Drug Administration currently requires that all licensed venom extracts contain the active enzymes, phospholipase and hyaluronidase, and that the vaccine be labeled with the weight of the protein in micrograms.

CLINICAL PRESENTATION

Hymenoptera stings can induce local and large local sting reactions, systemic allergic reactions, toxic reactions, and other uncommon reactions.

Normal Local Skin Reactions

A normal reaction to a Hymenoptera sting is characterized by pain and erythema at the site of the sting. Pruritus is common. These reactions are non–IgE-mediated and caused by the nonallergenic substances contained in venoms. The reaction usually subsides within a day or two. A fire ant sting results in the formation of a small vesicle, beginning 4 hours after the sting, which evolves into a sterile pustule over 24 hours. Because the pustule extends into the dermis and subcutaneous tissue, secondary infections can occur. Most pustules last 3 to 10 days and eventually resolve with crust formation. Sometimes residual scars and hyperpigmented macules form at the sting site.

Large Local Reactions

Large local reactions after Hymenoptera stings occur in 10% of the population. This reaction is characterized by swelling that extends well beyond the sting site and is usually 2 inches or more in diameter. Warmth, erythema, edema, pruritus, and pain occur. The swelling tends to peak at 24–48 hours but may continue to worsen for up to 72 hours after a sting. A large local reaction may persist for up to 7–10 days. Malaise and nausea may accompany such a reaction; however, the reaction is self-limited. The etiology of large local reactions is not understood. About 50% of patients with large local reactions have no detectable serum venom-specific IgE. Increased in vitro lymphocyte stimulation to venoms has been demonstrated in patients with large local reaction as compared with nonallergic individuals. These data suggest that a delayed cellular immune process, as well as tissue inflammation caused by nonallergenic substances, may be involved in the pathogenesis of the large local reactions. Patients who experience large local reactions have a tendency to develop the same kind of reaction with subsequent stings. There may be a small number of patients (3%–5%) who subsequently develop systemic reactions when they are re-stung. Whether this occurs by chance or whether these few individuals are predisposed to develop such a reaction in spite of their large local reaction remains unknown. Immunotherapy does not modify these reactions. Therefore, individuals with large local reactions should not be tested or placed on immunotherapy.

Systemic Reactions

A systemic or anaphylactic reaction is caused by an IgE-mediated mechanism. A systemic reaction to a sting develops abruptly and is manifested primarily by cutaneous, gastrointestinal, respiratory, and cardiovascular symptoms.

Systemic allergic reactions can be catego-rized as mild, moderate, or severe. Mild systemic reactions are usually limited to the skin, for example, generalized urticaria, erythema, and pruritus. Angioedema without respiratory compromise also can occur. Moderate reactions can be associated with the symptoms of a mild reaction but also manifest with mild respiratory symptoms such as acute bronchospasm, which is reversed with the use of an inhalational beta-agonist. Severe anaphylactic reactions can be associated with all of the above-listed symptoms and with life-threatening respiratory symptoms caused by laryngeal edema and acute bronchospasm, gastrointestinal cramping, nausea, vomiting, unconsciousness, hypotension, and cardiovascular shock. Most, but not all, anaphylactic reactions occur within minutes, usually within the first 30 minutes after a sting. Rarely, these reactions can occur as long as 72 hours following a sting. A prior history of a severe anaphylactic reaction to an insect sting is a risk factor for a subsequent similar reaction. Children and adolescents who are younger than 16 years of age and who have had a systemic reaction limited to the skin (generalized erythema, pruritus, and urticaria) are not at increased risk for a subsequent sting-induced life-threatening reaction.

Toxic Reactions

Toxic reactions occur from multiple insect stings. The African honey bee (*Apis mellifera scutellata*) was brought to Brazil in 1956 to replace the European honey bee (*Apis mellifera*) because it is more productive in a tropical climate. Interbreeding among the two species has resulted in a bee population termed Africanized honey bees, which have expanded northward from Brazil at a rate of 150 to 250 miles per year. In the fall of 1990, the Africanized honey bee entered the United States by way of south Texas. Africanized honey bees may cause toxic sting reactions that can be fatal even though a healthy adult may tolerate as many as 5000 stings without sequelae.

Other Reactions

Other reactions, such as neurologic sequelae, hemolytic anemia, glomerulonephritis, myocarditis, and, rarely, serum sickness also have been reported. Honey bee stings have been associated with an influenza-like syndrome with fever, myalgias, and chills approximately 8 to 24 hours after the sting. The pathophysiology of these reactions is unclear.

DIAGNOSIS

A clinical history with special attention to the timing and sequence of events helps to differentiate the immediate IgE-mediated reaction from other types of reactions. Documentation of the signs and symptoms as recorded during an emergency room visit can be helpful in better understanding the kind of reaction that occurred.

Most individuals do not know what insect stung them. A honey bee usually leaves a stinger at the sting site, and this may be useful information to suspect a honey bee sting-induced reaction. Fire ant stings cause the formation of a small vesicle that gradually evolves into a pustule 8 to 24 hours later. Additional information that can help make the diagnosis includes the location of the subject when the sting occurred. For example, a bare-footed patient is more likely to have been stung by a yellow jacket or honey bee than by a wasp. An individual who was working under the eaves of a home is more likely to have been stung by a wasp. Fire ants typically sting more commonly on the lower extremities. Honey bees are common in flowering fields. Yellow jackets tend to inhabit areas where garbage is stored.

Skin Testing and Radioallergosorbent Testing

Appropriately done skin tests are the most sensitive way to detect venom-specific IgE, and the results of testing are immediate. The wheal-and-flare reaction occurs if the test is positive. Radioallergosorbent tests (RAST) also can be used to confirm the presence of specific IgE to Hymenoptera venoms. It is important to remember that a positive skin test or RAST result simply denotes sensitization and prior exposure and is not predictive of a future sting response. Approximately 14% of

asymptomatic adults may have positive skin test results and yet have no history of Hymenoptera hypersensitivity.

Venom skin testing is associated with a 2% systemic reaction rate, 20% of which may be severe. Venom skin testing should be performed approximately 4 weeks or more after a systemic reaction and is not indicated for a person with a large local reaction. The RAST may be useful to demonstrate specific IgE when the results of the skin tests are equivocal, when the skin tests cannot be performed because of the interfering effect of medications or other conditions, or are part of a postmortem examination.

NATURAL HISTORY

The natural history of insect sting anaphylaxis is still under study. Approximately 50% of patients with a history of venom anaphylaxis and the presence of venom-specific IgE do not experience a systemic reaction when they are restung by the same insect. Insect sting allergy may be a self-limited disease. For example, of 220 patients with a history of insect sting-induced anaphylaxis who did not receive immunotherapy, 56% developed a systemic reaction when stung again by the same type of insect. The frequency of these reactions was higher in adults (74%) than in children (40%) and was unrelated to the time since the initial sting reaction. In another study, children who had experienced systemic allergic reactions were randomized to receive either immunotherapy or no treatment. In the untreated group, 9.2% of the children versus 1.2% in the treated group developed systemic reactions on re-sting. None of the reactions in either group were more severe than the previous ones.

Large local reactions also have a tendency to reoccur on re-sting. Repeat stings result in a large local reaction regardless of the presence of the venom-specific IgE or venom stinging insect immunotherapy. Determining the serum-specific IgE by RAST or skin testing does not aid in treatment or predicting prognosis in affected patients even though approximately 4% of them can develop anaphylaxis upon re-sting. Therefore, stinging insect immunotherapy is not indicated in patients with large local reactions.

In the southeastern United States, stings from imported fire ants are a common cause of Hymenoptera insect venom hypersensitivity. A survey by Stafford and co-workers in 1989, in cooperation with the American Academy of Allergy, Asthma, and Immunology Fire Ant Subcommittee, reported that approximately 20,755 patients are treated annually for reactions to fire ant stings. In a series by Adams and Lofgren, it was found that children and adolescents younger than 16 years of age living in an endemic area are most likely to be stung, having a sting rate of 32% to 52%. Tracy and co-workers reported in a prospective study involving 107 subjects that brief exposures (3 weeks) to imported fire ant-endemic areas by an unsensitized population resulted in a sting attack rate of 51% (55 individuals were stung out of 107 subjects who completed the study). In this group, imported fire ant-specific IgE developed in 13%, as shown by skin testing with whole body extract, and was more sensitive than imported fire ant venom-specific RAST, which converted in only 1.8%.

In children the natural history after an imported fire ant-induced mild systemic reaction is unknown. Thus, in contrast to a similar reaction induced by other Hymenoptera, children with systemic reactions limited to the skin require treatment with imported fire ant whole body vaccine.

To summarize, approximately half the patients with insect sting-induced anaphylaxis will not react to a subsequent sting and approximately half will react with symptoms similar to their previous reaction. A few will have a more severe reaction. The prognosis without treatment is excellent in children and adolescents younger than 16 years who have had mild systemic reactions to a bee, wasp, yellow jacket, or hornet sting. Large local reactions are usually self-limited.

TREATMENT

Large Local Reactions

Treatment of large local reactions consists of ice packs, elevation of the extremity, antihistamines, and pain medications. Most reactions are self-limited, peaking at 24 to 72 hours and lasting up to 7 to 10 days. A short course of

glucocorticosteroids may be helpful for individuals with severe large local reactions even though no controlled studies proving efficacy are available. Fire ant stings are treated by repeated cleansing of the site with soap and water, avoiding excoriation, and immediate treatment of any secondary infection.

Systemic Reactions

A systemic reaction to a Hymenoptera sting may evolve rapidly from a mild to a severe reaction. Early recognition and treatment are essential to prevent fatal outcomes. Therefore, an aggressive treatment program is preferred.

Treatment is the same as for any anaphylactic reaction, regardless of cause, epinephrine being the drug of choice (Table 21–1). Aqueous epinephrine 1:1000 (w/v), 0.2 to 0.5 ml, given subcutaneously or intramuscularly, should be administered immediately (0.01 ml per kg in children, not to exceed 0.3 ml per dose). Epinephrine 1:1000 (w/v), 0.1 to 0.3 ml, also may be injected directly into the sting site to delay absorption of venom. Repeated doses for protracted symptoms should be given as necessary or every 15 to 20 minutes. All patients, but especially those with a history of cardiac disease, should be carefully monitored. Intravenous epinephrine, 1:10,000 (w/v), given slowly, is indicated for anaphylactic shock that does not respond to therapy. Parenteral (intravenous or intramuscular) antihistamines, such as diphenhydramine hydrochloride (Benadryl, 5 mg per kg per 24 hours), in divided doses (maximal dose 400 mg per 24 hours in adults), also should be used for persistent symptoms of anaphylaxis.

Asthma should be treated with continuous inhalational beta-agonists. Intravenous fluid replacement, e.g., saline or colloid-containing solutions, is necessary for persistent hypotension. Pressor agents should be administered if shock persists; systemic glucocorticosteroids, if given early, may be useful to reverse protracted anaphylaxis or prevent delayed anaphylaxis. Oxygen therapy and airway patency are essential, and intubation or cricothyrotomy is indicated for severe upper airway edema that does not respond to therapy. In refractory cases that do not respond to epinephrine because a beta-adrenergic blocking agent is complicating the

Table 21–1. **Treatment of Anaphylaxis**

I. Immediate measures
 a. Aqueous epinephrine 1:1000 (w/v) (weight/volume); 0.01 ml/kg dose to a maximum dose of 0.2 to 0.5 ml by subcutaneous or intramuscular route and, if necessary, repeat every 15 minutes as necessary.
 b. Aqueous epinephrine 1:1000 (w/v), 0.1 ml in 0.9 ml of normal saline (1:10,000 (w/v)), IV over several minutes, and repeat as necessary for anaphylaxis not responding to therapy.
II. General measures
 a. Place subject in recumbent or Trendelenburg position and elevate lower extremities.
 b. Give oxygen.
 c. Maintain airway (endotracheal tube or cricothyrotomy may be required).
 d. Place a venous tourniquet above the reaction site to decrease absorption of the allergen.
III. Additional measures
 a. Aqueous epinephrine 1:1000 (w/v), 0.1–0.3 ml, at the reaction site will delay allergen absorption. (Should not be applied to digits.)
 b. Diphenhydramine (Benadryl®, 5 mg/kg/day) in divided doses, with the maximum dose per day being 300 mg per child and 400 mg per adult. Give slowly IV or give IM.
 c. For asthma, nebulized β_2-agonist, albuterol (Ventolin® or Proventil®), or metaproterenol (Metaprel®), 1.25–2.5 mg (0.25–0.5 ml of 5% solution) in 3 ml of saline. Repeat as needed every 20 minutes, or give by continuous nebulization (can use with ipratropium bromide).
 d. Ipratropium bromide, 0.5 mg in adults, 0.25 mg in children, in 3 ml of saline every 30 minutes for 3 doses, then every 2 to 4 hours (can use with β_2 agonist).
 e. Intravenous volume expanders (saline, colloids) at a rate of 20–50 ml/kg first hour for hypotension.
 f. If hypotension persists, dopamine, 400 mg in 500 ml D5W, should be given IV at an appropriate rate to maintain normal blood pressure. Children: 6 mg/kg of dopamine in 100 ml D5W; dose 2–20 μg/kg/min.
 g. Cimetidine (Tagamet®), 300 mg or ranitidine (Zantac®), 150 mg IV administered over 5 minutes, may also be useful. Adjust dose accordingly for children.
 h. Glucagon, 1 mg (1 unit) given IV as a bolus over 2 minutes, may be useful when a beta blocker is complicating anaphylaxis. Adjust accordingly for children.
 i. Glucocorticosteroids (i.e., methylprednisolone 1–2 mg per kg IV), is usually not helpful in acute anaphylaxis, but may be useful in delayed-onset or protracted anaphylaxis.

Adapted from Lockey RF, Rosenbach KP, Nelson RP: Insect sting hypersensitivity. *In* Rakel RE (ed): Conn's Current Therapy 1999. Philadelphia, WB Saunders, 1999, pp 786–791.

management, 1 mg (1 unit) glucagon given slowly intravenously over several minutes may be useful. A continuous infusion of 1 to 5 mg of glucagon per hour may be given if required.

REFERRAL TO A SPECIALIST

Any individual who has a mild, moderate, or severe systemic reaction should be evaluated by a specialist. All patients, regardless of age, who have mild, moderate or severe systemic reactions from ants should be evaluated. When in doubt, a referral is the best advice to assure proper evaluation and, if necessary, treatment.

STINGING INSECT IMMUNOTHERAPY

Stinging insect immunotherapy is a safe and effective method to prevent future sting-induced anaphylaxis in individuals who have experienced systemic reactions to an Hymenoptera insect. Three to 12% of individuals who undergo such therapy have systemic reactions during treatment. This rate of systemic reaction is no greater than that experienced with conventional inhalant immunotherapy. No fatalities have been reported with insect immunotherapy.

Indications

Which patients should be considered for immunotherapy? Currently, all adults, whatever the nature of their systemic allergic reactions, should be evaluated and considered for immunotherapy. More data are needed to determine whether adults who react to stings with only generalized pruritus, erythema, and urticaria are at lower risk if stung again than those with more severe systemic reactions not limited to skin (Table 21–2).

Even though the pathophysiology of a large local reaction may be mediated by an IgE mechanism, the natural history of a large local reaction, as previously discussed, makes immunotherapy unnecessary and, therefore, further evaluation is not indicated.

Stinging Insect Immunotherapy Regimen

Immunotherapy to stinging insects is safe, highly effective, and reduces the risk of re-

Table 21–2. **Indications for Stinging Insect Immunotherapy**

Classification of Sting Reaction by History	Venom Skin Test	Immunotherapy
Large local	Not indicated	No
Systemic (mild)	Positive	Patient–MD decision
	Negative	No
Children < 16 years	Positive	No
Systemic (moderate to severe)	Positive	Yes
	Negative	No
Toxic	Not indicated	Not indicated

sting anaphylaxis from 50%–60% to less than 5%. Individuals who still react to a second sting while on venom immunotherapy usually have mild reactions. The venoms used for immunotherapy are the same as those used for skin testing. There are different schedules for delivering increasing amounts of venom allergen until a maintenance dose of 100 μg is reached for each venom to which the individual is sensitive. Some investigators feel that only 50 μg of a specific venom is needed to achieve protection.

Whole-body vaccines are currently used for diagnosis and treating ant-induced systemic allergic reactions because ant venoms are not commercially available. Double-blind trials using a whole-body vaccine versus imported fire ant venom have yet to be conducted.

A maintenance dose of the appropriate vaccine is usually achieved over a 6- to 12-week period. Thereafter, the interval between injections can increase to every 4 weeks for the first year and subsequently to every 6 weeks.

Reactions Associated with Stinging Insect Immunotherapy

When venom vaccines were approved by the Food and Drug Administration in 1979, the question of the safety of venom immunotherapy was addressed by a long-term study. The Hymenoptera Venom Study, sponsored by the American Academy of Allergy, Asthma, and Immunology, followed 3236 subjects with Hymenoptera allergy for 3 years. The study demonstrated that skin tests and immunotherapy results in subjects with a history of systemic allergic reactions to Hymenoptera stings are safe when supervised by experienced physicians. Of the 3236 Hymenoptera-sensitive subjects who underwent skin testing, 0.25% had severe systemic reactions. Of the 1410 subjects who were given immunotherapy, 12% had systemic reactions while receiving the therapy, of which 9% of these systemic reactions were severe. There were no fatalities.

If patients are receiving venom immunotherapy in the primary care physician's office, he or she must be aware of the following. Since no initial warning sign has been identified as predictive of a severe outcome, all mild systemic reactions induced by immunotherapy should be regarded as potentially life-threatening and treated as such. Local redness and swelling at the site of injection is common, and one-fourth of patients may develop large local reactions from immunotherapy. Stinging insect immunotherapy has also been found to be safe for use during pregnancy. However, the risks and benefits of beginning such therapy during pregnancy should be discussed by a specialist and the patient or her family. All patients must wait 20–30 minutes in a physician's office after immunotherapy is given.

Duration of Immunotherapy

A position statement reported by the Committee on Insects of the American Academy of Allergy, Asthma, and Immunology outlines the following recommendations for continuing immunotherapy after 3 to 5 years. (1) The duration of further immunotherapy should be discussed by the physician specialist and the patient. Lifestyle issues, underlying medical conditions, repeat skin test results, and career or job requirements need to be considered. If a decision is made to stop such therapy, the pros and cons of carrying self-administered epinephrine should be reviewed carefully with the patient. (2) Although the conversion from positive test results to negative skin test results during insect immunotherapy is a criterion for stopping such therapy, there have been isolated reports of subsequent anaphylaxis after re-sting. In such cases, the issues outlined previously need to be discussed. (3) Patients with mild (cutaneous only) or moderate (mild with respiratory distress) reactions, in general, may discontinue stinging insect immunotherapy after 3 to 5 years. However, there is some minimal risk of re-sting reaction, and the severity of this reaction is usually, but not always, mild. (4) Treated patients with severe systemic reactions (symptoms of mild or moderate with hypotension, laryngeal edema, or bronchospasm) may have a higher risk for a similar kind of systemic reaction after insect immunotherapy is discontinued. Thus, these patients may benefit from treatment for 5 years or more.

In summary, unless the skin test response becomes negative, in which case immunotherapy can be discontinued, continuation of venom immunotherapy beyond 3 to 5 years should be decided by the physician and the patient. When in doubt, such therapy should be continued.

ARTHROPOD BITES AND STINGS

Arthropod bites and stings can be inflicted by different species of insects, arachnids (spiders), and acarids (mites). Several kinds of reactions are described: (1) trauma inflicted by the puncture of the skin, (2) reaction to the irritating toxic substances, and (3) allergic or IgE-mediated anaphylaxis. For example, the io caterpillar has stiff spines containing a poison that, when touched, pricks the skin and causes a severe local reaction. Proteins isolated from the saliva of various arthropods may play a role in the pathogenesis of local and systemic reactions. For example, the high molecular weight protein, F-1, of the mosquito, *Aedes aegypti*, seems to be the major skin-reactive substance.

Papular urticaria to flea bites is characterized by pruritic erythematous papules, vesicles, or bullae grouped in clusters. They are caused by multiple flea, mosquito, and bed bug bites. Papular urticaria develops in subjects with delayed reactions to such bites. It commonly occurs in children 2 to 7 years of age and usually involves the extremities.

Anaphylactic reactions from bites are rare, and they have been most commonly associated with insects of the orders Hemiptera and Diptera. Kissing bugs, cone-nose bugs, or assassin bugs of the order Hemiptera, genus *Triatoma*, are commonly found from Texas to California. A systemic allergic reaction has been reported secondary to a brown spider bite. Typically, these bugs bite at night when the victim is asleep; the bite is painless and the victim is awakened by itching, respiratory distress, and other allergic symptoms. Several deaths have been reported from anaphylaxis in the United States from biting insects, and there is evidence of IgE-sensitization to the insect's saliva with such reactions. IgE antibody-induced anaphylaxis also has been reported to the western black-legged tick, *Ixodus pacificus*, in California. The most commonly occurring insect bites are from the order Diptera, family Culicidae, or mosquitoes and appear to cause rare systemic reactions. The black flies (order Diptera, family Simuliidae) and horse flies have been associated with systemic reactions.

PROTECTION AND PREVENTION
Precautions for Insect Avoidance

Individuals who are insect allergic should be able to recognize the stinging insects (Table 21–3). Solitary outdoor activities should be avoided as much as possible. Recognition of nesting and foraging behavior is important. Avoid strong perfumes, lotions, or sprays that may attract insects. Insect repellents are not very effective. Patients should recognize fire ant colonies, which should be treated with ant bait insecticides to eliminate them.

Prescription of Emergency Treatment Kits

Patients who have experienced a systemic reaction following an insect sting should be given

Table 21–3.   **Measures for Prevention of Hymenoptera Stings**

What to Do	What Not to Do
Know the stinging insects	Do not use scented lotions or perfumes, which attract insects
Know nesting and foraging behaviors	
Remove or destroy nearby nests and hives: professionals do this	Do not provoke the insects, disturb a nest or hive
Wear ankle socks and ankle-high shoes	Do not go barefoot
Keep outdoor living area clean and free of refuse and garbage	Do not leave garbage cans of food uncovered
Insect repellents are useless for stinging insects	
For biting insects, midges, flies and mosquitoes, use deet*-containing repellents on clothes and skin, or apply Avon Skin-So-Soft.	

*N-N-diethyl-3-methylbenzamide: Most insect repellents contain this chemical. It is the only chemical insect repellent currently approved by the U.S. Food and Drug Administration.

a self-injectable epinephrine syringe. Instructions on the indications, use, and handling should be reviewed by the physician. Patient education is essential for correct delivery of the drug. In the United States, Epipen, Epi E-Z pen, Epipen Jr, Epi E-Z pen Jr, and the Ana-kit are brands of injectable epinephrine. Some of these devices automatically deliver, upon pressure activation, either 0.15 or 0.3 ml of epinephrine, subcutaneously. The Ana-kit contains two 0.3 ml doses of epinephrine, which are injected manually, an antihistamine, chlorpheniramine maleate, and a tourniquet. A Medic Alert bracelet or medallion (Medic Alert, 2323 Colorado Avenue, Turlock, CA 95382) should be worn at all times.

Suggested Reading

Bousquet J, Lockey RF, Malling H-J (eds.): WHO Position Paper. Allergen immunotherapy: Therapeutic vaccines for allergic diseases. Eur J Allergy Clin Immunol 53:1–42, 1998

deShazo RD, Butcher BT, Banks WA: Reactions to the stings of the imported fire ant [Review]. N Engl J Med 323:462–466, 1990

Graft DF, Golden DBK, Reisman RE, et al: The discontinuation of Hymenoptera venom immunotherapy. [Position statement: Report from the Committee on Insects]. J Allergy Clin Immunol 101:573–575, 1998

Hunt KJ, Valentine MD, Sobotka AK, et al: A controlled trial of immunotherapy in insect hypersensitivity. N Engl J Med 299:157–161, 1978

Lockey RF, Turkeltaub PC, Baird-Warren IA, et al: The Hymenoptera venom study I, 1979–1982: Demographics and history-sting data. J Allergy Clin Immunol 82:370–381

Lockey RF, Turkeltaub PC, Olive CE, et al: The Hymenoptera venom study. II. Skin test results and safety of venom skin testing. J Allergy Clin Immunol 84:967–974, 1989

Lockey RF, Turkeltaub PC, Olive ES, et al: The Hymenoptera venom study. III. Safety of venom immunotherapy. J Allergy Clin Immunol 86:775–780, 1990

Reisman RE: Natural history of insect sting allergy: Relationship of severity of symptoms of initial sting anaphylaxis to re-sting reactions. J Allergy Clin Immunol 90:335–339, 1992

Valentine MD, Schuberth KC, Kagey-Sobotka A, et al. The value of immunotherapy with venom in children with allergy to insect stings. N Engl J Med 323:1601–1603, 1990

Yunginger JW: Insect allergy. *In* Middleton EM, Reed CER, Ellis EFE, Adkinson NFA, Yunginger JWY, Busse WWB (eds.). Allergy Principles and Practice. 5th ed St. Louis, Mosby-Year Book, 1998, pp 1063–1072

Chapter 22

Latex Allergy

Dennis R. Ownby

During the late 1980s, immediate-type, or IgE antibody-mediated, allergic reactions to natural rubber latex became widely recognized. Most of these reactions were associated with health care, but some episodes occurred during other activities. Reports from the 1920s were consistent with allergic reactions to natural rubber latex, but it was not until 1979 that Nutter reported a woman with immediate contact urticaria from rubber gloves. Subsequently, latex allergy has been recognized with increasing frequency. The potential for fatal allergic reactions related to latex was first reported in 1991.

The word *latex* can have two different meanings. The first definition of latex in most dictionaries is of a milky, usually white, fluid derived from a variety of plants, which will coagulate on exposure to air. The second definition of latex is that of a water emulsion of finely divided particles of synthetic rubber or plastic, often used in paints and coatings. Thus, latex gloves are made from the latex of rubber trees and may cause allergic reactions, but latex house paint rarely contains natural rubber and will not cause allergic reactions in latex-allergic individuals. Frequently the phrase natural rubber latex is used to specify rubber made from latex that comes from the Brazilian rubber tree, *Hevea brasiliensis,* but in this chapter the word latex is used to refer to natural rubber latex unless further clarification is necessary to prevent confusion.

Natural rubber was originally discovered by native peoples of Central and South America. The first practical use of latex was the development of waterproof fabrics by MacIntosh, patented in 1823. This development was followed by the discovery of vulcanization by Goodyear in 1839. Vulcanization is the process by which latex is heated in the presence of sulfur, producing much better elasticity and thermostability. The first medical use of rubber gloves is attributed to Dr. William Halstead in the 1880s. With the increasing demand for rubber products, production of latex was increased by the cultivation of *H. brasiliensis* trees on large plantations. Today commercial rubber plantations are most common in southeast Asia, Malaysia, and Africa. In the last 20 years, glove manufacturing companies have moved production facilities to the countries where the latex is being produced to reduce costs.

CLINICAL MANIFESTATIONS OF LATEX ALLERGY

Adverse reactions to latex products, especially gloves, can typically be classified into one of three types: (1) irritant contact dermatitis, (2) delayed allergic-contact dermatitis, and (3) immediate or IgE-mediated allergic reactions.

Irritant contact dermatitis is a common problem, especially for persons frequently wearing latex or rubber gloves for long periods of time. The affected skin is dry and scaly. In severe cases the skin may thicken, crack, and bleed. Excoriation is often present. These reactions result from irritation and disruption of the epidermis by various agents and activities including repeated hand washing, use of strong detergents and antimicrobial cleaners, and hyper-hydration of the skin from occlusion under an impermeable barrier. Dusting powder in gloves may also contribute to irritation by increasing mechanical abrasion. The severity of the changes may wax and wane, gradually becoming chronic. Treatment of irritant contact dermatitis should focus on reducing the inciting elements, local skin care with moisturizers, and reducing the time spent under occlusion.

Allergic or delayed contact dermatitis can occur from contact with rubber in many different ways. The reaction consists of an erythematous, pruritic, and sometimes vesicular rash, appearing 12 to 36 hours after the rubber contact. The rash is caused by a cell-mediated, delayed-type hypersensitivity reaction to low-molecular–weight materials in the rubber. Most reactions are related to the chemical accelerators and antioxidants that are added during manufacturing. Thiuram compounds are the most common cause of dermatitis, but carbamate and paraphenylenediamine compounds cause similar reactions. A diagnosis of delayed contact dermatitis can be entertained from the history of the onset of the skin lesions in addition to the morphology and distribution of the lesions. Lesions will appear only where there has been direct contact with the rubber article. A clinical suspicion can be confirmed by patch testing with the appropriate rubber chemicals. Treatment of contact reactions is avoidance of the chemical causing the reaction. For workers who require barrier protection, this means finding a glove produced with lower levels of different chemicals. Although many persons switch from glove to glove trying to find one that does not cause a reaction, knowledge of the specific sensitizing agent, which can be gained from patch testing, can significantly ease the process.

Immediate or IgE-mediated allergic reactions also may be caused by latex. These reactions are caused by IgE antibodies specific for proteins or glycoproteins present in latex. Most, if not all, of these proteins are present in the latex as it comes from the tree. Reactions typically start within minutes of exposure to latex, but sometimes the interval between exposure and onset of symptoms can be an hour or more. As with other IgE-mediated reactions the cardinal signs are itching, erythema, and edema. The severity of immediate allergic reactions can range from mild local itching to fatal anaphylaxis. In some individuals, there seems to a progression from mild to increasingly severe reactions whereas in others the first reaction the person is aware of is severe. Some individuals continue to have mild reactions that do not appear to increase in severity over years of exposure.

Immediate contact urticaria is typically the first noticeable manifestation of IgE sensitization to latex. Individuals with latex allergy develop redness, itching, and hives 1 to 30 minutes after contact with latex. Swelling also may be prominent, especially if a mucosal surface such as the lips or tongue is involved. Without treatment, these local symptoms usually subside within a few hours. Many health care workers mistakenly attribute these symptoms to glove powder or to hand washing materials. Others may have noticed that immediately washing their hands after removing gloves reduces the intensity and duration of the reactions. Prompt hand washing may also prevent them from inducing ocular symptoms by touching or rubbing their eyes while there is still allergen on their hands. Simply rubbing the eyes can transfer sufficient allergen into the conjunctiva to cause a local reaction.

Rhinitis, conjunctivitis, and asthma also may be caused by direct or indirect contact with latex. During production of latex gloves, corn starch powder (dusting powder, U.S.P.) is placed on the surfaces of the glove to prevent the glove from sticking to itself and to aid in donning the glove. Although the powder is on the glove, latex allergens may be absorbed onto the surface of the starch particles. When gloves are donned or doffed, the allergen-coated starch particles may become airborne providing a mechanism for airborne allergen dispersion. Airborne latex may cause allergic rhinitis, conjunctivitis, and asthma in allergic individuals. In most health care workers it is difficult to determine the relative importance of airborne versus cutaneous latex contact in inducing symptoms; however, several case reports suggest that airway symptoms will continue if airborne exposure continues even after direct latex contact is halted. A case report also suggested that an emergency room clerk developed asthma from airborne exposure to latex even though she did not personally wear latex gloves. The clinical histories of some patients suggest that airborne exposure to latex may be related to recurrent sinusitis.

Latex allergy should be considered in any person occupationally exposed to latex with new onset of asthma or in any exposed person whose pre-existing asthma is increasing in severity. One study suggested that latex-related occupational asthma may be present in as many as 2.5% of health care workers. Latex-induced occupational asthma may be severe, requiring some individuals to discontinue working in environments where latex exposure could occur. The onset of latex-related asthma can be subtle. Many health care workers are unaware of wheezing or shortness of breath. They do notice increased fatigue and often relate it to stress on the job. They also may notice a sensation of chest tightness, especially when they are going to bed. Initially it may be hard to correlate these vague symptoms with work or latex exposure. The best method for establishing a diagnosis is to have the person's peak flow or spirometry monitored while at and away from work. Similarly, latex-related symptoms may be difficult to distinguish in persons with pre-existing asthma. The clinical course may be a slow or relatively rapid increase in the severity of asthma symptoms. When this change takes place over months or years, the relationship to latex can be found only when there is a high index of suspicion. Studies have documented the relationship between asthma and latex by environmental challenges, but routine diagnostic methods are not established.

Anaphylaxis can be induced in latex-allergic individuals either by direct contact or airborne exposure to latex. Fatal anaphylaxis has been related to latex balloons on catheters used to administer barium enemas. Latex-induced anaphylaxis has been reported in many settings including exposure to condoms or bladder catheters, intra-abdominal surgery, childbirth, dental examinations, vaginal or rectal examinations, or holding sports equipment with rubber grips. Anaphylaxis also can be triggered by blowing up rubber balloons or by being around rubber balloons, especially if they burst.

At present, there is no way to identify which latex-allergic individuals are at risk for anaphylaxis. Individuals with previous anaphylactic reactions are presumably at high risk as are individuals who have had severe symptoms with minimal exposure. Although the risk for other individuals with latex allergy may be lower, it cannot be dismissed, and all allergic individuals should be given detailed advice on latex avoidance and emergency procedures if avoidance fails. The risk of anaphylaxis appears to depend on the degree of allergic sensitivity and the amount and rate at which the allergen enters the body.

DIAGNOSIS OF LATEX ALLERGY

A diagnosis of latex allergy is based on a consistent medical history and demonstration of latex-specific IgE antibodies. Diagnostic challenges may be necessary in some cases, but challenge procedures are not well standardized. Observation of an acute reaction is helpful, but in most cases the severity of a reaction must be estimated from the patient's description. A consistent medical history includes signs and symptoms of allergic reactions shortly after exposure to latex. The more typical the signs and symptoms, and the more times these symptoms have occurred, the more likely the diagnosis. In most cases, the exposure to latex is obvious, such as when a person dons latex gloves; in other cases, however, the exposure is not as obvious. Having an adhesive bandage applied to the skin or standing with wet feet on a nonslip bath mat provide potential exposures to latex that may not be recognized. Symptoms usually appear first at the site of latex exposure, but this site may be difficult to discern when the onset of symptoms is rapid or when the exposure is airborne. Patients also need to be directly asked about symptoms in situations in which latex exposure is likely to occur, such as during dental or medical examinations, when blowing up balloons, or during surgical procedures. As discussed earlier, typical symptoms would be itching, swelling, and redness at the site of latex contact, such as swelling and itching of the lips during a dental examination. Rhinitis, conjunctivitis, and asthma also may occur. It is important to clearly establish the time sequence between the probable or known exposure to latex and the onset of symptoms. Symptoms occurring hours after exposure are not likely to be caused by allergy.

If a patient is seen during an acute episode, it is important for the treating physician to document the severity of the reaction. It is much more informative to know that the person's blood pressure was 80/40 mmHg during a reaction, than it is to have the patient state that they felt faint during a reaction. Important areas to document, in as much detail as possible, include visible swelling, respiratory rate, pulse, wheezing, blood pressure, and pulmonary function. Documenting the treatment given to the patient and the response to the patient to the treatment are equally important.

When evaluating a person for possible latex allergy the physician also must inquire about factors that are related to the risk of latex allergy. Individuals with other allergies are more likely to be allergic to latex, so patients should be questioned about allergic rhinitis, asthma, atopic dermatitis or other allergic problems. Particularly important is a history of adverse reactions to foods. Several common foods (Table 22–1) contain allergens that cross-react with allergens in latex; thus, a history of allergic symptoms following ingestion of one of these foods increases the probability of latex allergy. The patient's occupation is important, because frequent exposure to latex, especially occupational exposure, appears to increase the risk of latex allergy. Other potential exposures to latex such as surgical procedures, indwelling catheters, or use of rubber gloves for house work or hobbies should be evaluated. If a patient has undergone invasive surgical or diagnostic proce-

Table 22–1. **Foods Reported to Cause Reactions in Latex-Allergic Individuals**

Banana*
Avocado*
Kiwi*
European chestnut*
Apple
Cantaloupe
Celery
Fig
Papaya
Pear
Pitted fruits (cherry, peach, plum, etc.)
Potato
Spinach
Tomatoes
Turnip
Wheat

*These foods have the clearest and most frequent associations with latex allergy.

dures, he or she should be questioned about any unexplained adverse reactions. Although the history may be highly suggestive of latex allergy, a diagnostic impression must be substantiated by demonstration of latex-specific IgE antibodies. Incorrectly diagnosing a problem as latex allergy can be as dangerous to the patient as missing a diagnosis of latex allergy.

In most developed countries, skin testing is the optimal method for demonstrating latex-specific IgE antibodies. Several studies have shown that epicutaneous skin testing is sensitive, specific, and economical. In most studies, the sensitivity of epicutaneous skin tests approaches 100%. Skin testing has the advantage of providing information within minutes, and the results of the tests are clear to the patient. As with other allergens, epicutaneous testing with latex extracts has been associated with anaphylactic events. Because of the potential for adverse events, skin testing with latex should be performed only by physicians with substantial experience with the risks of skin testing and in a location in which prompt emergency medical care can be provided.

Currently, in the United States, there is no commercially available, Food and Drug Administration cleared, diagnostic latex extract for skin testing. This situation means that if a physician wants to perform skin testing, he must prepare his own latex extract. These homemade extracts are rarely well characterized, and, therefore, the diagnostic value of skin tests performed with these extracts is unknown. False-negative results are likely because of inadequate concentrations of constituent allergens, but false-positive reactions from irritants also could occur. Recently reported results with a candidate extract are promising, suggesting that a diagnostic extract may become available in the near future in the United States. In Canada, Bencard Allergy Laboratories (Missisauga, Ontario) and, in France, Stallergenes S.A. (Marseilles, France) provide latex extracts for diagnostic testing that appear to be reliable.

In addition to skin testing, latex-specific IgE can be demonstrated by serologic tests. Three companies now market FDA-cleared materials for *in vitro* detection of anti-latex IgE antibodies in the United States. Depending on the study population selected, these commercial tests appear to have sensitivities and specificities of between 80% and 90%. Although these values are relatively good for tests of specific IgE, they mean that 10% to 20% of persons with true latex allergy may be missed by these tests. Thus, a negative result of an *in vitro* test cannot be used to conclusively exclude the possibility of latex allergy. If a patient's history is highly suggestive, the patient should be cared for as if a latex allergy were present even if an IgE antibody test result is negative. Some commercial laboratories use reagents produced in-house when testing for anti-latex IgE antibodies or use alternative scoring systems. The results obtained by these commercial laboratories have rarely been critically examined in relation to clinical disease in a large number of patients; therefore, the diagnostic value of tests performed in these laboratories is unknown. Physicians ordering tests for anti-latex IgE antibodies should ask the laboratory whether the method used is cleared by the FDA and if testing is performed according to the manufacturer's instructions. If they are not, the physician should demand documentation of the diagnostic value and reproducibility of the testing results.

RISK FACTORS FOR LATEX ALLERGY

The group at highest risk for latex allergy is individuals with spina bifida. A survey of myelodysplasia clinics in 16 Shriners Hospitals (a total of 2925 children) found that between 0% and 22% of children in each clinic had latex allergy. The clinic reporting the 22% prevalence was the only one in which most of the families were directly interviewed. A serologic and skin test survey of patients with spina bifida revealed that 44% (51 of 116) had latex-specific IgE. Twenty-five of the 51 skin test–positive children had symptoms related to latex. The sensitivity of the skin tests (100%) was slightly better than the *in vitro* test (95.8%), and the specificity of the skin tests (82.3%) was also better than that of the *in vitro* test (68.9%). Other studies of children with myelodysplasia report latex allergy in up to 65% of children.

This high prevalence of latex allergy in persons with spina bifida is presumably secondary to the early and frequent surgical procedures these individuals typically undergo in addition to the recurrent contact with rubber urinary tract catheters and gloves used in other aspects of their care. Exposure to latex during chronic medical care is apparently the cause of the high prevalence of latex allergy in persons with spina bifida, so individuals with other conditions that require frequent surgery and chronic care, such as bladder exstrophy, cerebral palsy, and spinal cord injury, are probably also at increased risk. Individuals in these high-risk groups are probably best taken care of in environments in which latex exposure is kept to an absolute minimum. Reducing latex exposure should substantially reduce the risk of the individual developing latex allergy. Allergies, including latex allergy, may develop at any age so it is probably prudent to minimize the latex exposure of all individuals in risk groups. Health care workers and others who are occupationally exposed to latex also are thought to be at increased risk of latex allergy. Several studies have suggested that the risk of latex allergy or latex sensitization is from 2.8% to 17.1%. In Finland, 2.8% of workers (15 of 512) in clinical units and laboratories were allergic to latex. The highest incidence of latex allergy (4 of 54 persons, or 7.4%) was found in operating room physicians. During 1991, 49 health care workers at the Mayo Medical Center were referred to the Allergic Diseases Department for possible latex allergy; 36 had rhinoconjunctivitis and 13 experienced bronchospasm with latex exposure. Of these, 34 had positive skin test results and 19 had a positive result of the latex *in vitro* tests for anti-latex IgE antibodies. In a large urban hospital, 8.9% of 781 nurses were found to have latex-specific IgE antibodies. The prevalence of latex sensitization did not significantly differ between nurses working in the operating rooms or intensive care units when compared with those on general medical or surgical floors. The risk of sensitization appeared to be higher in those with histories of other allergic diseases and in non-Caucasians.

These estimates of the prevalence of latex allergy in health care workers are higher than the presumed prevalence of latex allergy in the general population. It is, however, difficult to determine the relative risk of latex allergy in health care workers because there are few comparable studies of individuals employed in other occupations. When health care workers are studied, the prevalence of latex allergy may be overestimated because of health care workers' knowledge and concern about latex allergy.

The prevalence of type I latex allergy in unselected populations is not clearly known. All of the currently used methods for detecting latex allergy have potential flaws. Histories of symptoms may be unreliable for many reasons, skin tests may detect sensitized but asymptomatic individuals, and *in vitro* tests may detect cross-reactive antibodies. When 1000 blood donors were screened using the FDA-cleared AlaSTAT method, 6.4% were seropositive for anti-latex IgE. In this study efforts were made to reduce the number of health care workers who were included among the blood donors. A similar study of 996 preoperative, adult patients, found a prevalence of 6.7%. When skin tests have been used as a screening tool, the prevalence of anti-latex IgE antibodies appears to be lower. In an outpatient allergy clinic, 3 of 44 atopic children had positive epicutaneous skin test responses to a latex glove extract. None of these children had histories of latex-associated reactions, and none of the 36 nonatopic children tested had a positive skin test response to latex. One of 130 (0.8%) non–health care workers at a university hospital in Finland was found to be allergic to rubber by prick test, whereas 3 of 100 atopic adults who were not occupationally exposed to latex were skin test–positive in a Canadian study.

LATEX PROCESSING AND ALLERGENS

Processing

Natural rubber latex is a processed plant product widely used in many different types of products. Among the important physical properties of natural rubber latex are its high degree of elasticity and impermeability to water. These properties have made latex valuable in many barrier applications, such as in gloves. Currently, over 99% of natural rubber is derived from the latex obtained from the commercial rubber tree *Hevea brasiliensis.*

Latex is collected from mature *H. bra-* *siliensis* trees by cutting a spiral groove into the bark of the tree and allowing the latex to drip from the groove down a spout and into a cup: a process called tapping. Ammonia, or another preservative, is placed in the collection cup to prevent autocoagulation and bacterial contamination of the latex. Ammonia disrupts the rubber particles and produces a two-phase product that is approximately 30% to 40% solids. Rubber particles contain cis-1,4-polyisoprene coated with a layer of protein and lipids. Natural rubber forms as the polyisoprene units polymerize into long and variably cross-linked chains. Many of the proteins in latex appear to have antifungal properties.

In a processing plant, the latex is mixed with various chemicals such as antioxidants (to protect the finished latex from oxygen in the air) and accelerators (to speed the process of vulcanization). After compounding, the latex is pumped into large vats where forms are dipped into the latex. The forms are usually coated with a coagulant to produce a thicker layer of latex and with releasing agents to help separate the product from the mold. After the form has been dipped, the product is leached in water before drying, vulcanization, and removal from the mold. The protein content of *Hevea* latex products, and presumably the allergen content, can be reduced considerably by extended washing, heat treatment, chlorination, or enzyme digestion. These processes can be used alone or in combination; however, each additional step in manufacturing adds additional cost. At the present time, it is not known whether there is a threshold of allergen content below which allergic sensitization will not occur.

Allergens

At least 10 individual proteins have been identified as allergens in latex from *Hevea* trees. By international convention, allergens are named using the first three letters of the genus, the first letter of the species and a numeral indicating order of discovery. Thus, allergens from *Hevea brasilenesis* are designated Hev b 1,2,3, and so forth. Some of these allergens (Hev b 1, Hev b 5, Hev b 6, and Hev b 7) are fully characterized and sequenced, whereas others are only partially sequenced. The molecular weights of these allergens range from 4.6 to 57 kDa, although aggregates and polymers of some of the allergens have been found.

Latex and Food Allergies

Many studies have shown that some foods contain allergens that cross-react with latex allergens. These foods are listed in Table 22–1. One study found that among 47 latex-allergic adults (mostly health care workers), 17 (36%) had clinical reactivity to at least one food. Fifty-three percent had a positive prick test result with avocado, and a smaller number were reactive to potato, banana, tomato, chestnut, and kiwi. These cross-reactions appear to be caused by the presence of highly homologous proteins or protein segments in the foods and latex. The presence of these homologous proteins does not appear to be related to close phylogenetic relationships between the foods and rubber trees. The clinical importance of these cross-reactions is variable. In some patients the presence of cross-reactive IgE antibodies appears to be an incidental finding with little or no clinical significance, whereas in others both latex and the cross-reactive food will cause clinically significant reactions. As with latex-induced reactions, reactions from the cross-reactive foods can range from mild to severe. The severity of the reaction to latex does not predict the severity of the reactions to the food nor does the severity of the reaction to food indicate the severity of the response to latex.

Two questions are frequently asked about latex and food allergies. What should latex allergic patients be told about eating cross-reactive foods? If a person has a reaction to one of the cross-reactive foods, should he or she be evaluated for latex allergy? Prospective studies to answer these questions have not been published. When trying to answer these questions, it is important to balance the patient's safety with the difficulties of needless dietary restrictions. Some would say that none of these foods are essential for a balanced and nutritious diet and therefore they should all be avoided. In the author's opinion, all patients with latex allergy should be cautioned about the risks of cross-reactivity between foods and latex; if a patient has been regularly eating the food without difficulty he or she may continue to eat the food. Patients should, however, be cautioned to stop eating the food at the first sign of any adverse reaction. At least with banana, the cross-reactive allergens appear to be heat stable, so that banana cooked in muffins or breads can still cause reactions in allergic individuals. Patients also should be cautioned that little is known about factors, such as degree of ripeness, country of origin, or plant variety, that may influence the presence of cross-reactive proteins.

The author also believes that a person with a probable allergic reaction to one of the frequently cross-reactive foods should be completely evaluated for latex allergy. The risks of failing to diagnose latex allergy are highly significant, and the effort involved in the evaluation should be modest. If a person has a food allergy to a food that is not clearly cross-reactive with latex, the physician should consider other risk factors. If the reaction to the food was minimal and the patient does not have other risk factors for latex allergy, careful observation may be all that is necessary. If, however, the patient has other risk factors for latex allergy, an evaluation for latex allergy is indicated.

TREATMENT

Avoidance

At present, the only effective method for managing latex allergy is avoidance. Although this is an easy concept to grasp, it can be extremely difficult to successfully put into practice. Latex avoidance can be thought of in four, related, but differing scenarios: (1) avoidance during health care, (2) avoidance in the workplace to allow allergic individuals to continue working, (3) avoidance to prevent latex allergy in high-risk individuals, and (4) avoidance in the home for allergic or high-risk individuals. Successful avoidance requires an appreciation for the types of products that may contain latex. Tables 22–2 and 22–3 list common household and medical items, respectively, that may contain latex. Persons trying to avoid latex also should be educated about how latex may enter the body from a latex-containing item and the relationship between the amount of allergen entering the body and the risk of reactions.

Latex avoidance during health care requires that the patient be cared for in a "latex safe" environment. In a latex safe environment, a patient should not come into direct contact with latex-containing products, the air within the patient's breathing space should be free of latex allergens, and any fluid or medication given to the patient must be free of latex contamination. To meet these goals physicians and other health care providers must develop procedures or protocols specific for their environment ahead of time. Suggested protocols have been published and appear on the Internet.

In a private office a latex safe environment starts by dedicating at least one patient care room to being latex safe. Ideally this room should be close to the waiting room, so that the patient does not need to travel far within the office suite. No latex items should be permitted in the room. This means obtaining a nonlatex blood pressure cuff, using only nonlatex examination gloves, and using only nonlatex items for blood drawing in this room. Persons who may have latex on their clothing

Table 22–3. Items in Health Care That May Contain Natural Rubber Latex*

Anesthesia masks
Bite blocks
Blood pressure cuffs
Catheters, e.g., Foley
Cervical caps
Cervical dilators
Dental dams
Elastic bands on face masks
Elastic bandages
Electrode pads
Endotracheal tubes and balloons
Esophageal dilators
Eye dropper bulbs
Feeding tubes
Finger cots
Gloves, examination and surgical
Hot water bottles
Implants
Instrument mats
Intravenous injection ports
Nasal-pharyngeal airways
Orthodontic elastics
Prophy cups
Reservoir breathing bags
Rubber sheeting or coverings
Syringe stoppers
Tooth protectors
Tourniquets
Ultrasound covers
Urine bags and straps
Ventilator bellows
Wound drains

*This list is not exhaustive; the items listed are merely common examples. Other items used in health care may contain natural rubber latex. If there is any question, the manufacturer should be consulted.

Table 22–2. Home and Workplace Items That Potentially Contain Latex*

Adhesives
Bandages
Baby bottle nipples
Backing of some rugs
Balloons
Condoms
Diaphragms
Douche bulbs
Elastic in clothing and disposable diapers
Erasers
Eye dropper bulbs
Hot water bottles
"Koosh" balls
Pacifiers
Rubber bands
Rubber hand grips on racquets, bicycles, garden tools, etc.
Rubber gloves
Rubber toys, such as soft doll heads, rubber balls
Shoes
Swim caps and goggles
Teething rings
Whoopee cushion

*This list is not exhaustive; the items listed are merely common examples. Other items in the home and workplace may contain natural rubber latex. If there is any question, the manufacturer should be consulted.

from wearing powdered latex gloves should not enter the room, and anyone setting up equipment or instruments in the room must use nonlatex gloves. Studies have suggested that airborne latex allergen tends to be on relatively heavy particles that settle out of the air in a few hours. Therefore, patients who are allergic to latex should be scheduled as the first patients in the morning so that the risks of airborne latex are minimized. A difficult issue in some types of practice is the problem of injection ports on intravenous tubing and the stoppers of multidose vials. Case reports have suggested that injecting through a latex injection port can cause a reaction in an allergic individual. The alternatives are the use of stopcocks or nonlatex, needleless, injection ports. A case report also suggested that vaccines drawn from multidose vials may cause allergic reactions. The problem of multidose vials may be solved by checking with the manufacturer to learn if the vial stopper is totally synthetic or contains natural rubber. An alternative is to obtain medications in single use, break open, vials. Latex-free disposable syringes are now available from some manufacturers.

When an individual with latex allergy is employed in health care or some other occupation where latex exposure is common, the workplace needs to be altered to prevent latex exposure. Although there are many barriers to removing latex from the workplace, latex safe work environments are possible. Changing the work environment starts with carefully evaluating the employee's role in the workplace to identify all potential sources of latex exposure. All latex-containing items must be identified. If there is a significant risk of the employee being directly or indirectly exposed to the latex in an item, the item must be removed and a nonlatex substitute obtained. The elimination of powdered latex gloves is probably the single most effective measure in the reduction of overall risk in health care.

Although no studies have demonstrated the effectiveness of latex prevention, it is rational to expect that reducing or eliminating latex exposure will reduce or eliminate latex allergy. Prevention is especially important for those in high-risk groups, such as infants born with spina bifida and similar anomalies. All medical care provided to such individuals should be in a latex safe environment. The parents of the child should be educated about the potential risks and benefits of prevention and about strategies for latex avoidance. For those occupationally exposed to latex, prevention efforts begin with efforts to reduce the latex exposure of all workers. The most obvious strategies are using nonlatex gloves when appropriate and using low-allergen, nonpowdered latex gloves when nonlatex gloves are inappropriate. Other large sources of latex exposure should be identified and reduced or eliminated if possible.

Latex avoidance in the home and other everyday environments is necessary for allergic and desirable for other individuals at high risk. Avoidance starts with eliminating items such as those listed in Table 22–2 from the home. If the item is absolutely essential in the home, efforts must be made to prevent the item from coming into contact with the affected person.

Outside of the home, persons must be cautious about other environments. One of the most common exposures that causes reactions is rubber balloons. As balloons are blown up, allergen-coated particles are released into the air, and if a balloon pops, large amounts of allergen become airborne. Stores or homes using balloons as decorations must be avoided. Indirect latex exposure also can occur in restaurants. Allergic reactions appear to have been elicited by the ingestion of food contaminated with allergens from the food handler's latex gloves.

Emergency Planning

Patients who are allergic to latex should be advised to wear emergency identification indicating their latex allergy. They also may need to carry written documentation of their allergy to show other health care providers, who might otherwise not believe the patient. Despite efforts to avoid latex, patients may accidentally be exposed to latex. Patients should be given epinephrine for self-administration (Epi-Pen, AnaKit) and instructions on how and when to use epinephrine. They should be advised to seek emergency medical care at the first sign of a significant reaction.

Pretreatment

Beyond avoidance, patients may ask about pharmacologic prophylaxis to prevent allergic reactions. Prophylaxis with prednisone and diphenhydramine can reduce reactions from radiographic contrast material. An essential distinction is that reactions to contrast material are not IgE mediated, whereas reactions to latex are. Limited trials evaluating prednisone and diphenhydramine have not shown reductions in latex-related reactions. A concern about using prophylaxis is that it may create a false sense of security and result in reduced vigilance toward latex avoidance. Although prophylaxis may be of little risk to the patient, the lack of demonstrated benefit and potential risks mitigate against its use. There is no evidence to justify long-term treatment to prevent latex-induced reactions.

Immunotherapy

In theory, immunotherapy (allergy shots) should effectively control the symptoms of latex allergy in many patients. Before immunotherapy can be used, however, it must be carefully evaluated in controlled trials, with well characterized extracts. No matter how well intentioned, the use of immunotherapy outside of careful clinical trials cannot be accepted at the present time.

Natural History of Latex Allergy

Unfortunately, no long-term follow-up studies have been performed with persons who are allergic to latex. Some individuals appear to have a progression of their latex allergy from mild local itching to mild systemic symptoms such as conjunctivitis and rhinitis to anaphylaxis. Others appear to have symptoms from latex exposure that do not change over years of exposure. When individuals with latex allergy avoid latex, some gradually become less reactive to latex over months or years, whereas the reactivity of others persists. An important area for future research is the clinical outcome of avoidance.

WHY HAS LATEX ALLERGY BECOME A PROBLEM NOW?

Limited anecdotal evidence suggests that latex allergy was present, but rare and generally unappreciated until the late 1980s. The most obvious change during the mid-1980s was the adoption of universal precautions in health care. Universal precautions dramatically increased the exposure to latex gloves for both health care workers and persons receiving health care. The increased exposure to latex gloves may have contributed to the current problem of latex allergy.

Questions have arisen about the quality of gloves produced in the mid-1980s. As companies increased production to keep up with demand, and as new companies began to produce gloves, allergen levels in gloves may have increased. Since no one has been able to study the allergen content of a representative sample of gloves produced prior to 1985, this question has not been answered.

One of the changes that occurred in the late 1970s and early 1980s was the movement of latex glove production from the United States to latex-producing countries such as Thailand and Malaysia. This change may be important, because latex is usually collected into ammonia to preserve it, and the ammonia remains in the latex until processing. While in the latex, ammonia accelerates hydrolysis of latex proteins. Thus, if latex was harvested in Asia and shipped to the United States, ammonia may have remained in the latex for several months. When glove production shifted to latex-producing countries, latex was used to make gloves within weeks of harvesting, reducing the chance for protein hydrolysis and, perhaps, increasing the level of allergenic proteins in the finished gloves.

Additional theories have been proposed to explain the recent recognition of latex allergy. One theory is that more frequent tapping of the trees during the 1980s may have resulted in higher allergen concentrations in latex. Another theory is that plantation managers began to use agents on the rubber trees to increase the yield of latex per tree. As part of the response to these yield-enhancing agents, the concentration of allergens in latex may have increased. It is also possible that by genetically selecting rubber trees for maximum latex yield, trees also were unknowingly selected for increased levels of allergens. Little information is available to judge the merits of these theories at the present time.

CONCLUSION

Latex allergy is rare, but can have devastating effects, including loss of the ability to work and death. Just as with antibiotics, all individuals should be questioned about previous adverse reactions to rubber products prior to latex exposure during health care. Patients in high-risk groups should be educated regarding potential risks and evaluated if they have symptoms suggestive of latex allergy. Individuals identified as having latex allergy should be given instructions and epinephrine for emergency care in addition to education about avoiding latex exposure.

KEY POINTS

▶ IgE-mediated allergic reactions to natural rubber latex can be severe.

▶ Individuals with spina bifida and health care workers appear to be at increased risk for latex allergy, but latex allergy has also been severe in other individuals.

▶ A diagnosis of latex allergy depends on a consistent history and demonstration of latex-specific IgE antibodies.

▶ The best treatment for latex allergy is avoidance of direct or indirect (airborne) exposure to latex.

▶ Several common foods may cause allergic reactions in individuals who are allergic to latex through cross-reactive allergens.

▶ Pharmacologic prophylaxis has not been shown to be effective in preventing latex-induced reactions.

▶ Individuals with latex allergy must be given appropriate instructions for emergency situations and epinephrine for self-administration.

Suggested Reading

Allmers H, Brehler R, Chen Z, et al: Reduction of latex aeroallergens and latex-specific IgE antibodies in sensitized workers after removal of powdered natural rubber latex gloves in a hospital. J Allergy Clin Immunol 102:841–846, 1998

Cohen DE, Scheman A, Stewart L, et al: American Academy of Dermatology's position paper on latex allergy. J Am Acad Dermatol 38:98–106, 1998

Fisher AA: Allergic contact reactions in health personnel. J Allergy Clin Immunol 90:729–738, 1992

Hamilton RG, Adkinson NF Jr, Multi-Center Latex Skin Testing Study Task Force: Diagnosis of natural rubber latex allergy: Multicenter latex skin testing efficacy study. J Allergy Clin Immunol 102:482–490, 1998

Ownby DR: Manifestations of latex allergy. Immunol Allergy Clin North Am 15:31–43, 1995

Ownby DR, Tomlanovich M, Sammons N, McCullough J: Anaphylaxis associated with latex allergy during barium enema examinations. Am J Roentgenol 156:903–908, 1991

Preventing allergic reactions to natural rubber latex in the workplace. NIOSH Alert 1997; Cincinnati, Ohio: National Institute for Occupational Safety and Health. DHHS (NIOSH) Publication Number 97-135: pp. 1–11

Sussman G, Tarlo S, Dolovich J: The spectrum of IgE-mediated responses to latex. JAMA 265:2844–2847, 1991

Vandenplas O, Delwiche J-P, Evrard G, et al: Prevalence of occupational asthma due to latex among hospital personnel. Am J Respir Crit Care Med 151:54–60, 1995

Yunginger JW: Natural rubber latex allergy. In Middleton E Jr, Ellis EF, Yunginger JW, Reed CE, Adkinson NF Jr, Busse WW (eds): Allergy: Principles and Practice. 5th ed. St. Louis, Mosby, 1998, pp 1073–1078

Chapter 23

Immunotherapy

Ann M. Wanner

There are three ways to treat allergic disease: allergen avoidance, medications, and immunotherapy. This chapter defines the types of immunotherapy available, the immune mechanisms involved, indications, contraindications, methods of administration, costs, benefits, side-effects, and treatment of immunotherapy injection reactions.

Noon and Freeman first used injections of grass pollen extracts to treat grass-allergic patients at the turn of the century. After the series of injections, clinical symptoms caused by allergen exposure decreased. This seminal observation led to the use of allergen immunotherapy. Over time, our understanding of IgE-mediated reactions has increased, specific antigens have been identified, standardized allergenic extracts have been developed, and immunotherapy has been significantly refined.

Pollens, animal danders, dust mites, molds, foods, and venoms from stinging insects have been used as antigens for immunotherapy. Technical considerations limit the utility of each class of antigen. With the exception of grasses, pollens are not uniformly standardized. Wide variability exists in the potency of nonstandardized lots of pollen allergens from different manufacturers. Cat and dog allergens are the only animal danders that have been well studied for immunotherapy, yet clearly there are many other danders that cause clinical allergic disease for which immunotherapy is unproved. Two types of dust mite allergens, dust mite *Dermatophagoides farinae* and dust mite *Dermatophagoides pteronyssinus,* are commercially available for testing and therapy. Additional important species of dust mites are known to exist but are not available for testing or therapy. Mold extracts are difficult

to characterize and standardize because the antigens in mold spores vary greatly depending on the culture media and culture conditions of temperature and humidity. Commercially prepared food extracts are available for a wide range of ingestants; however, testing with a fresh food extract may be more accurate because food allergens can be degraded by the manufacturing process. Testing with the food in question is the only option for unusual foods that are not available as a commercial extract.

Allergic diseases for which immunotherapy has been studied include asthma, conjunctivitis, rhinitis, urticaria, atopic dermatitis or eczema, food allergies, and stinging insect hypersensitivity. Controlled studies have shown that immunotherapy is effective in the treatment of pollen-, mold-, dust mite-, and animal dander-related asthma, conjunctivitis, and rhinitis. Immunotherapy treatment for atopic dermatitis and urticaria has shown variable results. Immunotherapy studies for food allergens are limited, considered experimental, and have been associated with a high incidence of systemic reactions. Stinging insect venom immunotherapy has been well studied. Studies using purified venom extracts have shown good efficacy, with protection from subsequent stings in 98% of cases. Inhaled insect allergens such as cockroach, which has been shown to be a major allergen in asthma, are currently being evaluated in immunotherapy trials.

WHAT IS IMMUNOTHERAPY?

Allergen immunotherapy is the repeated subcutaneous injection of specific allergenic extracts. Testing to relevant allergens must first be performed using prick and, if needed, intradermal skin tests. The patient's history and knowledge of regional and local allergens should be used to guide the selection of antigens for testing. Accurately identifying the antigens that are causing the allergic disease is crucial for successful immunotherapy. The clinical response to immunotherapy is antigen-specific. If irrelevant antigens are tested and subsequently placed into an extract, the risk of reactions will increase and the benefits that would have been derived from more important allergens will decrease. When important allergens are omitted or not identified, then symptoms caused by these allergens will not improve despite treatment of other relevant allergens. Ideally, testing should be performed with single, pure allergenic extracts. Antigen mixes should be used for screening only when cross-reactivity has been well documented. Whole house dust extracts, which are crude mixtures, should not be substituted for dust mites either for testing or treatment. Radioallergosorbent (RAST) testing for serum IgE antibodies should be used only when cutaneous testing cannot be performed because it is more costly and less reliable.

Once the relevant allergens are identified, they are combined typically into one or two mixtures for injection administration. Treatment is initiated with a build-up phase, which begins with a very low antigen dose and is increased stepwise over the course of a series of injections until a high antigen dose, also called a maintenance dose, is reached (Table 23–1). The maximum or maintenance antigen dose is ideally the highest dose tolerable that minimizes systemic reactions. The higher the dose of maintenance injections, the greater the success in achieving a disease remission and possible long-term cure. Very high-dose immunotherapy is associated with an increased rate of systemic reactions. Low-dose immunotherapy is no more effective than placebo. Controlled studies with ragweed and dust mites have determined the optimal therapeutic dose of allergen to be 5 to 20 micrograms or 200 to 400 biologic activity units (BAU) per injection. The optimal doses for other inhalant antigens have been extrapolated from these studies and would be generally equivalent to a

Table 23–1. **Typical Dosing Schedule for Allergen Immunotherapy***

	Dose (ml)	Injection Number
Vial #1	.05	1
1:100,000	.10	2
Wt/Vol Concentration	.20	3
	.40	4
Vial #2	.05	5
1:10,000	.10	6
	.20	7
	.30	8
	.40	9
Vial #3	.05	10
1:1000	.10	11
	.20	12
	.30	13
	.40	14
Vial #4	.05	15
1:100	.10	16
	.20	17
	.30	18
	.40	19
	.50	20

*Schedule will vary depending on physician preference and patient factors.

1:100 to 1:10 weight/volume dilution of non-standardized allergen. The recommended maintenance dose for standardized venom immunotherapy is 100 micrograms of each venom.

During the build-up phase of immunotherapy, patients can receive injections once to several times a week. There is no greater incidence of adverse reactions when injections are given daily versus weekly. The time to reach maintenance therapy can vary from 3 to 12 months. Maintenance injection doses can be given once a week to once a month. Recent experience with extended maintenance therapy protocols has found that giving maintenance injections every 6 to 8 weeks is both safe and efficacious.

Injections should be administered using a 27- or 30-gauge needle with a 0.5- to 1.0-ml syringe to ensure accuracy. Allergy injections are typically administered subcutaneously in the posterior upper arm. It is important to aspirate before the injection is administered to ensure that the antigen is not given intravenously, which increases the risk of a systemic reaction.

An adjustment in the antigen dose must be made when immunotherapy injections are missed. During the build-up phase, injections should be no more than 7 days apart. The following recommendations are general guidelines for missed doses. If the treatment lapse is between 1 and 2 weeks, the last dose should be repeated. If the last injection was more than 2 weeks ago, the dose should be decreased by one dose for every week missed. When a patient has a systemic reaction, a dosage adjustment also must be made. The injection dose following the reaction should be half the dose that resulted in the systemic reaction. Close observation for a longer time interval after allergen injection and pretreatment with medications such as antihistamines, bronchodilators, and steroids can be considered for patients with a history of systemic reactions.

Immunotherapy has been used seasonally. This schedule requires administering frequent injections several weeks to several months before and into the start of the pollen season. The injections are then discontinued and resumed the following year. The benefit from preseasonal immunotherapy is much less than when shots are given continuously, and this form of treatment is no longer used.

Rapid desensitization or rush immunotherapy protocols have been developed. This approach consists of a build-up phase of allergen injections over hours to days. An increased frequency of local and systemic reactions is seen with rush immunotherapy. Premedication combined with very careful monitoring either as an inpatient or outpatient is required.

A small percentage (~5%) of patients do not respond to allergen immunotherapy. Treatment efficacy should be assessed after approximately 18 months of therapy. A decision should be made whether to stop treatment, modify, or continue the current therapy. Improvements in pulmonary, ocular, nasal, and skin symptoms, measured as reduction in severity or duration of symptoms or by reduced medication usage, are the best clinical measures of efficacy. There are no reliable laboratory parameters that can be used to predict when to discontinue immunotherapy for inhalant allergy. For venom immunotherapy there are more objective parameters for discontinuing treatment. Repeat skin testing to measure changes in immediate hypersensitivity, serum levels of IgG blocking antibodies, and RAST serum IgE levels to venoms can be used to guide discontinuation of venom immunotherapy at a date earlier than 3 to 5 years. However,

the decision to stop or continue immunotherapy must be individualized.

On the basis of venom immunotherapy experience, it is currently recommended that maintenance immunotherapy for inhaled allergens be given for a minimum of 3 to 5 years. Generally the longer the duration of therapy, the less chance of a relapse. After 3 to 5 years, approximately 30% of patients will achieve a permanent cure of their allergies, 35% will achieve a long-term remission lasting several years to decades, and the remaining 35% will achieve a remission lasting months to a few years. Patients who relapse after their first course of immunotherapy can choose to resume injection treatment indefinitely at an extended maintenance interval.

HOW DOES IMMUNOTHERAPY WORK?

Allergen immunotherapy results in diverse immunologic changes. The World Health Organization has recommended changing the term allergen extract to allergen vaccine to reflect the fact that immunotherapy is used as an immune modifier. Inflammatory cell recruitment into tissues, activation of immune effector cells, and mediator release from immune modulating cells are all decreased. Of the known altered immunologic parameters it is not clear which is most responsible for efficacy (Table 23–2). There is no immunologic effect studied to date that is a predictor of responsiveness to immunotherapy or an indicator of which patients will achieve a long-term versus a short-term remission. Changes that are known to occur include a decrease in the levels of IgE produced to specific allergens, an increase in the level of IgG blocking

Table 23–2. **Immunologic Changes Associated with Immunotherapy**

Decreases total IgE to specific allergen
Blunts the seasonal rise in IgE to antigens
Increases blocking antibodies IgG_1 (peaks 2–3 months) and IgG_4 (peaks 2 years)
Increases activation of T suppressor cells
Decreases basophil histamine release
Decreases eosinophil chemotactic factors

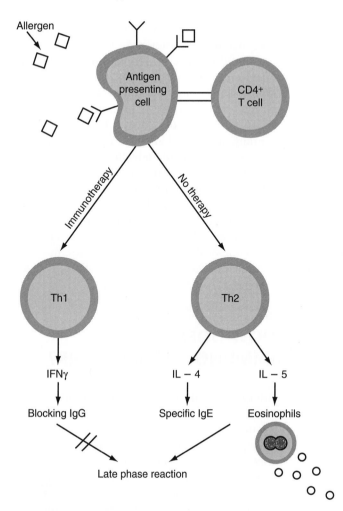

Figure 23–1. Effects of immunotherapy on T-cells.

antibody to allergens, a decrease in the production of interleukins (IL) 4, IL-5, and IL-10, an increase in IL-13, an increase in allergen-specific IgA and IgG in nasal secretions, induction of specific T suppressor cells, a decrease in lymphocyte responsiveness to specific allergens, induction of anti-idiotypic antibodies, and a decrease in the numbers of respiratory eosinophils and mast cells. Not all of these immunologic changes occur in all individuals. The specific changes in the immune response are dependent on the individual patient, the allergens involved, the allergic disease, and the route, dose, and duration of immunotherapy. There is clearly a dose-response relationship between the total dose of antigen administered and changes in IgE and IgG levels. IgG_1 blocking antibody levels peak and then plateau within several months, whereas IgG_4 levels peak and plateau after 2 years of therapy. IgG blocking antibody levels are higher at the end

of the first year when maintenance doses are given weekly instead of monthly, although they fall when maintenance shots are subsequently spread out to monthly intervals. These antibodies block basophil histamine release. Suppression of both the immediate and late allergic response correlates with the cumulative dose of extract administered.

The decrease in serum of specific IgE and increase in IgG blocking antibodies to an allergen were initially thought to be the sole mechanism of immunotherapy. Subsequent studies have found that the observed changes in antibody levels are a reflection of alterations in cytokine production by two T-cell subgroups, T helper 1 (Th1) and T helper 2 (Th2) cells (Fig. 23–1). These cytokines have a complex relationship to antibody production and recruitment of inflammatory cells to mucosal surfaces. The immediate allergic reaction occurs when allergen cross-links specific IgE bound to mast cells, resulting in mediator release. This release is followed by a late phase reaction mediated by eosinophils and T-cells. Allergen-specific T-cell clones in atopic individuals produce increased amounts of IL-4, which promotes B-cell production of IgE, and IL-5, which enhances eosinophil differentiation and activation. This is a Th2-type response. Immunotherapy results in a switch from a Th2-type response to a Th1-type response (see Fig. 23–1). Thus, T cell–derived cytokines play a major role in both the antibody and the cell-mediated components of allergic inflammation. Further defining the T-cell changes that occur in patients on immunotherapy will be essential to an improved understanding of clinical outcomes.

Although immunotherapy causes a decrease in allergen-specific IgE, it does not routinely result in loss of skin test reactivity. Thus, repeated skin testing to allergens is not a reliable indicator of successful immunotherapy. Retesting is indicated only if there is a change in clinical allergy symptoms that suggests a change in sensitization. Repeat skin testing to allergens can be helpful when individuals move between distinctly different geographic areas of the country.

TYPES OF EXTRACTS AVAILABLE

A good quality allergen vaccine is essential for diagnosis and treatment. The majority of inhalant extracts are crude mixtures of whole pollen grains, mold spores, and animal danders. Over the past 85 years, there have been many attempts to standardize extracts. The goal of standardized extracts is to provide better quality control of antigen concentration and potency, decrease lot-to-lot variability, and decrease local and systemic reactions. Unfortunately many allergens remain poorly defined. Allergen standardization has proved to be a complicated process that requires identification of the most relevant allergenic proteins from each individual antigen.

Standardized allergenic extracts have their potency defined in BAU. One-hundred thousand BAU is defined as the amount of extract at a 1:5 million dilution that produces a specified skin test response. Nonstandardized extracts are defined in either protein nitrogen units (PNU), where 1 PNU = .00001 mg protein nitrogen, or weight to volume (w/v) concentration; neither of these measures correlates reliably with potency. There is significant lot-to-lot variation in nonstandardized extracts. Standardized and nonstandardized extracts are compatible for mixing. Standardized extracts are currently available for both dust mite *D. farinae* and dust mite *D. pteronyssinus,* cat, dog, grasses, *Alternaria* and *Cladosporium* molds, and Hymenoptera venoms. The most commonly used extracts are aqueous. Alum-precipitated extracts, available for a limited number of antigens, delay antigen absorption, resulting in fewer systemic reactions. Experimental studies with polymerized extracts have demonstrated efficacy with a reduction in the rates of systemic reactions. Polymerized extracts are not yet commercially available. Future advances in allergy vaccine technology are likely to improve the quality of allergenic immunotherapy. Extracts using modified antigens, recombinant antigens, adjuvants, and peptides are currently being studied.

The potency of stored allergenic extracts is affected by time, temperature, and concentration. Proteolytic enzymes from the allergen tend to degrade the stored antigens, but are inhibited in the presence of stabilizers and preservatives. Storage at 4°C minimizes the loss of potency. Concentrated extracts such as 1:10 and 1:100 w/v dilutions lose potency at the same rate as the concentrated allergen stock bottle. Over a 12-month period loss of potency averages around 10%. The more dilute extracts 1:1000, 1:10,000, and 1:100,000 w/v dilutions expire within a few weeks to a few months. Dry powder extracts are reconstituted either with human serum albumin or glycerol as stabilizers to prevent antigen adsorption to the inner surface of the vial. Most diluents also contain an antibacterial agent, most commonly phenol.

ALTERNATIVE TYPES OF IMMUNOTHERAPY

The effect of immunotherapy by other routes of administration has been studied in the hope of finding an easier method of administration, improving efficacy, and decreasing side-effects.

These regimens are still considered experimental.

Nasal immunotherapy delivers allergens directly to the nasal mucosa by means of a nasal inhaler. Studies have been done with pollens and dust mites. Universal side-effects with this delivery system are pruritus, sneezing, rhinorrhea, and congestion. Nasal side-effects can be blunted by premedication with cromolyn sodium nasal spray. In double-blind placebo-controlled studies, nasal and eye symptom scores and medication use improved to a variable degree in the treated groups. No long-term studies of nasal immunotherapy have been carried out. The benefits of nasal immunotherapy are thought to be derived only locally. The efficacy for asthma, conjunctivitis, or allergic skin diseases is uncertain.

Oral immunotherapy has been used in an attempt to reduce systemic allergic symptoms. Initial studies showed no efficacy, presumably because of significant gastrointestinal degradation of the antigen. Even enteric-coated and encapsulated allergens are digested. Susceptibility to enteric digestion varies with the unique properties of each individual allergen. Calculating the effective antigen dose is difficult. In subsequent studies, it required up to 100-fold higher doses of antigen than that used for standard subcutaneous immunotherapy to achieve a decrease in symptoms. Using such high doses makes the cost of therapy prohibitive for most antigens. For other antigens available supplies would not meet demand. Systemic reactions were frequent in treated patients; they consisted of nausea, vomiting, diarrhea, and abdominal pain.

Sublingual immunotherapy studies have shown variable efficacy. Although some initial European studies showed a decrease in symptoms, a 3-month high-dose double-blind placebo-controlled U.S. study showed no efficacy for sublingual immunotherapy.

There are limited data on treating asthma with bronchial immunotherapy. Antigens are delivered by means of a dry powder inhaler. Further studies will be needed to evaluate this form of therapy.

Immunotherapy should not be used for undefined allergens such as bacteria, foods, and yeast because of lack of efficacy.

WHO IS A CANDIDATE FOR IMMUNOTHERAPY?

There is no age restriction for immunotherapy. Efficacy is actually greater in children and young adults; however, data are limited in children under the age of 5 because of the inherent aversion to injections in this age group. Systemic reactions in the under 5 age group are slightly increased. The benefits and risks must be weighed on a case by case basis.

Allergic Rhinitis and Allergic Conjunctivitis

Immunotherapy should be considered in patients with moderate to severe seasonal or perennial allergies when avoidance is not feasible, medications are either ineffective or not well tolerated, and prednisone is required to control symptoms. Complete avoidance of allergens can be difficult. Exposure to certain allergens such as animal danders occurs at school and work environments where animals are not present. The animal danders are deposited from clothing in contact with animals. Dander levels measured in schools and work areas can be high enough to cause allergy symptoms including asthma. Immunotherapy offers an alternative to medications for patients in climates where there is a prolonged pollen season or for patients who are sensitized to multiple pollens or nonpollen inhalants or both and would require prolonged or perennial medication usage. Patients who are averse to medication use or are concerned about long-term medication side-effects are also good candidates for immunotherapy. Other factors to consider include whether or not the symptoms interfere with daytime activities or sleep, cause lost time from work or school, or result in frequent office visits. The severity and complexity of disease, duration of symptoms, response to medical therapy, and side-effects of medications must be weighed against the cost, side-effects, and time commitment of effective immunotherapy.

Good efficacy has been demonstrated by means of double-blind placebo-controlled trials for immunotherapy treatment of allergic rhinitis and conjunctivitis caused by pollens, dust mites, animal danders, and molds. Immunotherapy and avoidance are the only available therapies that can impact the natural course of allergic disease. In patients with allergic rhinoconjunctivitis the risk of developing asthma is three times higher than in the general population. Retrospective studies on immunotherapy suggest that it can prevent the onset of asthma in patients with allergic rhinitis. Further well-controlled studies will be needed to confirm this finding.

Asthma

Asthma is a complex multifactorial disease. Nonspecific factors such as cold air, exercise, and irritants can cause bronchial obstruction and inflammation. Exposure to allergens also can cause and exacerbate acute and chronic asthma. The goal of treatment is to reduce symptoms and decrease inflammation and bronchial hyper-reactivity. Accurate testing of pertinent allergens, correlation with asthma symptoms, and proper patient selection are needed to ensure successful immunotherapy. Randomized, double-blind placebo-controlled immunotherapy trials have shown good efficacy for the treatment of asthma as measured by symptom scores, medication use, pulmonary function test results, and specific and nonspecific bronchial hyper-reactivity. The dose of an allergen required to provoke an asthmatic response increases with immunotherapy treatment. Nonspecific bronchial hyper-reactivity as measured by methacholine and histamine provocation improves with allergen injection therapy. Both the acute asthmatic response and the late asthmatic response to an allergen are inhibited by immunotherapy.

Analysis of therapeutic immunotherapy trials in patients with asthma has demonstrated clinical effectiveness for dust mites, cat dander, grasses, and the standardized molds *Alternaria* and *Cladosporium*. Very few studies have shown efficacy for animal danders if animals remain in the home. Immunotherapy provides maximal benefit in conjunction with allergen avoidance. Mold extracts other than standardized *Alternaria* and *Cladosporium* are of poor and variable quality, which limits their usefulness for immunotherapy.

Individuals with seasonal or perennial allergic asthma, those with asthma that requires medications year round, and those who are averse to using medications are all candidates for immunotherapy. Immunotherapy should be considered in patients with multiple systems affected such as the eyes, nose, skin, and lungs and in those who require multiple medications to control symptoms. Other factors to consider are whether symptoms interfere with daytime activities or sleep, cause time lost from work or school, or result in emergency room visits or hospitalizations, and whether extracts are available to treat the allergens involved. The severity of disease, duration of symptoms, and response to medical therapy must be weighed against the cost, complexity, and side-effects of medications. Although medications will control symptoms, immunotherapy is the only treatment that modifies the disease and induces a remission or long-term cure.

Venom Immunotherapy

Immunotherapy for venom allergy has been well studied. Initial studies used whole body extracts. Double-blind placebo-controlled studies with whole body extracts showed no efficacy. Subsequent trials with pure wasp, yellow jacket, and white-faced and yellow hornet venoms showed excellent protection from stings in 98% of treated patients. Immunotherapy protection for honey bee allergy is slightly lower at 80%. Venom immunotherapy for severe stinging insect allergy is now the standard of care. Venom immunotherapy side-effects are similar to those of inhalant immunotherapy. Systemic reactions are more common with wasp or honey bee venoms, but no fatalities have been reported in patients treated with venom immunotherapy. Recent experience with extended maintenance immunotherapy has found it safe and efficacious to extend the maintenance interval to 6 to 8 weeks after the first 6 months of therapy.

Standardized venom extracts are available for honey bee, wasp, white-faced hornet, yellow hornet, and yellow jacket. The maintenance dose is 100 micrograms for each venom. All venoms that elicit positive skin test responses are used for injection therapy. A mixed vespid venom extract is also available, containing quantities of yellow jacket, yellow hornet, and white-faced hornet venoms in a single mixture. Mixed vespid venom extract can be used in patients with multiple venom sensitivity to decrease the number of separate injections needed. An exception to venom extracts is fire ant immunotherapy. Whole body fire ant extracts confer protection similar to fire ant venom except for a mild increase in local reactions. Whole body extracts are currently the only therapy available for fire ant allergy.

The option of venom immunotherapy should be offered to individuals who have had an anaphylactic or a systemic reaction to stinging insect venom. In children, isolated cutaneous symptoms such as pruritus or hives do not appear to progress to systemic reactions. Accordingly, testing and immunotherapy are not indicated. Large local reactions to stinging insects in children and adults are common. Routine testing and immunotherapy are not recommended for patients with large local reactions because they do not usually progress to systemic reactions.

Insect sting challenge studies on patients treated with venom immunotherapy for various time intervals have found good long-term protection from stings after 3 to 5 years of therapy. Most patients will neither lose skin test reactivity nor lower serum IgE concentrations to venoms despite a lack of clinical reactions. Repeating skin tests to measure changes in immediate hypersensitivity, measuring serum IgG blocking antibody, and RAST venom-specific IgE levels can be used to guide discontinuation of therapy at a date earlier than 3 to 5 years. The decision to stop or continue immunotherapy must be individualized.

CONTRAINDICATIONS TO IMMUNOTHERAPY

Although there are no absolute contraindications, there are some relative contraindications to allergy injections. Individuals with unstable asthma are at higher risk for systemic reactions from immunotherapy. Ideally asthma should be stabilized before treatment with immunotherapy is initiated. It is generally not advisable to initiate immunotherapy during pregnancy because of the higher risk of systemic reactions during the build-up phase of immunotherapy. Systemic reactions during pregnancy incur the potential risk of fetal hypoxia or uterine contractions leading to premature labor. It would be preferable to have the pregnancy completed before the initiation of immunotherapy. It is safe to continue maintenance immunotherapy in patients who become pregnant at either the regular maintenance dose or a reduced maintenance dose.

Individuals on beta blockers and immunotherapy are at higher risk for fatal reactions. In the presence of oral or topically administered beta blockers the response to epinephrine, which is first-line therapy for anaphylaxis, is blunted. The beta blocker can usually be discontinued in favor of alternative medications that do not increase the risk of anaphylaxis. Immunotherapy should not be administered to those patients taking beta blockers except in rare instances in which the beta blockers cannot be stopped and the benefits of immunotherapy clearly outweigh the risks.

Theoretically, patients with immunodeficiencies may not respond to immunotherapy. Careful consideration should be given before placing an individual with a chronic infectious disease on immunotherapy because of the increased risks to those administering the allergy injections. There is no evidence that immunotherapy is harmful to administer to patients with concomitant autoimmune disease. The risks and benefits must be carefully weighed in any patient who has a chronic medical condition, including cardiac, vascular, liver, or renal disease, or poorly controlled asthma or other chronic lung diseases that would make the patient less likely to tolerate an episode of anaphylaxis. Poorly compliant patients or those with significant psychosocial disorders should not be placed on immunotherapy without careful consideration.

WHAT ARE THE SIDE-EFFECTS OF IMMUNOTHERAPY?

Before initiating immunotherapy, the patient must be informed of the pros and cons, costs, time commitment, and side-effects of treatment. The most common side-effect of immunotherapy is a local reaction of redness, swelling, itching, and warmth at the injection site. Local reactions can occur immediately, within 20 to 30 minutes after an injection, or can be delayed, occurring 30 minutes to hours later. Immediate local reactions usually subside in a few hours. Delayed local reactions can require 48 hours or more to resolve. Local injection reactions can be minimized by premedicating with antihistamines or by applying ice packs at the injection site. If the local reaction is large, for example the wheal is more than 2 cm, then a dose reduction should be considered. Alternately, the same dose can be divided into two injections and given at different sites. Patients should be educated to inform their physician or the office staff of delayed reactions, so that dose adjustments can be made. Local reactions tend to diminish over time. In general, local reactions do not predict systemic reactions.

Systemic reactions can vary from symptoms of allergic rhinoconjunctivitis, mild cutaneous pruritus, or urticaria to anaphylaxis. The major risk of allergen immunotherapy is anaphylaxis. Allergen immunotherapy should be administered under the supervision of a physician. The physician and medical staff who administer immunotherapy should be trained to recognize early signs of anaphylaxis and implement appropriate therapy (Table 23–3). Staff should have medical equipment available to maintain an open airway, insert intravenous lines, perform cardiopulmonary resuscitation, and administer nebulizer therapy and injectable drugs, especially epinephrine. Epinephrine is the first-line drug for treatment of anaphylaxis. Patients should be instructed to wait in the physician's office for 20 to 30 minutes after an injection. Before the patient leaves the office, the injection site should be checked. The size of the local reaction should be recorded in the patient's shot record (Table 23–4). High-risk patients, such as those with unstable asthma or those with a history of prior shot reactions, should be observed longer.

Preventing reactions requires good staff training to minimize errors in administration of injections. Patients should be assessed at the time of the injection for the presence of fever, an acute viral illness especially with a cough, increased asthma, or allergic rhinitis symptoms. If present, these conditions would warrant withholding the injection or giving a reduced dose. Dose adjustments should be made depending on the severity of symptoms. In patients with asthma, allergy injections

Table 23–3. **Anaphylaxis Protocol**

Stay calm
Quickly determine the seriousness of the reaction by assessing the patient for:
    Breathing or swallowing difficulty, wheezing, rapid respiratory rate
    Skin rash, swelling or hives, and local reaction size at injection site
    Vagal reaction: slowed heart rate, clammy skin, faint, or nauseated
For **Hives** only, administer a quick-acting antihistamine (e.g., diphenhydramine, 50 mg po or IM or 5 mg/kg) followed
    by a long-acting antihistamine (e.g., 50 mg hydroxyzine elixir or 1 mg/kg) or repeat diphenhydramine every 4 hours
    for 8–12 hours. Observe the patient until hives subside to ensure no further symptoms develop. Alternatively,
    epinephrine can be administered IM at a dose of .15 ml (child) or .30 ml (adult) 1:1000.
For **Vagal** reactions, have the patient sit or lie down, then administer smelling salts or atropine .30 mg (child)/.60 mg
    (adult) IM/IV. Be prepared to set up IV; monitor blood pressure and heart rate until normal
For **Systemic** reaction with airway involvement or anaphylaxis:
    Have patient sit down. Do not have a patient who is having difficulty breathing lie down
    Place tourniquets above injection site(s)
    Administer epinephrine 1:1000 .01 ml/kg up to .30 ml (child) to .30–.50 ml (adult) IM, ¼ of dose at injection site
        and ¾ of dose above tourniquet. Epinephrine can be repeated every 3–5 minutes
    Set up nebulizer. Administer via nebulizer, for both children and adults, albuterol .50 ml in 2.5 ml saline or with
        epinephrine 1:1000 .50 ml with or without atropine 1 ml (1 mg/ml) or ipatropium bromide 2.5 ml. If patient is
        cyanotic or has a low pulse oximetry reading, administer nebulizer solutions via an oxygen tank run at a flow rate
        greater than or equal to 6 L per minute.
    Other medications:
        Diphenhydramine 50 mg po/IM or 5 mg/kg, H2 blocker, e.g., ranitidine 75 mg po/25 mg IV (to age 6)—150 mg
            po/50 mg IV (age 6 and over)
        Prednisone 0.5–1 mg/kg po or methylprednisolone 0.5–1 mg/kg IV
    Be prepared to set up IV for administering fluids or medication. Have a crash cart available if needed to maintain an
        open airway. Be prepared to call 911 for severe reactions not responsive to the above medications.

Table 23–4. **Antigen Dosage Record (ml)**

Name: _____ **DOB:** _____ **MD:** _____ **Antigen:** _____

Medications: _____

Premedication: [   ]N   [   ]Y _____

Schedule: Injections 1–5 times per week during build-up until at maintenance dose of 1:100 .50 ml. Once maintenance is reached, give injections once a week for 2 doses, then every 2 weeks for 2 doses, then every 4 weeks.

Vial #1 1:100,000 Dose #1–.05	Date	Dilution	Dose (ml)	Wheal/ Erythema, cm	Comments	√Premedication	Nurse Initials
2–.10							
3–.20							
4–.40							
Vial #2							
1:10,000							
5–.05							
6–.10							
7–.20							
8–.30							
9–.40							
Vial #3							
1:1000							
10–.05							
11–.10							
12–.20							
13–.30							
14–.40							
Vial #4							
1:100							
15–.05							
16–.10							
17–.20							
18–.30							
19–.40							
20–.50							

should generally be withheld if the peak expiratory flow rate (PEFR) or forced expiratory volume in 1 second (FEV_1) is less than 70% of the predicted normal value.

Surveys of immunotherapy fatalities have found 46 deaths between 1945 and 1987, 17 deaths from 1985 to 1989, and 10 deaths from 1991 to 1992. Overall the fatality rate from allergy injections remains low at one per two million doses. Analysis of these observations revealed that patients at highest risk for anaphylaxis had severe or unstable asthma. Other identifiable risk factors were undergoing the build-up phase of injections, changing to a new vial of extract, home administration of injections, and having seasonal exacerbations of allergies or asthma. Patients who are highly allergic by skin testing and those on higher dosage regimens were also at higher risk. The rates of systemic reactions caused by venom and inhalant immunotherapy are the same, but there have been no fatalities with venom immunotherapy. Screening patients for increased respiratory symptoms before an injection and administering injections in a medical facility minimizes the frequency of serious reactions. Under unusual circumstances when allergen immunotherapy cannot be administered in a medical facility, very careful consideration must be given to the benefits of therapy versus the risks of home administration. The American Academy of Allergy, Asthma, and Immunology (AAAAI) and the American College of Allergy, Asthma and Immunology (ACAAI) position statements on immunotherapy do not support the administration of allergy injections outside of a medical facility.

WHAT ARE THE COSTS AND TIME COMMITMENTS?

Two factors contribute to the cost of allergen immunotherapy: the expense of the antigen extract mixture and the cost of each individual injection. The cost of preparing the antigen mixture depends on the price of each individual allergen, the number of antigens used, and whether all antigens can be combined into one vial or more than one vial is required. These expenses are small compared with the cost of the professional time of administering the extract during the build-up phase. Costs are markedly reduced once maintenance therapy is reached and the frequency of injections is reduced. Studies comparing immunotherapy expense with medications have found immunotherapy to be very cost-effective.

The time commitment for allergen immunotherapy can be divided into two components, the build-up phase and the maintenance injections. The time required to complete the build-up phase is dependent to a large degree on the patient's compliance with frequent injections and the level of the patient's allergic sensitivity. The primary reason for discontinuing treatment is inconvenience. When injection doses are frequently missed, it will increase the time to reach maintenance. Difficulty with local or systemic reactions may require a longer build-up phase. Once the maintenance dose is reached, a time commitment of 3 to 5 years is recommended to achieve long-term remission of allergies. Immunotherapy can be continued longer or indefinitely.

WHY DOES IMMUNOTHERAPY FAIL?

There are many reasons why immunotherapy fails. First and foremost is patient selection. Clearly documented IgE-mediated disease must be identified by accurate and skillful allergy testing. With good patient selection, a 5% failure rate exists. Treating the right patient for the wrong allergen or treating the wrong disease, such as non–IgE-mediated vasomotor rhinitis, with immunotherapy can lead to treatment failure. Excessive environmental exposure to allergen, low allergenic extract potency, insufficient duration of immunotherapy, patient noncompliance, and coexistent medical problems also can contribute to immunotherapy failure.

Suggested Reading

Bousquet J, Lockey RF, Malling HJ: WHO position paper. Allergen immunotherapy: Therapeutic vaccines for allergic diseases. Eur J Allergy Clin Immunol 53:1–42, 1998

Bousquet J, Michel FB: Specific immunotherapy in allergic rhinitis and asthma. *In* Busse W, Holgate S (eds): Asthma and Rhinitis. Cambridge, Blackwell Science, 1995, pp 1309–1324

Durham S, Till S: Immunologic changes associated with allergen immunotherapy. J Allergy Clin Immunol 102:157–164, 1998

Nelson H: Immunotherapy for inhalant allergens. *In* Middleton E, Reed C, Ellis E, et al (eds): Allergy Principles and Practice, Vol II. St. Louis, Mosby, 1998, pp 1050–1062

Reisman R: Insect sting allergy. *In* Lieberman P, Anderson J (eds): Allergic Diseases: Diagnosis and Treatment. Totowa, NJ, Humana Press, 1997, pp 65–75

Weber R: Immunotherapy with allergens. *In* Primer on Allergic and Immunologic Diseases. JAMA 1997, 1881–1887

Yunginger J: Insect allergy. *In* Middleton E, Reed C, Ellis E, et al (eds): Allergy Principles and Practice. St. Louis, Mosby, 1998, pp 1063–1072

Index

Note: Page numbers in *italics* indicate figures; those followed by t indicate tables.

ISBN 0-7216-8166-2

90038

DATE DUE
